DIAGNOSIS AND ASSESSMENT IN AUTISM

CURRENT ISSUES IN AUTISM
Series Editors: Eric Schopler and Gary B. Mesibov

University of North Carolina School of Medicine
Chapel Hill, North Carolina

DIAGNOSIS AND ASSESSMENT IN AUTISM

Edited by
Eric Schopler
and
Gary B. Mesibov

University of North Carolina School of Medicine
Chapel Hill, North Carolina

PLENUM PRESS • NEW YORK AND LONDON

Library of Congress Cataloging in Publication Data

Diagnosis and assessment in autism / edited by Eric Schopler and Gary B. Mesibov.
    p.   cm. — (Current affairs in autism)
    Includes bibliographies.
    Includes index.
    ISBN 0-306-42889-X
    1. Autism. I. Schopler, Eric. II. Mesibov, Gary B.
RJ506.A9D53   1988   88-19675
618.92′8982 — dc19   CIP

10 9 8 7 6 5 4

© 1988 Plenum Press, New York
A Division of Plenum Publishing Corporation
233 Spring Street, New York, N.Y. 10013

Printed in the United States of America

For our children and adults touched by the disorganization of autism, with the hope that this volume will help them toward fuller understanding and better coping

Contributors

MARY AKERLEY, 10609 Glenwild Road, Silver Spring, Maryland 20901

LORIAN BAKER, Neuropsychiatric Institute, University of California at Los Angeles, Los Angeles, California 90024

SUSAN BOSWELL, Millbrook Elementary School, Raleigh, North Carolina 27609

DENNIS P. CANTWELL, Neuropsychiatric Institute, University of California at Los Angeles, Los Angeles, California 90024

DONALD J. COHEN, Child Study Center, Yale University, New Haven, Connecticut 06510-8009

SUSAN FOLSTEIN, Department of Psychiatry and Behavioral Science, Johns Hopkins University, School of Medicine, Baltimore, Maryland 21205

JAMES J. GALLAGHER, Frank Porter Graham Child Development Center, The University of North Carolina at Chapel Hill, Chapel Hill, North Carolina 27599-8040

SANDRA HARRIS, Applied and Professional Psychology, Rutgers University, Piscataway, New Jersey 08854

NANCY M. JOHNSON-MARTIN, CHILD Project, Duke University Medical Center, Durham, North Carolina 27705

MICHAEL L. JONES, Bureau of Child Research, University of Kansas, Lawrence, Kansas 66045

ANN Le COUTEUR, Department of Child and Adolescent Psychiatry, Institute of Psychiatry, University of London, London SE5 8AF, England

CATHERINE LORD, Department of Pediatrics, University of Alberta, and Department of Psychology, Glenrose Rehabilitation Hospital, Edmonton, Alberta T5G 0B7, Canada

HOPE MACDONALD, Department of Child and Adolescent Psychiatry, Institute of Psychiatry, University of London, London SE5 8AF, England

LEE M. MARCUS, Division TEACCH, The University of North Carolina at Chapel Hill, Chapel Hill, North Carolina 27599-7180

GARY B. MESIBOV, Division TEACCH, The University of North Carolina at Chapel Hill, Chapel Hill, North Carolina 27599-7180

SUSAN L. PARKS, Villa Maria Residential Treatment Center, Timonium, Maryland 21093

MICHAEL D. POWERS, Preschool Autism Project, Department of Special Education, University of Maryland, College Park, Maryland 20742

DANIEL J. RAITEN, Department of Behavioral Medicine, Children's Hospital, National Medical Center, Washington, D.C. 20010

PATRICIA RIOS, Department of Child and Adolescent Psychiatry, Institute of Psychiatry, University of London, London SE5 8AF, England

MICHAEL RUTTER, Department of Child and Adolescent Psychiatry, Institute of Psychiatry, University of London, London SE5 8AF, England

ERIC SCHOPLER, Division TEACCH, The University of North Carolina at Chapel Hill, Chapel Hill, North Carolina 27599-7180

MARIAN TROXLER, Millbrook Elementary School, Raleigh, North Carolina 27609

FRED R. VOLKMAR, Child Study Center, Yale University, New Haven, Connecticut 06510-8009

LINDA R. WATSON, Division TEACCH, The University of North Carolina at Chapel Hill, Chapel Hill, North Carolina 27599-7180

JOHN S. WERRY, Department of Psychiatry, School of Medicine, University of Auckland, P. B., Auckland, New Zealand

LORNA WING, MRC Social Psychiatry Unit, Institute of Psychiatry, University of London, London SE5 8AF, England

Preface

Division TEACCH, located in the School of Medicine at the University of North Carolina at Chapel Hill, was one of the first programs in the country to understand that autism was an organic rather than a biologic condition. We were also one of the earliest programs to recognize the enormous variability in characteristics and behaviors of children described as autistic. For these reasons, the processes of diagnosis and assessment have always been important and central to our program. We are therefore extremely pleased to have a volume representing the most current thinking of the field's leaders in these important areas.

As with the preceding books in our series, *Current Issues in Autism,* this volume is based on one of the annual TEACCH conferences held in Chapel Hill each May. The books are not simply published proceedings of the conference papers, however. Rather, conference participants are asked to develop a full chapter around their presentations. Other international experts whose work is beyond the scope of the conference, but related to the major theme, are asked to contribute chapters as well. These volumes are designed to provide the most current knowledge in research and professional practice available on the most important issues defining and clarifying autism.

This volume is designed to advance our understanding of issues in diagnosis and assessment. The latest and most pertinent instruments are presented along with some cogent analyses of their contributions to the field. Several chapters devoted to current, special issues are also included to inform the reader of certain of today's state of the art practices, that may become tomorrow's scientifically established procedures. We expect this volume will be useful to students, professionals, and parents concerned with understanding and assisting individuals with autism.

Eric Schopler
Gary B. Mesibov

Acknowledgments

We are indebted to many people for their cooperation and generous assistance, and it is our great pleasure to acknowledge each of them. First, our thanks to Helen Garrison, who organized the conference that was the starting point for this book. Her continuing attention to detail and ability to organize these major events are greatly admired and appreciated. Our secretarial staff, including Judy Carter and Vickie Weaver, was always cooperative and provided competent typing and secretarial assistance.

We also want to thank our many TEACCH colleagues for their ongoing help and assistance. Though too numerous to name individually, their insights and understanding of the diagnostic and assessment processes are a continuing source of information and inspiration to us. As with all our efforts in the TEACCH Program, this book would not have been possible without the assistance of the families of autistic people in North Carolina, the University of North Carolina at Chapel Hill School of Medicine, and the North Carolina State Legislature. Their continuing ability to cooperate and coordinate their efforts is the most important reason for optimism on the part of those struggling with this most difficult handicap.

Contents

Chapter 7

THE CONTINUUM OF AUTISTIC CHARACTERISTICS   91

Lorna Wing

Chapter 8

MULTIAXIAL DIAGNOSTIC APPROACHES   111

Dennis P. Cantwell and Lorian Baker

Chapter 9

PSYCHOMETRIC INSTRUMENTS AVAILABLE FOR THE
ASSESSMENT OF AUTISTIC CHILDREN   123

Susan L. Parks

Part III: General Assessment Issues

Chapter 10

BEHAVIORAL ASSESSMENT OF AUTISM   139

Michael D. Powers

Chapter 11

INTELLECTUAL AND DEVELOPMENTAL ASSESSMENT OF
AUTISTIC CHILDREN FROM PRESCHOOL TO SCHOOLAGE:
CLINICAL IMPLICATIONS OF TWO FOLLOW-UP STUDIES   167

Catherine Lord and Eric Schopler

Chapter 12

ASSESSING THE QUALITY OF LIVING ENVIRONMENTS   183

Michael L. Jones

Chapter 13

FAMILY ASSESSMENT IN AUTISM   199

Sandra Harris

Chapter 14

NUTRITION AND DEVELOPMENTAL DISABILITIES: CLINICAL
ASSESSMENT   211

Daniel J. Raiten

Part IV: Special Issues

Chapter 15

DIAGNOSIS AND ASSESSMENT OF AUTISTIC ADOLESCENTS
AND ADULTS   227

Gary B. Mesibov

Chapter 16

DIAGNOSIS AND SUBCLASSIFICATION OF AUTISM: CONCEPTS
AND INSTRUMENT DEVELOPMENT   239

Michael Rutter, Ann LeCouteur, Catherine Lord, Hope Macdonald,
Patricia Rios, and Susan Folstein

Chapter 17

ASSESSMENT IN THE CLASSROOM   261

Gary B. Mesibov, Marian Troxler, and Susan Boswell

Chapter 18

DIAGNOSIS AND ASSESSMENT OF PRESCHOOL CHILDREN   271

Linda R. Watson and Lee M. Marcus

Chapter 19

ASSESSMENT OF LOW-FUNCTIONING CHILDREN   303

Nancy M. Johnson-Martin

1

Introduction and Overview

Introduction to Diagnosis and Assessment of Autism

ERIC SCHOPLER and GARY B. MESIBOV

INTRODUCTION

With our superabundance of tests, scales, and questionnaires evaluating and reducing to numbers our performance in every sphere of life from school and work to sex, evaluation has come under attack in many quarters. On the other hand, our 20+ years of experience in the *T*reatment and *E*ducation of *A*utistic and related *C*ommunication handicapped *CH*ildren (TEACCH) program has taught us that careful and appropriate evaluation can be crucial components of our intervention programs for autistic youngsters and their families. We therefore considered it especially important and worthwhile to devote our sixth volume in this series on autism to diagnosis and assessment and to distinguish some common misunderstandings and misuses of diagnosis and assessment from valid and needed evaluation, especially with such complex disorders as autism.

As some of the chapters in this volume are rather technical, it bears keeping in mind that most of our daily activities, especially those requiring some planning, are based on appropriate assessments of the situation. At the simplest level, it may mean checking the flow of traffic before crossing the street. For more complex situations, such as building a house, flying a plane, or understanding an autistic child, it means taking into account many different factors through the best techniques, preferably objective and measurable, that are available. Because this is the process most of us—except the impulse driven—use in our daily lives and also try to teach our children, normal or handicapped alike—to size up a situation before acting on it—the question arises: Why are appropriate diagnostic and assessment procedures not used more consistently?

In our TEACCH program (Schopler *et al.*, 1984) we have always placed a strong emphasis on diagnosis and assessment. We are convinced that this process is essential for finding the most rational basis for any intervention, whether in the area of research, education, teaching communication, social skills, parent counseling, medical care, vocational training, or related issues. Thoughtful assessment increases the likelihood for implementing effective individualized treatment plans and for developing thoughtful and effective staff.

ERIC SCHOPLER and GARY B. MESIBOV • Division TEACCH, The University of North Carolina at Chapel Hill, Chapel Hill, North Carolina 27599-7180.

Why, then, do not all our colleagues share our commitment to this evaluation process? In this introductory chapter, we consider some of the reasons offered by professionals against using diagnostic and assessment strategies. We follow this with an example of how the emphasis on both formal and informal assessment is implemented in our TEACCH program, in which this emphasis plays a critical role in the effectiveness and viability of the program. Finally, we orient the reader to the organization of this volume and to the unique contribution of each chapter to the process of better understanding the child and his condition.

MISUSE OF FORMAL DIAGNOSTIC EVALUATION

Most objections against the use of diagnostic assessment are directed against formal evaluation, that is, the use of classification systems or instruments established and recognized for providing an ''objective'' evaluation. Such objections can readily be illustrated from any number of professional disciplines.

Psychiatric Diagnosis

For psychiatry, the Diagnostic and Statistical Manual of Mental Disorders (DSM-III-R 1987) has been developed after repeated revisions to offer a diagnostic classification system. Here one of the common criticisms arises from the requirement in many psychiatric clinics to assign an appropriate diagnostic number from the manual to each patient seen in the clinic. Critics rightly point out that a number or an equivalent word label is not a meaningful description of a patient or of the complaints bringing that patient to the clinic. Assigning such numbers is therefore a useless exercise.

While few would argue that a complex syndrome such as autism can be adequately summarized by a number, it should be remembered that such reductionism was not the primary purpose of the diagnostic manual. It was originally developed to enable psychiatrists to count the sort of patients they see as a way of demonstrating how they spend their time. This is not at all a useless exercise. On the contrary, it forms the statistical basis for planning a clinic's budget and research focus. However, this is not at all the same as expecting such diagnostic labels to represent the optimum understanding or treatment for a patient. Clearly, no diagnostic number or label can mean any more than what is known about the condition represented by that label. But even for conditions that are not well understood—and even misunderstood—the clinic still has to count them and group them, however rough or general the category may be. In other words, it is not necessarily the diagnostic process that is flawed; it is rather the inappropriate expectations and uses of it.

Psychological Evaluation

Parallel dissatisfaction has been directed at psychological and intelligence testing. For example, it is widely recognized that the degree of mental impairment is one of the greatest sources of heterogeneity in autism. Austic children with severe degrees of mental retardation are significantly different from autistic children with above-average intellectual functioning. Their problems of education and of social and vocational adjustment are all quite different. However, parallel to the criticism of psychiatric labeling, the complaint with IQ tests has been that placement and other treatment decisions are often made on the basis of specific IQ cutoff scores. For example, an autistic boy with an IQ of 69 may be eligible for a particular group home, yet be excluded if his IQ is 70. Clearly, the difference of only a few IQ points is not a meaningful basis for a treatment decision. Few would disagree with this observation. The important point is that some of the critics overlook that the difficulty is not with the psychological assessment itself, but rather with its use.

Administrators use cutoff points in order to place or refer applicants, according to criteria that are objective and set by someone other than themselves. We would much rather have clinical or educational decisions made according to treatment needs rather than arbitrary cutoff numbers. Unfortunately, such treatment decisions have more individual variation and therefore appear less objective. All too often, administrators have a conservative bent. They are likely to see IQ cutoff numbers as a better protective shield for their decisions than the more variable individual recommendation. Another line of administrative defense is sometimes a financial consideration. It is obviously cheaper to use arbitrary exclusion numbers than it is to admit that a particular applicant has a valid group home placement need, a need that could be met by developing an additional group home rather than by removing a referral with artificial and meaningless cutoff numbers. Here, as with the psychiatric diagnostic manual, the diagnostic groupings are caricatured for administrative use or misuse, rather than being themselves flawed.

Educational Assessment

Another variation of this theme can be illustrated from school systems in which special classrooms have been set up for special educational needs. In the case of autism, these are often small classrooms of four to six students with a teacher and an assistant teacher. Some school authorities have let their teachers know that they are placing two additional students in their classrooms by having these two additional students suddenly appear one morning without previous notification. The administrative explanation often runs like this: "We found two autistic children. You have our autistic classroom. You must take these children." This is one more instance in which the teacher comes away convinced that diagnosis is useless, when it is actually an autocratic school-placement procedure that is threatening the integrity of the classroom structure and teaching morale.

Research Categories

Disdain for diagnostic evaluation can also be found on occasion in the research arena. Sometimes, federal agencies set funding priorities for certain diagnostic categories. Researchers uninformed on the agency's priority basis can become quite critical of the diagnostic grouping. Their disdain for diagnostic grouping combined with their high pressured need for research funding may cause them to be indifferent and casual about making accurate diagnostic distinctions.

Another example from the research area can be found among some behaviorists who deny the value of using any diagnostic or assessment procedures. They are committed in principle to the proposition that only behavioral units are clinically meaningful and argue that these units can be suppressed or increased according to the scientific laws of behavior modification. They regard other diagnostic considerations as mere interference with behavioral analysis. This point of view has prompted some behaviorists to avoid all intelligence testing (Lovaas 1977) and to foster unrealistic expectations and promises for improvement. There have been instances in which normal development for preschool autistic children was promised and maintained by avoiding IQ testing and comparison before and after treatment (Schopler, Short, & Mesibov, in press). The resulting frustration for many children and parents could have been avoided, if the limits of behavioral intervention were acknowledged and understood and if diagnostic evaluation and assessment had been used. While narrow and oversimplified interpretations of behavior theory are gradually becoming less frequent, there is still too much misunderstanding and avoidance of diagnostic procedures by some behaviorists.

There are no doubt additional reasons why diagnostic assessment is often avoided. It requires individual attention, which can be both time consuming and intellectually taxing. However, in our work with autistic children in Division TEACCH, we have placed a heavy emphasis on diagnostic assessment from the beginning of the program in 1966 (Reichler & Schopler, 1976). After more than 20 years experience, we still rely on this process. Some of the formal tests have changed, and the available information to be evaluated has increased, but most of our primary program objectives have remained viable. We still need to know the diagnostic features of each new child referred, as well as how these compare with established diagnostic categories. What is the child's unique set of adaptational strengths and problems? What are the child's effects on parents and siblings and on their social life? How can family coping and the children's development be supported and enhanced? In a similar vein, how effective is the school experience? How can it be enhanced through the teacher, the curriculum, and the administration? Effective and viable resolution of such questions is largely dependent on the thoughtful analysis of the relevant assessment information.

FORMAL AND INFORMAL DIAGNOSIS AND ASSESSMENT

Because the TEACCH program has demonstrated its effectiveness in helping autistic children and their families (Marcus, Lansing, Andrews, & Schopler, 1978; Schopler, Mesibov & Boker, 1982; Schopler, 1987; Short, 1984), our evaluation procedures can be used as examples of those that have worked well and continue to do so. From the outset, we recognized that an important distinction was to be made between diagnosis and assessment. In the case of autism, the former referred to those features of a child shared by others, qualifying them for the classification of autism. These same children, however, have a number of other individual characteristics that are not part of the autism syndrome. The evaluation of these unique characteristics is every bit as important as the diagnostic classification, because without understanding them it is most unlikely that an effective treatment program can be developed. In order to maintain this important distinction, we use the term diagnosis to refer to the grouping of common features under the same diagnostic label, while assessment is used to evaluate the unique and individual characteristics of each client.

Diagnosis

A number of different systems for the diagnosis of autism have been published. These include the original Kanner (1943) criteria, the Creak (1961) points, Rutter's (1978) definition, the Rutter and Schopler update (see Chapter 2), that of the National Society for Autistic Children (NSAC, 1978), and the DSM-III-R (APA, 1987). Although widely used for clinical diagnosis and research, these five systems have not been developed into a formal rating scale or checklist. Instead, they have been widely used informally for clinical and research classification. There are minor differences among the systems (Schopler, 1978), but these do not overwhelm their commonalities. Professionals are often upset by these differences. They seem to forget that the children share a complex set of empirically demonstrated characteristics. This fuzziness might be ironed out by semantic or theoretical precision. However, success in this enterprise usually means only that an intellectual barrier has been erected between scientist and children.

Historically, the Kanner (1943) definition was the primary system for diagnosing autism. It was followed by the nine Creak (1961) points, intended to evolve a broader definition that would also incorporate childhood schizophrenia. These Creak criteria were based on behavioral observations rather than theory. Nevertheless, they were difficult to use for research because they were never quantified. In addition, their lack of developmental perspective made them particularly difficult to use with young children. Although the Creak points included autism with schizophrenia, De Meyer, Churchill, Pontius, and Gilkey (1971) found that Creak's main points for childhood schizophrenia corresponded more closely to autism than to schizophrenia. Kolvin's (1971) research demonstrating the distinction between autism and childhood schizophrenia had not yet been published.

The next three diagnostic systems were of more recent origin, with slight differences among them reflecting the different purposes for which they were evolved. Rutter's (1978) definition (updated in Chapter 2) was based on the evaluation of empirical research published since the Kanner (1943) and Creak (1961) criteria. The NSAC (1978) definition was intended for use in shaping social policy, legislation, and public awareness. DSM-III-R (1987) represents the most recent classification system formulated by the American Psychiatric Association. All three of these systems agree on three basic features of autism: (1) onset during infancy or childhood, (2) certain pervasive lack of responsiveness to other people, and (3) impairment of language and cognitive function.

At the beginning of the TEACCH Program, we saw the need to develop a formal diagnostic system (Reichler & Schopler, 1971) and we constructed a set of 15 scales to be rated for the diagnosis of autism. The psychometric properties of this Childhood Autism Rating Scale (CARS) have been established (Schopler, Reichler, DeVellis & Daly, 1980) and refined (Schopler, Reichler & Renner, 1986). The scale is described further in Chapter 16.

While this diagnostic category does not permit anything like an individualized treatment plan, it does lead to several general conclusions about such a child's educational needs, including the following:

1. The use of a small classroom with individual teaching, emphasizing structure and visual teaching techniques
2. Curriculum focus on enhancing communication and social skills in various modalities
3. Special training in leisure, and prevocation skills
4. The appropriate use of behavior theory for managing behavior problems
5. Special attention to problems of generalization to other settings

The autism diagnosis and the general educational principles derived from it, however, do not offer information necessary for developing an individualized educational program.

Assessment of Unique Characteristics

In the field of education, individualized evaluation and teaching is often regarded as a luxury found only in costly private programs. However, it is hard to work with autistic children without recognizing that differences in mental skills and behavior characteristics are sufficiently great to make individualized programming a cost effective necessity with them rather than a luxury.

Because of their uneven motivation patterns and intellectual functioning these children were often unresponsive to standard testing. They were considered untreatable, and this in turn resulted in misunderstanding and mismanagement. Their lack of test response was interpreted too often as the willful lack of cooperation of potentially normally functioning children.

To reverse this trend, we developed the Psychoeducational Profile (PEP) (Schopler & Reichler, 1979), designed to assess a variety of characteristics and behaviors not central to the definition of autism. It had already become evident that autistic children could be tested if lower or easier test items were administered (Alpern, 1967) and that autism and mental retardation could and did coexist.

In the PEP, we included several provisions designed to reduce or eliminate untestability. First, we selected test materials that we knew from our clinical experience were of intrinsic interest to autistic children. Second, to overcome the problems encountered by autistic children because of failure to respond to standardized text instructions, we built a flexible structure for administration into the test. Test items did not have to be administered in predetermined order or according to standard instructions. Third, because language problems are characteristic of these children, the PEP was designed for minimum language and maximum communication flexibility. Fourth, in addition to scoring responses as "pass" or "fail," one can also take into account partially completed responses by scoring them as they emerge. It is, in fact, the *emerge* category that is central to planning individualized treatment.

This formal assessment instrument has proved to be most useful for austistic children and has made virtually all autistic children testable. This formal evaluation was then combined with the informal assessment data from home and school in order for us to develop the most optimum individualized treatment program possible from available information.

More recently, we extended the PEP through adolescence into adulthood (with the Adolescent and Adult Psychoeducational Profile (AAPEP) (Mesibov, Schopler, Schaffer & Landrus, 1988). This was needed not only to assess new adolescent skills, but also because of the shifting emphasis required from school to residential and vocational placement. The AAPEP includes the same *pass, emerge, fail* scoring system so useful for planning educational programs with the younger children. It also extends the formal assessment data by systematically evaluating data from the home, the school, or the workplace, in addition to the direct observation of the youngster responding to test items. All three of these test areas included items grouped into six function areas: (1) vocational skills, (2) independent functioning, (3) leisure skills, (4) vocational behavior, (5) functional communication, and (6) interpersonal behavior. These were designed to assess those skills necessary for successful functioning in either a group home and sheltered workshop settings, or both. By using a formal system of evaluating these six function areas independently across the individual's three main life domains, it is possible to achieve a reliable and valid decision making process (Mesibov *et al.*, 1988).

In addition to extending the PEP to an upward age range, we have also found the need to extend it downward. This is primarily because of the increase in our referrals of children functioning below the 2-year level. Moreover, we found that the existing edition of the PEP did not have a sufficient number of items for the first 2 years of life to permit clinically meaningful bases for establishing developmental levels for the earliest developmental functions. This revision (Schopler, Reichler & Lansing, in press) will soon be available.

Formal diagnostic and assessment procedures like those discussed above are needed for research and are especially useful at major decision points affecting the client's life. Those include the parents' first inquiry about what is wrong with their child, what to do about first entrance into school, and transition from one school to another or to the workplace. Although formal evaluations offer valuable guidelines to families, teachers, and other professionals involved in the day-to-day life of autistic people, there are also daily problems and variations not covered in the formal evaluation process. These can best be dealt with if the staff has been trained in the informal assessment of daily problems.

Informal Assessment

During more than 15 years of training parents, teachers, group home personnel, and others to improve their ability to foster development in their complex and challenging roles, we have been teaching them how to conduct informal assessments from their daily life observations. In order to develop our assessment curriculum, we wrote an informal survey of the management problems most frequently of concern to parents and professionals. These included aggression, ineffective discipline, eating difficulties, inadequate play skills, lack of initiative, sleeping problems, tantrums without known cause, and toilet-training problems.

We have found that the process of informal assessment can best be discussed and visualized around the image of an iceberg, only one ninth of which appears above the water, while the remainder is out of sight. The specific behavior problems encountered with the autistic client are represented by the portion of the iceberg visible above the water, while the possible reasons triggering these behaviors are out of sight or only partially visible. The process can be illustrated using the behavior problem of aggression as an example.

Aggression

Specific behaviors such as spitting, biting, kicking, pushing, and throwing are visible at or above the water line, while the reasons may seem mysteriously unknown, out of sight beneath the water line. They could include reasons common to autism: that the child relates poorly to others, has impaired communications, is unaware of others' feelings, has inappropriate sensory preference—likes noise or movement, inadequate play skills and is bored, and so on. These explanatory mechanisms show a great deal of individual variation, and often vary for the same individual in different environments.

This iceberg metaphor can appear risky for autism because it could invite unbridled speculation about causal mechanisms. It was only a short time ago that widespread misunderstandings of autism were generated by wild speculative and unproved psychoanalytic (causal) theories about the child's strange behaviors. However, such high-inference theories need not be used. They can be replaced by low-inference causal explanations that can be tested or verified.

For example, if we think the child's pushing comes from an inability to relate to others, the child can be taught some alternate method of relating, such as holding hands. If we think the child hits from lack of communication, perhaps the child can be taught a verbal greeting. If the problem is unawareness of others' feelings, this can sometimes be improved by teaching how to read certain facial expressions. If the child throws and spits from boredom, this behavior can be changed by restructuring activities.

Each explanatory mechanism should be based on direct inference rather than theory. It should be based on knowing the individual child and on familiarity with the child's background and reactions to different circumstances. This helps focus the range of explanations. Moreover, each explanatory hypothesis can be tested with a related intervention. If the child's learning to raise a hand as a signal for attention replaces hitting, the attention-getting explanation was on target. If the hand-raising does not reduce the child's hitting, a different causal mechanism is involved.

Although the informal assessment process does not guarantee an effective intervention in all cases, in our experience, it has been instrumental in reducing reliance on the rise of aversives, and it has been effective in most cases. We have reviewed the importance of both formal and informal evaluation from our TEACCH experience. The excellent chapters in this volume cover several issues: overview of labeling autistic children, diagnostic concerns, assessment, and special problems.

INTRODUCTION AND OVERVIEW

Part I of this volume deals with the many aspects of diagnosing autistic youngsters. Rutter and Schopler begin this section with a superb discussion of current trends and diagnostic issues related to childhood autism. Their discussions of the basic cognitive deficit, current rating instruments, boundaries between autism and related disabilities, and etiological heterogeneity within autism syndromes will give readers of this volume a much better understanding of current directions in the diagnosis and classification of autism.

Gallagher follows with an informal discussion of the political implications of the autism diagnosis. Diagnostic labels have helped parents in the United States to identify others with similar needs and concerns. This has led to strong political advocacy, which was responsible for P.L. 94-142 and other important legislation that has been the impetus for the current improvement in services to handicapped people across the United States. Labeling has also been important for furthering research efforts that have provided more insight into the causes, nature, and potential treatments for conditions like autism.

Werry provides a thoughtful discussion of classification systems, their strengths and weakness. He describes the characteristics of good classification systems in general as being therapeutic, prognostic, etiologic, pathologic, symptomatologic, communicative–heuristic, preventative, and explanatory. With particular reference to autism, he then describes how one might evaluate the diagnostic criteria. Are they reliable among different raters in different places over time? Is there covariation of the elements in that the defining characteristics are almost always found together? Do they discriminate between autism and other conditions? Finally, he discusses validity that speaks to the value of such a diagnosis. For example, does the diagnostic system help professionals with the selection of appropriate treatments, or to predict outcomes? The remainder of his thought-provoking chapter deals with an analysis of different classification systems and ways to select the most appropriate ones.

Mary Akerley, an attorney and parent of a young man with autism, concludes this section by describing some important advantages of labeling children as autistic from a parent's perspective. Although she acknowledges that labels can be abused and in fact, "Deceptive labels can be killers," she still sees an important function for them if properly used. In her chapter, Akerley poignantly describes her search for answers when she knew her child had a problem, as well as the importance for a parent of knowing what one is dealing with. The label of "autism" also suggests certain treatments or programs that parents would not routinely find without proper diagnosis of their children.

DIAGNOSTIC ISSUES

Part II of this volume is organized around current diagnostic issues. Volkmar and Cohen begin with a critical analysis of classification issues in autism with discussions of some of the major factors, including age of onset, developmental level, social dysfunction, and communication. Their discussion provides a nice historical perspective as well as a better understanding of related diagnostic classifications, such as Asperger's syndrome and atypical pervasive developmental disorder.

Lorna Wing was among the first professionals in the field to argue for a broader conceptualization of the autism syndrome. Her chapter describes the continuum of autistic characteristics, with a good discussion of the wide range of possibilities. She then describes the relationship of autism to other developmental disorders and concludes with a fine presentation of the clinical implications of her work.

Cantwell and Baker review an important international approach to classification, the multiaxial diagnostic systems. They describe the conceptual and pragmatic appeal of these systems for researchers and clinicians dealing with children and then provide some excellent case examples. The chapter ends with an excellent discussion of specific axes and their application to the diagnostic classification of autism.

Susan Parks concludes the section with a review of available diagnostic instruments. Focusing on the most widely used instruments for this purpose, she describes the strengths and limitations of the Rimland Diagnostic Checklist, the Ruttenberg *et al.* BRIAAC, the Freeman, Ritvo, and Searles, BOS, and the ASIEP. There is also a discussion of several assessment instruments as well as a thoughtful analysis of the reliability, validity, and other published data relating to these instruments. Readers wanting a careful assessment of the uses and limitations of these widely distributed instruments will find this chapter extremely interesting and informative.

GENERAL ASSESSMENT ISSUES

Part III covers important issues in the assessment of individuals with autism. Michael Powers begins this section with a comprehensive overview of the area of behavioral assessment. Behavioral techniques have been extremely influential in work with autistic individuals. Powers does a fine job summarizing this broad area and demonstrating its relevance for those in the field of autism.

The chapter by Lord and Schopler presents a most interesting perspective on intelligence testing in autism. After reading this chapter, one will develop a healthy skepticism about the universality of such concepts as intelligence especially as it relates to autistic youngsters. The chapter also documents the relative consistency of IQ measures over time and their value as predictive measures. This chapter is also helpful in its analysis of IQ tests and its explanation of inconsistencies between tests based on some strengths and weaknesses of autistic youngsters.

Although much of the work in this field emphasizes assessments of autistic children, professionals are becoming more aware of the role of environmental factors. The chapter by Jones is extremely helpful in providing a systematic approach to analyzing living environments and demonstrating their potential for improving or interfering with outcomes for autistic youngsters. Practical applications of this systematic approach are described and examined.

Sandra Harris provides a helpful framework for assessing families of autistic children. Her systematic approach should prove useful for those analyzing family dynamics with an eye toward developing effective intervention strategies. Harris presents a nice balance between understanding the normal concerns and issues facing families of handicapped children, without ignoring the additional stresses presented by a handicapped youngster. Without overemphasizing the pathology, Harris provides some helpful guidelines for working with these families.

The last chapter in this section involves nutritional assessments. The early work by Rimland on megavitamins has alerted researchers to the importance of nutritional issues. Raiten reviews this important work, followed by some important insights and techniques in the dietary assessment process.

SPECIAL ISSUES

The final section of this book relates to special issues in diagnosis and assessment. Although most of the work in the field began more than a decade ago with young autistic children, many of them have grown up and are remaining in community-based programs. As they grow older, issues related to adolescence and adulthood are becoming more important. In his chapter, Mesibov describes adjustments in the TEACCH Program's diagnostic and assessment instruments to meet the needs of the older age group. Professionals interested in this group will find these instruments most useful.

The chapter by Rutter and co-workers also presents some refreshing new approaches to the assessment process. Focusing on the social deficits of these youngsters, the chapter presents some interesting approaches to assessing the nature of these fundamental deficits. Investigators interested in higher functioning autistic people will find these techniques especially helpful.

Although we generally think of assessment as relating to standardized tests, teachers of autistic children are constantly involved in a less formal assessment process in their classrooms if they are to work effectively with their youngsters. Special issues in assessing autistic children in the classroom are described by Mesibov, Troxler, and Boswell. This chapter should be especially useful for classroom teachers of autistic children.

Current interest in the early identification of handicapped children and preschool programs makes the chapter on assessment of preschool children by Watson and Marcus extremely timely. They begin with a discussion of diagnosis with very young children and then describe the earliest manifestations of the most common impairments in autistic youngsters such as social relatedness and communication. The chapter has a strong emphasis on parent involvement, consistent with most current conceptions in the field. The clinical applications at the end of the chapter will be of particular relevance to practitioners in the field.

The final chapter in the book, by Nancy Johnson-Martin, deals with the assessment of extremely low functioning children. This has been of concern to those working with profoundly retarded autistic youngsters, and Johnston-Martin has some excellent ideas and strategies for working with this group. Her review of diagnostic and assessment instruments and their appropriateness for this population will be extremely helpful, as are her practical suggestions for appropriate adaptations.

Overall, we are delighted with the breadth and variety of approaches to the timely issues of diagnosis and assessment represented by the contributions to this volume. Although we were unable to include all investigators who have contributed to this important area, our contributors include leading national and international figures in the study of autism and related handicaps. Researchers and clinicians alike should find some systematic reanalyses of ongoing issues as well as some new ideas and approaches. The integration of research and clinical perspectives is always healthy and adds a special dimension to this work.

REFERENCES

Alpern, G. D. (1967). Measurement of "untestable" autistic children. *Journal of Abnormal Psychology, 72*, 478–96.

American Psychiatric Association. (1987). *Diagnostic and statistical manual of mental disorders* (3rd ed., rev.). Washington, DC Author.

Creak, M. (1961) Schizophrenia syndrome in childhood: Progress report of a working party. *Cerebral Palsy Bulletin, 3*, 501–4.

DeMyer, M. K., Churchill, D. W., Pontius, W., & Gilkey, K. M. (1971). A comparison of five diagnostic systems for childhood schizophrenia and infantile autism. *Journal of Autism and Childhood Schizophrenia, 1*, 175–89.

Kanner, L. (1943). Autistic disturbances of affective contact. *Nervous Child, 2*, 217–50.

Kolvin, I. (1971). Psychoses in childhood—a comparative study. In M. Rutter (Ed.), *Infantile Autism: Concepts, characteristics and treatment.* (pp. 7–26). London: Churchill Livingstone.

Lovaas, O. I. (1977). *The autistic child.* New York: Irvington.

Marcus, L. M., Lansing, M., Andrews, C., & Schopler, E. (1978). Improvement of teaching effectiveness in parents of autistic children. *Journal of the of the Academy of Child Psychiatry, 17*, 625–39.

Mesibov, G., Schopler, E., Schaffer, B., & Landrus, R. (1988) *Individualized assessment and treatment for autistic and developmentally disabled children. Vol. 4. Adolescent and adult psychoeducational profile (AAPEP).* Austin, TX: Pro-Ed.

National Society for Autistic Children. (1978). National Society for Autistic Children definition of the syndrome of autism. *Journal of Autism and Childhood Schizophrenia, 8*, 162–7.

Reichler, R. J., & Schopler, E. (1971). Observations on the nature of human relatedness. *Journal of Autism and Childhood Schizophrenia, 1*, 283–96.

Reichler, R. J., & Schopler. E. (1976). Developmental therapy: A program model for providing individual services in the community. In E. Schopler & R. Reichler (Eds.), *Psychopathology and Child Development: Research and treatment* (pp. 347–72). New York: Plenum.

Rutter, M. (1978). Diagnosis and definition of childhood autism. *Journal of Autism and Developmental Disorders, 8*, 139–161.

Schopler, E. (1978). National Society for Autistic Children definition of the syndrome of autism: Discussion. *Journal of Autism and Childhood Schizophrenia, 8*, 167–9.

Schopler, E. (1987). Specific and nonspecific factors in the effectiveness of a treatment system. *American Psychologist, 42*, 376–83.

Schopler, E., Mesibov, G. B., & Baker, A. (1982). Evaluation of treatment for autistic children and their parents. *Journal of the American Academy of Child Psychiatry, 21*, 262–7.

Schopler, E., Mesibov, G. B., Shigley, R. H., & Bashford, A. (1984). Helping autistic children through their parents: The TEACCH model. In E. Schopler & G. B. Mesibov (Eds.), *The effects of autism on the family* (pp. 65–81). New York: Plenum.

Schopler, E., & Reichler, R. J. (1979). Individualized assessment and treatment for autistic and developmentally disabled children. *Psychoeducational Profile* (Vol. I). Austin, TX: Pro-Ed.

Schopler, E., Reichler, R. J., DeVellis, R. F., & Daly, K. (1980). Toward objective classification of childhood autism: Childhood Autism Rating Scale (CARS). *Journal of Autism and Developmental Disorders, 10*, 91–103.

Schopler, E. Reichler, R., & Renner, B. (1986). *The childhood autism rating scale (CARS)*. New York: Irvington.

Schopler, E., Reichler, R. J., & Lansing, M. D. (in press). *The new psychoeducational profile*. Austin, TX: Pro-Ed.

Schopler, E., Short, A., & Mesibov, G.B. (in press). Relation of behavioral treatment to ''normal functioning'': Comment on Lovaas. *Journal of Consulting and Clinical Psychology*.

Short, A. B. (1984). Short-term treatment outcome using parents as co-therapists for their autistic children. *Journal of Child Psychology and Psychiatry and Allied Disciplines, 25,* 443–58.

2

Autism and Pervasive Developmental Disorders
Concepts and Diagnostic Issues

MICHAEL RUTTER and ERIC SCHOPLER

INTRODUCTION

Ten years ago, we presented a review of the growing body of research developing on the diagnosis, understanding, and treatment of autism (Rutter, 1978; Schopler, 1978). The definition of autism developed by the National Society for Autistic Children was published along with that review. Although informed by scientific research, the NSAC definition was developed to shape favorable social policy rather than scientific synthesis, and so some anticipated differences between the two definitions arose. Since that time research has continued to accelerate. While these past 7 years have brought new information, they have also generated some new confusion and disputes. This review presents our synthesis of the accumulated research and provides our best assessment of the evidence for resolving some of these disputes.[1]

For more than 100 years, there have been isolated case reports of very young children with severe mental disorders that have involved a marked distortion of the developmental process (Maudsley, 1867). Nevertheless, the general recognition of these conditions is a much more recent phenomenon. During the first half of this century there were a variety of descriptions of syndromes of this type; these included dementia precocissima (De Sanctis, 1906, 1969), childhood schizophrenia (Bender, 1947), and dementia infantilis (Heller, 1930, 1969). The terminology used reflected the general assumption that these represented the very early onset of adult-type psychoses. Kanner's (1943) incisive description of the syndrome of infantile autism was somewhat of an exception in that he set forth the diagnostic criteria in terms of specific child behaviors as he observed them rather than in terms of modifications of adult criteria. Nevertheless, the overall climate of psychiatric thinking led to an acceptance that autism, too, was an unusual form of schizophrenia that happened to begin very early in life. (See Schopler, 1983, for a fuller account of the ways in which diagnostic concepts of

MICHAEL RUTTER • Department of Child and Adolescent Psychiatry, Institute of Psychiatry, University of London, London SE5 8AF, England.   ERIC SCHOPLER • Division TEACCH, The University of North Carolina at Chapel Hill, Chapel Hill, North Carolina 27599-7180.

autism have varied over time in relationship to changing theories, therapeutic approaches, and empirical knowledge.)

For some years, there was a confusing proliferation of diagnostic terms and sub-classification under the broad umbrella of "childhood schizophrenia" (Eisenberg, 1972; Kolvin, 1974; Makita, 1974; Rutter, 1972, 1978). Then, during the 1970s, there came a growing recognition that it was necessary to differentiate between severe mental disorders arising during the infancy period, of which autism is the prototype, and the psychoses arising in later childhood or adolescence, of which schizophrenia is the prototype (Rutter, 1985*a*). The latter group of conditions involve a *loss* of reality sense in individuals who have previously functioned normally or near normally and hence may properly be termed *psychoses* (insofar as that word has any precise meaning). However, the former are more usefully considered as a serious abnormality in the developmental process itself—an abnormality present from early in life. It is for that reason that the American Psychiatric Association (1980) classification, DSM-III. used the term *pervasive developmental disorders.*

The adoption of the term *pervasive developmental disorders* was important in its empha-sis on the developmental aspects or characteristics of the abnormalities and in its highlighting of the differentiation from mental illnesses as they occur in adult life. The adjective *pervasive* was meant to draw attention to the widespread distortion of the developmental process (involving communication, socialization, and thought processes)—a breadth of abnormality that makes autism different from the specific developmental disorders of speech or language, in which the problems are much more restricted in scope, even though associated socioemo-tional difficulties are relatively common (Cantwell & Baker, 1985). Nevertheless, not every-one has been satisfied with the term because, although the disorders affect a wide range of developmental processes, some are unimpaired. The disorders are pervasive, but they are not all-pervasive. Indeed, it is the very fact that general intelligence may be relatively spared (perhaps a fifth of autistic children have performance IQs within the normal range) that underlines the need to separate autism from global mental handicap.

DISTINCTIVENESS AND VALIDITY OF THE AUTISM SYNDROME

There is continuing dispute over both the boundaries and the subdivision of pervasive developmental disorders, but questions on diagnosis and classification are best considered by first examining the narrower issue of whether autism constitutes a syndrome that is mean-ingfully different from acute psychiatric conditions (such as emotional and conduct disor-ders), from the psychoses of later childhood (such as schizophrenia), from general mental retardation, and from the specific developmental disorders of speech and language. As the evidence has been fully discussed previously (Rutter, 1978; Rutter & Gould, 1985), the findings may be summarized quite briefly.

The likely discontinuity between autism and schizophrenia is strongly indicated by the sharply bimodal distribution of age of onset (Rutter, 1974). Severe mental disorders of a kind that might possibly be linked with either autism or schizophrenia rarely begin in middle childhood. There is a peak in infancy made up of autisticlike disorders and a peak in adolescence made up of schizophrenialike disorders, but a marked trough in between. This finding in itself makes it improbable that autism and schizophrenia constitute subvarieties of the same basic condition. However, in addition, autism and schizophrenia differ sharply in family history (a familial loading of schizophrenia is rare with autism), in phenomenology (delusions and hallucinations are rare in autism), in course (often episodic with periods of normality or near-normality in schizophrenia, but persistent in autism), and in the association with epileptic seizures (rare in schizophrenia but present in about a quarter of cases of autism).

Initially, Kanner (1943) asserted that autistic children all had a normal cognitive potential. That is now known not to be the case; to the contrary, more than three fourths of autistic children are also mentally retarded (Rutter, 1979). Nevertheless, autistic children have been found to differ sharply from nonautistic mentally handicapped children of comparable mental age. Thus, although seizures occur in about one fourth of children in both the groups, there is a marked difference with respect to the age of onset (usually in early childhood in mental retardation but in adolescence in autism—Deykin & MacMahon, 1979; Richardson, Koller, Katz & McLaren, 1980), in medical correlates (e.g., Down's syndrome is the most common cause of mental handicap but is very rarely associated with autism—(Wing & Gould, 1979), in sex distribution (a slight male preponderance in mental retardation—Birch, Richardson; Baird, Horobin & Illsley, 1970, but a 4 : 1 sex ratio in autism—Rutter, 1985a), in patterns of cognitive disability (autistic children are more likely to fail on tasks that require skills in abstraction, language, and the use of meaning—Hermelin & O'Connor, 1970; Rutter, 1983), and in their discrimination of socioemotional cues (markedly impaired in autism but not in mental handicap—Hobson, 1987).

On the face of it, autism might seem to be very similar to the most severe developmental disorders of receptive language. Indeed, there are similarities and some overlap (Paul, Cohen & Caparulo, 1983; Paul & Cohen, 1984). However, there also are marked differences (Rutter, 1979). Autism is distinctive in terms of its sex distribution (specific developmental disorders of expressive language show a male preponderance but the disorders of *receptive* language, which are closest to autism, do not—although autism does), its worse prognosis (Cantwell, Baker, Rutter & Mawhood, 1987), its pattern of cognitive disabilities (both wider and more severe in autism, even after equating for level of language handicap—Bartak, Rutter & Cox, 1975), and its persisting pattern of socioemotional–behavioral abnormalities (Cantwell *et al.*, 1987).

Although there have been claims that autism arises on the basis of fear over social contacts (Tinbergen & Tinbergen, 1983) or of parental rejection (Bettelheim, 1967), the available evidence does not support either concept. It is true, of course, that abnormalities in rearing can lead to serious social problems, but the nature of the social abnormalities differs markedly from that found in autism. Thus, institution-reared children tend to be clinging and excessively friendly in an indiscriminate fashion (Rutter, 1981), and abused children show marked insecurities in their personal attachments (Mrazek & Mrazek, 1985). Neither feature is characteristic of autism.

Autism differs in so many ways from the ordinary run of emotional and behavioral disorders of childhood that its distinctiveness is beyond dispute. Thus, it stands out in terms of its strong association with mental retardation and with organic brain dysfunction, as well as in its worse prognosis, and its persisting differences in symptomatology (Rutter, 1979).

We may conclude that there is no doubt that autism constitutes a valid and meaningfully different psychiatric syndrome; indeed, the evidence on its validity is stronger than for any other psychiatric condition in childhood. Nevertheless, as we shall see, that does not mean that there are no crucial diagnostic and classification issues that await resolution. We consider these issues in some detail below.

DIAGNOSTIC CRITERIA FOR AUTISM

Before proceeding further, it is necessary to pause to outline the diagnostic criteria for autism. Not surprisingly, these have varied in emphasis over the years as concepts have varied in their focus and preoccupations. When autism was viewed as an infantile psychosis, most attention tended to be paid to bizarre behaviors. As clinicians and researchers began to appreciate the importance of the cognitive deficits, the spotlight shifted to impairments in language and in social development. Most recently, it has come to be realized that what differentiates autism from other disorders of development is the *deviance*, rather than the delay, in the developmental process. It is essential to understand that these shifts in concept have *not* meant that the term *autism* has come to be applied to different conditions. Autistic children usually show an admixture of bizarre behaviors, developmental delay, and developmental deviance. What has happened is that research findings have led people to recognize that, although the first two groups of features are indeed common in autism, it is the third group that most sharply sets it apart from other conditions. Thus, schizophrenic children also show an assortment of bizarre behaviors but generally do not exhibit the same deviance of language and social development characteristic of autism. Similarly, impaired language and socialization is found in many developmental disorders (especially general mental retardation), but the particular pattern of deviance found in autism is distinctive to that syndrome.

For these reasons, both the major systems of classification, ICD9 (World Health Organization, 1978) and DSM-III (American Psychiatric Association, 1980) have tended to concentrate on four main sets of diagnostic criteria (see Rutter, 1984; Schopler, 1983). First, there is the requirement that the disorder be manifest before 30 months of age. This stipulation has led to some confusion because of the ambiguity as to whether this means that there must be evidence of developmental impairment or distortion before 30 months, or rather that the specifically autistic features must be apparent before 30 months. As the latter vary appreciably in the age at which they are detectable (i.e., the disorder may have an onset in early infancy yet not be recognized until sometime later), it is clear that the first approach is the most appropriate one. Two main diagnostic issues arise with respect to age of manifestation. The first query is how to classify disorders that appear indistinguishable from autism but which differ in terms of development, the children having been apparently normal until after the age of 30 months. This problem most often applies to children for whom the information on early development is inadequate for certainty on the timing of onset of abnormality. A lifting of the cutoff from 30 months to 3 years removes most of these difficulties without altering the basic concept of the syndrome. Occasional cases of autisticlike disorders do occur after the age of 3, but they are rare and usually due to acquired brain disease (or genetic disorders of later manifestation, such as the cerebral lipoidoses). For the moment, at least, it seems useful to separate those late onset conditions from "classic" autism.[1]

The second query is whether autism that seems to have been preceded by a period of definitely normal development differs in any fundamental way from autism in which development has been abnormal from the outset. General principles suggest that the two are likely to differ in etiology; nevertheless, research so far has failed to demonstrate any such differences. Indeed, one pair of monozygotic (MZ) twins were concordant for autism but

---

[1]We have used the adjective *classic* in quotes to make clear that there is no assumption that Kanner's original diagnostic criteria should have precedence. The whole burden of our argument is that the choice of criteria should be based on empirical evidence regarding validity of diagnostic distinctions. Nevertheless, because the term *autism* has come to be used in rather varied ways, it has been necessary to have some way of indicating when we are using it in Kanner's original sense.

markedly discordant for age of onset (Folstein & Rutter, 1977). This remains one of many areas requiring further investigation.

The second set of diagnostic criteria concerns various aspects of deviance in the development of social relationships. The accurate delineation of the social abnormalities characteristic of autism were impeded for many years by two tendencies. First, for many years investigators tended to ignore the need to take account of the mental retardation that so often accompanies autism. Some delay or impairment in social development is likely to occur as a result of the mental handicap quite independently of the autism. It is now appreciated that it is crucial to define the social abnormalities in terms of *deviance* in relation to the child's mental age; this means that diagnostic assessment must include a careful and systematic cognitive evaluation (Rutter, 1984). Second, until recently, there was a lack of an adequate conceptualization or vocabulary of social features. Accordingly, the social abnormalities of autism tended to be defined in terms of vague descriptors such as "aloofness" or "social withdrawal," or in terms of nonspecific features such as "lack of eye-to-eye gaze" that may arise from a variety of causes (e.g., very anxious or very shy children are likely to avoid visual contact).

Gains in knowledge of normal social development, as well as an improved understanding of autism, have recently led to a better specification of the particular social abnormalities that characterize autism. These are thought to reflect a basic deficit in the capacity to form relationships. This is evident in autistic children's inadequate appreciation of socioemotional cues and in their lack of response to other people's emotions and a lack of modulation of behavior according to social context; in their poor use of social signals and weak integration of social, emotional, and communicative behaviors; and especially in their lack of socioemotional reciprocity. These deficits are shown in features such as (1) a failure to use eye-to-eye gaze, facial expression, body posture, and gesture to regulate social interaction; (2) rarely seeking others for comfort or affection; (3) rarely initiating interactive play with others; (4) rarely offering comfort to others or responding to other people's distress or happiness; (5) rarely greeting others; and (6) no peer friendships in terms of a mutual sharing of interests, activities, and emotions—despite ample opportunities. In each case, these behaviors should be assessed in terms of difference from those appropriate for the child's *mental* age.

The third set of diagnostic criteria comprises abnormalities in communication. At one time these tended to be framed in terms of speech or language impairment, but it is clear that the characteristic features involve deviance rather than delay (although delay in development is also usual), and the abnormalities extend beyond speech to many aspects of the communicative process. Indeed, the strictly linguistic features (i.e., the use of grammar) are least affected. Rather, there appears to be a basic deficit in the capacity to use language for social communication. This is evident in the relative lack of *social* usage of such language skills as are possessed and in the poor synchrony and lack of reciprocity in conversational interchange, a poor flexibility in language expression and a relative lack of creativity and fantasy in thought processes, an inadequate response to other people's verbal and nonverbal overtures, and an impaired use of variations in cadence or emphasis to reflect communicative modulation. These features may be shown by (1) a delay in, or total lack of, the development of spoken language that is not compensated for by use of gesture or mime as alternative modes of communication (often preceded by a lack of communicative babbling); (2) a failure to respond to the communications of others, such as (when young) not responding when called by name; (3) a relative failure to initiate or sustain conversational interchange in which there is a to and fro and responsivity to the communications of the other person; (4) stereotyped and repetitive use of language; (5) use of *you* when *I* is meant; (6) idiosyncratic use of words; and (7) abnormalities in pitch, stress, rate, rhythm, and intonation of speech. The lack of creativity and spontaneity in autistic children's use of social language is paralleled by a similar deficit in preverbal skills. Thus, a lack of varied spontaneous "make-believe" play is especially characteristic.

It is evident that, because these features concern abnormalities in the communicative process and not just speech, they can be manifest both before the child can talk and after language competence has reached normal levels. Thus, normal infants use sounds to communicate well before they can talk. and these vocalizations exhibit conversational synchrony and reciprocity; this is not so with autistic infants. Moreover, deaf children who lack speech nevertheless succeed in communicating by other means; autistic children do not. Also, autistic adults who are able to speak fluently are likely still to show abnormalities in the flow of conversational interchanges, a formality of language, a lack of emotional expression in speech, and a lack of fantasy and imagination.

The fourth set of diagnostic criteria concerns restricted, repetitive, and stereotyped patterns of behavior. The meaning of this tendency to impose rigidity and routine on a wide range of aspects of day-to-day functioning remains obscure. However, it does appear to be a general tendency since it applies to novel activities and not just to familiar habits and play patterns (Frith, 1971). In part, the stereotypy probably reflects the lack of creativity associated with autism, but it seems to be more than that in that it applies so widely even in the least intellectually handicapped individuals. The ways in which the stereotyped patterns may be shown include (1) an encompassing preoccupation with stereotyped and restricted patterns of interest, (2) attachments to unusual objects, (3) compulsive rituals, (4) stereotyped and repetitive motor mannerisms, (5) preoccupations with part-objects or nonfunctional elements of play materials, and (6) distress over changes in small details of the environment.

NATURE OF THE BASIC DEFICIT

It is clear from this account of the diagnostic criteria for autism that over the last two decades there have been progressive attempts to move from abnormal behaviors, expressed in general terms, to *qualitatively* distinct features that are syndrome specific, to the reformulation of those features in terms of the particular psychological processes thought to be affected. Such attempts are essential if the nature of the basic deficit is to be identified. Once this is accomplished, the usual procedure in medicine is to redefine the condition in terms of the underlying abnormality rather than the signs and symptoms that first identified the syndrome. Thus, thyrotoxicosis is defined in terms of the abnormality in thyroxine production and not the palpitations, loss of weight, and exophthalmos that the abnormality tends to produce. Patients with such symptoms who do not show abnormalities in thyroxine production are not diagnosed as suffering from thyrotoxicosis. It should be emphasized that this identification of the basic abnormality is *not* synonymous with discovery of the cause. Not only may the cause not be known but also a single abnormality may have more than one cause. That would be the case, for example, with many blood dyscrasias and also with immune disorders.

It should be added that there need not necessarily be any unitary basic deficit. For example, that applies to cerebral palsy. There is a general sort of unity in terms of abnormalities in motor functioning but such abnormalities take several rather different forms. Athetosis, spasticity, and apraxia reflect rather different neurophysiologic abnormalities. The particular pattern of motor deficit depends on the distribution of brain damage and on the type of abnormal brain functioning with which that damage happens to be associated. There is no one basic deficit because the disorder reflects varying patterns of organic brain dysfunction rather than any single disease state. Inevitably, when that is the state of affairs, there is an essential ambiguity over the boundaries of the disorder in question.

A further point that needs to be made is that this delineation of the basic deficit need not be an all-or-none affair. Thus, for example, mental retardation is comparable to cerebral palsy insofar as it constitutes a general syndrome (characterized by a deficit in intellectual development) rather than by a specific unitary abnormality of one underlying process. Nevertheless, this general syndrome is gradually being broken down as specific disease entities become identified. Thus, Down's syndrome is defined by particular chromosomal anomalies. In this instance the delineation is not made in terms of a particular type of cognitive deficit; nevertheless, the cognitive pattern associated with Down's syndrome tends to have some distinctive features (Anwar, 1983).

The key question is: What sort of disorder does autism constitute? At one level it must be a general syndrome like cerebral palsy or mental retardation. This is because it is known that many children with severe mental handicap show some autistic features, because the autistic pattern is rather variable, and because it may be found with a variety of medical conditions (Wing & Gould, 1979). Thus, conditions that give rise to widespread organic brain dysfunction may sometimes cause patterns of brain pathology that affect the systems underlying the autistic abnormalities. However, that does not seem to be a satisfactory general answer for several different reasons. In the first place, there are very marked differences in the rate of autism between medical conditions that commonly give rise to mental handicap (Rutter, 1979). For example, autism is quite rare in children with Down's syndrome or with cerebral palsy; by contrast, it is relatively common in those with infantile spasms or congenital rubella. It appears that there must be something particular about the pathologic processes that give rise to autism, although what that is remains obscure.

Second, most autistic individuals do not show any gross structural abnormalities of the brain—at least not as evident on the basis of the data available from the techniques used so far. Thus, computed tomography (CT) scans have not revealed any consistent abnormality (Damasio, Maurer, Damasio & Chui, 1980; Caparulo et al., 1981; Gillberg & Svendsen, 1983; Rumsey et al., 1983; Rosenbloom et al., 1984; Prior, Tress, Hoffman & Boldt, 1984), nor apparently is there any diagnostically distinctive metabolic pattern as reflected in positron emission tomography (PET) findings (Rumsey et al., 1985; Herold, Frackowiak, Rutter & Howlin, 1985). There have been very few neuropathologic studies, but these, too, have shown either quite subtle histologic changes or no detectable abnormalities (Bauman & Kemper, 1985; Coleman, Romano, Lapham & Simon, 1985; Darby, 1976; Williams, Hauser, Purpura, Delong & Swisher. 1980). Moreover, although autistic children show a modest increase in perinatal complications (Finegan & Quadrington, 1979; Deykin & Mac-Mahon, 1980; Torrey, Hersh & McCabe, 1975; Gillberg & Gillberg, 1983), the increase is *not* mainly in the more severe complications commonly associated with brain damage (such as very low birth weight or extreme prematurity). Third, so far, the identified medical causes account for a tiny proportion of cases of autism. The one possible exception to that statement is provided by the fragile-X phenomenon, which may account for as many as 5–17% of cases (Blomquist et al., 1984), although several investigations have found very few cases of fragile-X in substantial series of cases of autism (see below for a fuller description of the fragile-X disorder).

We must conclude that it appears that the majority of autistic cases do not fall into the nonspecific organic brain syndrome pattern, in spite of the strong evidence that autism has an organic basis. That is to say, unlike the case with severe mental retardation or cerebral palsy, autism is *not* usually associated with gross abnormalities of brain structure or histology. Moreover, it is *unusual* for generalized brain damage to give rise to autism. The organic basis of autism must be of some more subtle, less easy to detect, variety. Most autistic individuals are physically normal, do not exhibit any evidence of overt structural brain pathology, and have not experienced hazards known to be likely to cause brain damage. That is particularly so with respect to autistic individuals without general mental retardation. Whereas certainly we do not know that there *is* any unitary basic deficit in autism (whether defined in neuropsychologic, neurophysiologic, or neuropathologic terms), it is possible that there may be one. Accordingly, it is most important that research continue to be directed toward its possible identification.

A good deal of progress has been made in this connection. Thus, it is now clear that in most cases there is a basic cognitive deficit that involves impaired language, sequencing, abstraction, and coding functions (Dawson, 1983; Rutter, 1983). Moreover, it has also been shown that autism is *not* particularly associated with abnormalities in perceptual discrimination, in the appreciation of visuospatial perspectives, or in self-recognition (Ferrari & Matthews, 1983; Spiker & Ricks, 1984). These findings constitute highly worthwhile progress. Not only have they been crucial in demonstrating the basic importance of cognitive deficits as usual (if not essential) parts of the syndrome, but they have also gone a long way toward demonstrations of just what sort of cognitive deficit is particularly associated with autism.

Nevertheless, it is equally apparent that much remains unexplained. Most especially, it is far from clear *how* these cognitive deficits give rise to the abnormalities in social functioning, or even *whether* they do so. In recent years experimental approaches have been directed to the elucidation of which psychological processes relevant to socialization might be impaired. So far, three possibilities appear to be leading contenders: (1) discrimination of emotional cues, (2) differentiations of age and gender, and (3) ability to appreciate what other people are thinking. Hobson (1983, 1987), in a series of well-planned experiments (mainly using the paradigm of matching videos with labeled pictures), has shown that autistic children differ markedly from both normal and mentally retarded children of comparable mental age in their ability to discriminate either emotional cues or differentiations based on age and gender. It would seem plausible that if autistic individuals cannot perceive when other people are happy, angry, or sad, they are likely to be handicapped in their social relationships. Hobson (1987) postulates that this lack of emotional discrimination may reflect a deficit in empathy. It is not clear what is involved in autistic children's poor discrimination of adults and children, males and females—is it that such differentiations lack salience for them or are they unable to appreciate the significance of the behavioral differences associated with age and gender? Also, is this the same dificit that underlies the failure in emotional discrimination or is it different?

The third possibility stems from an experiment by Baron-Cohen, Leslie, and Frith (1985) in which the task involved a doll-play setup in which a hidden object was moved while a doll figure was ''out of the room.'' The experiment tested whether the subject reported that the doll figure would look for the hidden object where she had last seen it or rather in the place where it now was (a place known to the subject but not to the doll figure). Autistic children differed from controls in being more likely to report that the object would be looked for in its present location—a finding interpreted as meaning that autistic individuals are impaired in their capacity to appreciate what another person is thinking. Again, this raises the question of whether this deficit (if confirmed by further research) is part of the already demonstrated impaired ability to appreciate emotional and gender cues.

These studies have moved us an important step toward a better understanding of autistic individuals' socioemotional disabilities, but it is by no means self-evident just what neuropsychological functions underlie the skills being tapped. Nor is it clear whether the findings reflect one deficit that encompasses these various skills or rather whether we are dealing with a constellation of associated deficits. In view of the crucial importance of the cognitive deficits associated with language and the abstraction of meaning, it may be supposed that these socioemotional deficits are in some way part of, or linked with, the other cognitive problems, but how and in what way do they interlink?

A further query is whether the autistic children's impaired ability to discriminate socioemotional cues or appreciate how another person is thinking are *necessary* features of autism. In other words, are these deficits so basic that if they are not found the diagnosis of autism should not be made? Or, alternatively, does their presence or absence serve to differentiate meaningful subcategories of autism? As we have argued above, that is an essential question to put. Nevertheless, it is obvious that we are far from ready to provide an answer. The *degree* of difference between autistic and mentally retarded groups of comparable mental age suggests the probable importance of the function being examined. But the deficits were least apparent in the intellectually normal individuals. It remains uncertain how far that observation was a reflection of a ceiling effect in the test used and how far a real difference in pattern of handicaps in the intellectually most able autistic individuals, an issue that also has been apparent with the study of other functions, such as the use of meaning in memory processes (Fyffe & Prior, 1978).

A further query concerns the *specificity* of these deficits to autism. So far, the direct comparisons have been between autism and mental handicap, but do the deficits also differentiate autism from, say, schizophrenia or other psychiatric disorders associated with social impairment? The question is pertinent and important both because the deficits might constitute a nonspecific accompaniment of any form of severe social disability and because somewhat comparable (although apparently lesser) deficits have been reported in schizophrenia (Walker, Bettes & McGuire, 1984; Novic, Luchins & Perline, 1984). This area of research is a most promising one; it carries with it the tantalizing possibility of defining the basic psychological deficit in autism—but that definition remains as yet some way away.

An alternative approach to the possible identification of the basic deficit in autism has been through the use of neurophysiological rather than psychological techniques. Thus, there have been investigations using EEG measures, contingent and noncontingent sensory evoked responses, autonomic reactivity, and vestibular responses (Ornitz, 1978; James & Barry, 1980). The findings have been quite inconsistent and inconclusive; also, in many cases, inadequate or inappropriate control groups have been used (Yule, 1978)—nevertheless, various abnormalities have been reported (see James & Barry, 1980; Rutter, 1985a). Perhaps those most likely to be associated with autism are the indicators of increased brain stem transmission times (Rosenblum *et al.,* 1980; Skoff, Mirsky & Turner, 1980; Fein, Skoff & Mirsky, 1981), of defective information storage (Novick, Kurtzberg & Vaughn, 1979), and of impaired development of hemispheric dominance (James & Barry, 1983). Further research on these functions, together with investigations of attentional processes, should prove rewarding. So far, however, the meaning of the neurophysiologic findings in autism remains obscure, and it is not at all clear how they might be linked to the findings on psychological deficits.

RATING INSTRUMENTS

The major problems inherent in research based on varying approaches to diagnosis have led to a variety of attempts to devise standardized rating instruments from which individual diagnoses can be derived (Parks, 1983). Broadly speaking, these fall into three main groups: (1) those based on questionnaires completed by parents or teachers, such as the checklist devised by Rimland (1984) and by Krug, Arick, and Almond (1980); (2) those based on structured observations of the child, such as BRIAAC (Ruttenberg, Dratman, Fraknoi & Wenar, 1966), BOS (Freeman, Ritvo, Guthrie, Schroth & Ball, 1978; Freeman *et al.*, 1984), and CARS (Schopler, Reichler, DeVellis & Daly, 1980; Schopler, Reichler & Renner, 1985); and (3) those based on a standardized interview of the parents (Wing & Gould, 1978).

Most of these instruments have been shown to have satisfactory reliability and to discriminate among autistic, mentally retarded, and normal samples. Moreover, they provide a useful way of recording various items of behavior needed both for diagnosis and for the planning of treatment and provision of services (see Schopler & Rutter, 1978; Schopler, 1983, for an account of how different approaches to classification may be needed for different purposes). Nevertheless, it is doubtful whether they provide a satisfactory solution to problems of individual diagnosis. In the first place, most are devised for severely handicapped children and appear likely to be less applicable to the more intellectually able individuals. Also, many of the items reflect a *lack* of particular skills rather than the deviance characteristic of autism. Not surprisingly, therefore, many of the items reflect intellectual handicap as much as autism. Also, the parental questionnaires cannot satisfactorily tap the distinctions on the *quality* of behaviors needed for diagnosis. The instruments based on observation are potentially more satisfactory, but they are necessarily limited to the behaviors likely to be manifest during a relatively brief period in a single setting; the consequence is that they most readily detect the gross abnormalities seen in the most handicapped children. The detailed interview schedules should be able to tap a wider range of behaviors, but the items tend not to reflect some of the key distinctions contained in the diagnostic criteria: moreover, they fail to use the professional observational skills necessary for some of these distinctions. The rating instruments constitute a valuable set of tools for behavioral assessment, but as yet they fall short of a comprehensively satisfactory approach to diagnosis. We suggest that what is needed for specific diagnostic purposes is a combination of a detailed standardized parental interview designed to elicit the key diagnostic features, together with a standardized observation system. The main limitation regarding the latter is that it is unlikely that a single structured interaction could be equally appropriate for a mute mentally handicapped autistic child and a verbal autistic individual within the normal range of general intelligence. Nevertheless, such an observation could be devised to tap a predetermined set of social, conversational, and behavioral qualities, using a standard set of ratings that reflect the key diagnostic features. The CARS approach provides a well-tested route toward that end.

BOUNDARIES OF AUTISM

Five main areas of controversy remain with respect to the boundaries of autism as a valid diagnostic entity: (1) autisticlike syndromes in children with severe mental handicap; (2) autisticlike disorders in individuals of normal intelligence without gross developmental delay, general or specific; (3) later-onset autisticlike disorders following a prolonged period of normal development; (4) severe disorders arising in early or middle childhood characterized by grossly bizarre behavior; and (5) the overlap between autism and severe developmental disorders of receptive language.

It is all too apparent that there is no readily recognizable separation point between "true" autism and other disorders that share some behavioral features but which do not fulfill the complete set of accepted diagnostic criteria. In reality, such a differentiation could only truly be based on some unequivocal indication of some specifically and uniquely autistic feature. Such a feature has yet to be identified. Moreover, many behavioral disorders are best conceptualized in dimensional rather than categorical terms; accordingly, it should not be assumed that there will prove to be any pathognomonic defining feature for autism. For the present, the nearest approach to validation or invalidation of the distinctions must rely on those features that have been shown most clearly to differentiate autistic children from nonautistic children of comparable mental age. These features include (1) abnormalities in the appreciation of socioemotional cues (as identified through the experimental studies of Hobson), (2) cognitive deficits in the abstraction of meaning (as derived originally from the studies of Hermelin & O'Connor), (3) the differential association with particular medical syndromes (e.g., strong with congenital rubella and weak with Down's syndrome), (4) the association with seizures that develop in adolescence rather than in early childhood, (5) concordance in monozygotic pairs of twins, and (6) familial loading on language and language-related cognitive impairments. Such "tests" have not yet been systematically applied to any of the "boundary" conditions mentioned.

The differentiation from autism is most problematical of all in the case of children who are very seriously retarded (say those with an MA below about 2 years). In their general population survey, Wing and Gould (1979; Wing, 1981) found that about one half of all children with severe mental handicap (IQ <50) showed the autistic-type triad of social and language impairments and repetitive behaviors. It is clear that this triad parallels the diagnostic criteria for autism as described earlier in the chapter; the difference lies in the emphasis on *impairment* rather than on a specific type of deviance. The consequences of this difference are most evident in the group of children with an IQ below 20; 82% of these showed the triad, but only 2% showed typical autism. The comparable figures for children in the 35–49 IQ range was 40% and 14%. Overall, the triad children showed medical condition associations similar to those characteristic of autism (e.g., infantile spasms common but Downs' syndrome rare), but no data are available on the other possibly discriminatory features.

The second area of difficulty concerns the differentiation between autism and autisticlike disorders in individuals of normal intelligence. These include both the disorders termed Asperger's syndrome (Wing, 1981) and those sometimes classified as schizoid disorder of childhood (Chick, Waterhouse & Wolff, 1979; Wolff & Barlow, 1979; Wolff & Chick, 1980). As ordinarily diagnosed, Asperger's syndrome requires the presence of lack of empathy, deviant styles of communication, constricted intellectual interests, and (often) idiosyncratic attachments to objects. The features all suggest that the condition represents mild autism without associated mental handicap, as do the findings on recognition and production of emotions (Scott, 1985). However, it seems that sometimes this clinical picture can occur without the language delay and impairment usually found with autism; the observation raises the interesting possibility that although such language deficits are usual in autism, perhaps they may not constitute a necessary feature (Rutter & Garmezy, 1983). The possibility warrants further study. As used by Wolff and colleagues, the diagnosis of schizoid disorder clearly includes cases that would be diagnosed by others as Asperger's syndrome. By contrast, the frequency of schizoid disorders in the Wolff clinic sample (3–4% of psychiatric clinic referrals) suggests that it must extend more broadly than that. It remains quite unknown whether such cases represent subclinical varieties of autism or some quite different condition. Again, the possibility demands systematic investigation.

The third type of clinical picture that gives rise to difficulties in diagnostic differentiation is that in which there is a profound regression and behavioral disintegration following some 3–4 years of apparently normal development—a syndrome that roughly follows

Heller's (1930, 1969) account of dementia infantilis but which now tends to be termed *disintegrative psychosis* (Rutter, 1985a). Often there is a premonitory period of vague illness, during or following which the child becomes restive, irritable, anxious, and overactive. Over the course of a few months there is an impoverishment followed by a loss of speech and language. Comprehension of language deteriorates and intelligence often declines, although an intelligent facial expression is usually retained. There is a loss of social skills, impairment of interpersonal relationships, a general loss of interest in objects, and the development of stereotypies and mannerisms (Rutter, 1985a).

Clearly there is a substantial overlap in symptomatology with autism, and it seems likely that some cases represent atypical forms of autism. Nevertheless, the gradual and severe loss of cognitive skills (often with loss of bowel and bladder control as well) after some years of normal development is not the picture usually seen in autism even when the onset seems to have followed initially normal early development. The apparently good cognitive potential implied by the normality of the first 3 years in these disintegrative disorders is unfortunately misleading. In most cases, the prognosis is poor, with the children usually remaining without speech and severely mentally handicapped. The importance of these late-onset cases lies in the frequency with which they are associated with progressive neurologic disorders, either congenital or acquired, such as the lipoidoses or leukodystrophies (e.g., Corbett, Harris, Taylor & Trimble, 1977; Malamud, 1959). In girls, there is also the special need to identify Rett's syndrome (a progressive dementing disorder associated with loss of facial expression and of interpersonal contact, stereotyped movements, ataxia, and loss of purposeful hand use), which can be mistaken for autism in its early stages (Hagberg, Aicardi, Bias & Ramos, 1983). Nevertheless, it is clear that in some cases the cause is unknown, without any unambiguous evidence of brain disease or damage; this is probably especially the case when the regression occurs at about 2½ to 3 years following the pattern seen in some cases of autism at a slightly earlier age (Evan-Jones & Rosenbloom, 1978).[2] Occasionally, the deterioration seems to follow some life event (such as hospital admission), but such events are in any case very common during the preschool years and it is dubious whether they play any essential part in etiology. These later-onset disintegrative disorders are much less common than autism and less is known about their characteristics. Nevertheless, it is our very ignorance regarding their meaning that makes it important to recognize their existence and to accept that as yet we do not know how far they overlap with the more usual early-onset autistic disorders.

The fourth major area of diagnostic controversy and uncertainty concerns conditions arising in early or middle childhood in which there is the onset of grossly disturbed behavior together with abnormalities in language and thought processes. There is no doubt that some of these conditions represent schizophrenic disorders of particularly early onset. This is best demonstrated for those beginning in the years leading up to adolescence, but there are undoubtedly cases with an onset as early as age 6 (Eggers, 1978; Green *et al.*, 1984; Kolvin, 1971; Kydd & Werry, 1982). Such children show many of the features associated with schizophrenia occurring in adult life, and both the course and family history are also similar. However, there are three main problem issues. First, Cantor, Evans, Pearce, and Pezzot-Pearce (1982) argued that schizophrenia can begin in infancy, with the disorders differing from autism in terms of (1) relatively good social relationships, (2) thought disorder, (3) sometimes the presence of delusions and hallucinations, (4) marked hypotonicity, and (5)

---

[2]In autism it is relatively common for parents to report a regression in language after initial acquisition of some speech. In most cases, however, it is clear that the early development was never fully normal (although, occasionally, it seems to have been so).

often a family history of schizophrenia. For obvious reasons there are major difficulties in the recognition of thought disorder and delusions in infants or very young children, and the nosologic validity of schizophrenia beginning in infancy has not been established. Nevertheless, it may be accepted that there are serious nonautistic disorders of development manifest at that age.

Second, there are severe disorders that arise in middle childhood in which there is a loss of reality sense and severe distortions in behavior and in thinking, but in which the specific diagnostic features of schizophrenia are lacking. There is a lack of evidence on the nature of these serious psychiatric disturbances and it is quite likely that they constitute a heterogeneous group. In most cases the diagnostic uncertainty concerns the question of schizophrenia rather than autism, but occasionally the picture can be somewhat autisticlike. For example, this was so with two published cases of children subjected to gross abuse and/or neglect (Curtiss, 1977; Skuse, 1984). In both instances, it remains unclear whether the disorder stemmed from the severe environmental distortions, from some constitutional deficit, or from a combination of the two.

Third, there are isolated reports of young children who were diagnosed autistic who later appeared to manifest schizophrenic symptomatology (Petty, Ornitz, Michelman & Zimmerman, 1984; Howells & Guirguis, 1984). It is difficult to know what weight to attach to these reports in that the systematic studies of children diagnosed as autistic according to traditional criteria have *not* found this transition (Rutter, 1970; Eisenberg, 1956; Kanner, 1973). It may be that the supposed autism-to-schizophrenia change reflects a broader concept of autism, of schizophrenia, or a difference in the interpretation of the odd thinking that is quite common in older autistic individuals. Alternatively. these unusual cases may represent a small subgroup that requires separate categorization. So far the data needed for a choice between these alternatives are lacking. Nevertheless, Tanguay (1984) used these cases together with a potpourri of other reports of varying quality to argue for the invalidity of the diagnosis of autism. His argument ignores contrary evidence and relies on a misinterpretation of the findings that are quoted. For example, it is wrongly asserted that the medical conditions associated with autism are the "very same" as those linked with nonautistic forms of mental retardation—an incorrect statement, as we have already noted. What is needed is a systematic testing of alternative explanations rather than a moving back to nondiscriminating models of developmental failure.

The final area of uncertainty over the boundaries of autism concerns the overlap with severe developmental disorders of receptive language. The systematic comparative studies of autistic and dysphasic children by Bartak et al. (1975) showed that most children with specific developmental receptive language disorders differed sharply from autistic children in linguistic, cognitive, and behavioral features. The same study also demonstrated that there was a small group with mixed features. A further follow-up by Cantwell et al. (in press) was informative in showing that as they got older, some dysphasic children showed severe behavioral and social difficulties, even though the two groups tended to remain distinctive. The Paul et al. (1983) follow-up of 28 children with severe developmental language disorders also showed that many exhibited autisticlike features; however, progress in social relationships was as much a function of the severity of the deficit in language comprehension as of initial autisticlike features. Both twin (Folstein & Rutter, 1977) and family (August, Stewart & Tsai, 1981) studies have also shown that some cases of autism are associated with a familial loading of language and intellectual retardation. The three diagnostic/classification issues are as follows: (1) How do the cases of autism associated with language problems in the family differ from those without this familial component? (2) What is the nosologic status of the cases with mixed autistic and developmental language disorder features? (3) As presumably only some types of developmental language disorder are linked with autism, what are the features that distinguish those associated with autism?

ETIOLOGIC HETEROGENEITY WITHIN AUTISM SYNDROMES

The last issue concerns the question of etiological heterogeneity within the field of autism syndromes. We have already noted that there *is* undoubted heterogeneity. The very fact that the clinical picture of autism can arise from diseases as diverse as congenital rubella (Chess, Fernandez & Korn, 1978; Chess, Korn & Fernandez, 1971), tuberous sclerosis (Creak, 1963; Lotter, 1974), encephalopathy (Wing & Gould, 1979), infantile spasms with hypsarrhythmia (Taft & Cohen, 1971; Riikonen & Amnell, 1981), cerebral lipoidosis (Creak, 1963), and neurofibromatosis (Gillberg & Forsell, 1984) makes that clear. However, even when all these conditions are combined, they account for a tiny minority of cases of autism. In the vast majority of instances there is no identifiable medical cause. Accordingly, it remains quite uncertain whether the minority of cases with a known pathologic cause represent phenocopies of some other unitary disorder with (an as yet undiscovered) single etiology, or whether the behavioral syndrome of autism represents just the final common pathway for a diverse range of organic brain conditions that happen to impinge on similar brain systems. In order to decide between these two contrasting alternatives, it is essential to have systematic research that focuses on the question of heterogeneity within autistic syndromes. It will be appreciated that such research must go well beyond the mere noting of heterogeneity. It is crucial that it be designed to determine the ways (if any) in which the diversity on one parameter coincides with diversity on other dimensions. The investigation of heterogeneity should include studies based on several different starting points.

First, the research may start with some identified medical condition. For example, the Swedish multicenter study of infantile autism (Blomquist *et al.*, 1984) found the fragile-X phenomenon in 16% of the 83 boys studied (but in none of the 19 girls). As the Yale group (Watson *et al.*, 1984) found the fragile-X in only 5% of 75 autistic males, and as there were no instances of fragile-X in the 57 cases studied by Venter, Hof, Coetzee, Van der Walt, and Retief (1984), in the 18 cases with either dysmorphic features or a family history of mental retardation studied by Pueschel, Herman, and Groden (1985), or in the 37 cases studied by Goldfine *et al* (1985), the evidence is contradictory as to whether the incidence of fragile-X in autism exceeds that in mental retardation (4–7%, Blomquist *et al.*, 1982, 1983). Nevertheless, either way there is a need to compare cases of autism with and without the fragile-X—do they differ, for instance, in phenomenology, course, or cognitive characteristics? Similarly, within a mentally retarded population does the phenomenon relate to behavioral features (thus, Levitas *et al.*, 1983, and Largo & Schinzel, 1985, suggested an association with autistic features even in individuals without classic autism)?

Comparable questions arise with respect to other genetic factors (Folstein & Rutter, 1988). Folstein and Rutter (1977) found an MZ–DZ difference in concordance that pointed to

---

[3]Ritvo and his colleagues (1985a,b) have used their twin and family study data to argue for autosomal recessive inheritance. However, their data are based on biased samples (e.g., a marked excess of MZ over same sex DZ pairs) and inappropriate analyses (e.g., the inclusion of opposite sex DZ pairs). Accordingly, little weight can be attached to their findings; moreover their own data include some that are inconsistent with their hypothesis (Spence *et al.*, 1985). It is quite premature to postulate specific models of inheritance before the necessary data for such models are available.

an important genetic factor in etiology.[3] The August *et al.* (1981) finding that some 15% of the siblings of autistic children, compared with only 3% of siblings of Down's syndrome individuals, had language disorders, learning disabilities, or mental retardation also suggested the likely role of an inherited predisposition to language and cognitive abnormalities of which autism constitutes one important part. Several rather different issues arise with respect to this possibility. In the first instance it is necessary to check whether or not the twin concordance and familial loading are a function of the fragile-X phenomenon. Isolated case reports suggest that it may be in some instances (August & Lockhart, 1984: Gillberg, 1983). However, if it does prove to be a general explanation of the familial findings, it is crucial to go on to use genetic family studies to examine heterogeneity within autism. For example, does the familial loading apply preponderantly to autistic children who are also mentally handicapped? (The August *et al.* findings suggested that it might.) Does it vary according to the sex of the autistic child, to the development of seizures in adolescence, or to pattern of phenomenology?

The same "search for heterogeneity" strategy may be applied to other biological features associated with autism. Thus, for example, how do the autistic children who develop seizures during adolescence differ from those who do not? It seems that the risk of seizures is substantially higher in those with associated mental handicap (Bartak & Rutter, 1976), but does the risk vary according to medical correlates, sex, phenomenology, or course? Research is needed in order to find out.

Second, the research may begin with some behavioral feature or some phenomenologic constellation. Rimland (1971, 1984) has repeatedly argued that scores on his E2 scale serve to differentiate a distinctive biochemically different syndrome of autism. However, the study on which he bases his claim (Boullin, Coleman, O'Brien & Rimland, 1971) could not be replicated by the same biochemical investigator when using a different sample (Boullin *et al.*, 1982). While the claim is premature, the research strategy is pertinent. We need to know, for example, whether there are meaningful differences (on some external criterion) according to age of onset, typical versus atypical clinical pictures, deterioration in adolescence (Gillberg & Schaumann, 1981), etc.

Third, it is important also to consider the ways in which male and female autistic individuals differ. It is well established that autism is much more common in boys than in girls, in a ratio of 3 or 4 : 1. Furthermore, it seems that autistic girls tend to be more seriously affected and possibly more likely to have a family history of cognitive problems (Tsai, Stewart & August, 1981: Lord, Schopler & Revick, 1982; Wing, 1981). These findings need replication. but also extension, in order to determine whether there are any other differences in pattern between autism in boys and that in girls.

Finally, response to treatment may be used as a differentiating factor. It appears that, on the whole, behavioral and educational methods of treatment are most effective (Bartak, 1978; Hemsley *et al.*, 1978; Howlin & Rutter, 1987; Rutter, 1985*b;* Schopler, Mesibov & Baker, 1982). The marked individual differences in treatment response mainly relate to the severity of intellectual and language impairment. That finding, of course, raises the possibility that autism in children of normal general intelligence may differ from autism associated with severe mental handicap. On the whole, the weight of findings suggests that the differences reflect variations on a continuum of degree of severity of disorder. However, the matter is far from resolved. Drug response constitutes, perhaps, a potentially better candidate for the investigation of diagnostic heterogeneity. Unfortunately, to date, although the major tranquilizers may serve to reduce agitation, tension, and overactivity (Corbett, 1976; Campbell, 1978), there is no evidence of any autism-specific drug effect. Rather premature excitement was generated by a case study of just three children (Geller, Ritro, Freeman & Yuwiler, 1982) in which it was suggested that fenfluramine, a drug that lowers serotonin levels, might be of benefit in autism. The excitement arose over the possibility that the improvements in autism might be a consequence of a specific biochemical change, i.e., a reduction in serotonin. That did not seem a likely possibility in that although serotonin levels are indeed raised in about a third of autistic children, so also are they in severe mental handicap and a host of other neurological conditions. In the event, further studies (August *et al.*, 1984; Ritvo, Freeman, Geller & Yuwiler, 1983) suggest that whatever benefits there may be from fenfluramine administration, they do not result from normalization of pathologically high serotonin levels. Nevertheless, although unrewarding so far, the use of differences in therapeutic response to specific treatments remains a worthwhile research strategy.

CONCLUSIONS

Of all the psychiatric syndromes that arise in childhood, autism is much the best validated by empirical research. It stands out from the bulk of common psychiatric conditions in terms of its strong association with both cognitive deficits and evidence of organic brain dysfunction. Also, it is differentiated from both general and specific developmental disorders of cognition in terms of psychological features (including the pattern of language-related cognitive deficits and also the serious impairment in the discrimination of socioemotional cues) and medical correlates (including the age of onset of seizures and the types of medical disorder with which it is associated). Nevertheless, uncertainties remain on the boundaries of this behaviorally defined syndrome, on its links with other disorders, on the extent to which within undoubted pathologic heterogeneity there is a single etiologically homogeneous core condition, and on the ways (if any) in which the concept of autism should be either broadened or subdivided. In this report we have sought to indicate the possible avenues of research that might serve to resolve these issues. Ultimately, the answers must rely on identification of the nature of the brain deficit that defines autism—whether in neuropsychologic, neurophysiologic, or neuropathologic terms. While that identification is not yet in sight, several promising leads are available.

ACKNOWLEDGMENT. This chapter was originally prepared for an NIMH Research Workshop to examine research issues in relation to the assessment, diagnosis, and classification of child and adolescent psychiatric disorders. Adapted with permission from M. Rutter, A. H. Tuma, and I. Lann (eds). *Assessment and Diagnosis in Child Psychopathology,* Guilford Press, New York, 1988. This chapter originally appeared in *The Journal of Autism and Developmental Disorders, 17,* 159–186.

REFERENCES

American Psychiatric Association. (1980). *Diagnostic and statistical manual of mental disorders (DSM-III)* (3rd ed.). Washington, D.C.: Author.
Anwar, F. (1983). The role of sensory modality for the reproduction of shape by the severely retarded. *British Journal of Developmental Psychology, 1,* 317–28.

August, G. J., & Lockhart, L. H. (1984). Familial autism and the fragile-X chromosome. *Journal of Autism and Developmental Disorders, 14,* 197–204.

August, G. J., Raz, N., Papanicolaon, A. C., Baird, T. D., Hirsch, S. L., & Hsu, L. L. (1984). Fenfluramine treatment in infantile autism: Neurochemical, electrophysiological, and behavioral effects. *Journal of Nervous and Mental Disease, 172,* 604–12.

August, G. J., Stewart, M. A., & Tsai, L. (1981). The incidence of cognitive disabilities in the siblings of autistic children. *British Journal of Psychiatry, 138,* 416–22.

Baron-Cohen, S., Leslie, A. M., & Frith, U. (1985). Does the autistic child have a "theory of mind"? *Cognition, 21,* 37–46.

Bartak, L. (1978). Educational approaches. In M. Rutter & E. Schopler (Eds.), *Autism: A reappraisal of concepts and treatment* (pp. 423–38). New York: Plenum.

Bartak, L., & Rutter, M. (1976). Differences between mentally retarded and normally intelligent autistic children. *Journal of Autism and Childhood Schizophrenia, 6,* 109–20.

Bartak, L., Rutter, M., & Cox, A. (1975). A comparative study of infantile autism and specific developmental receptive language disorder. I. The children. *British Journal of Psychiatry, 126,* 127–145.

Bauman, M., & Kemper, T. L. (1985). Histoanatomic observations of the brain in early infantile autism. *Neurology, 35,* 866–74.

Bender, L. (1947). Childhood schizophrenia. Clinical study of one hundred schizophrenic children. *American Journal of Orthopsychiatry, 17,* 40–56.

Bettelheim, B. (1967). *The empty fortress: Infantile autism and the birth of the self.* New York: Free Press.

Birch, H. G., Richardson, S. A., Baird, D., Horobin, G., & Illsley, R. (1970). *Mental subnormality in the community: A clinical and epidemiological study.* Baltimore: Williams & Wilkins.

Blomquist, H. K., Bohman, M., Edvinsson. S. O., Gillberg, C.. Gustavson, K-H., Holmgren, G.. & Wahlstrom, J. (1984). Frequency of the fragile X syndrome in infantile autism: A Swedish multi-center study. *Clinical Genetics, 27,* 113–17.

Blomquist, H. K., Gustavson, K-H., Holmgren, G., Nordenson, I., & Palsson-Strae, U. (1983). Fragile X syndrome in mildly mentally retarded children in a northern Swedish county. A prevalence study. *Clinical Genetics, 24,* 393–9.

Blomquist, H. K., Gustavson, K-H., Holmgren, G., Nordenson, I., & Sweins, A. (1982). Fragile site X-chromosomes and X-linked mental retardation in severely retarded boys in a northern Swedish county. A prevalence study. *Clinical Genetics, 21,* 209–14.

Boullin, D. J., Coleman, M., O'Brien, R. A., & Rimland, B. (1971). Laboratory predictions of infantile autism, based on 5-hydroxytryptamine efflux from blood platelets and their correlation with the Rimland E2 scores. *Journal of Autism and Childhood Schizophrenia, 1,* 63–71.

Boullin, D. J., Freeman, B. J., Geller, E., Ritvo, E., Rutter, M., & Yuwiler, A. (1982). Toward the resolution of conflicting findings. (Letter to the editor.) *Journal of Autism and Developmental Disorders, 12,* 97–98.

Campbell, M. (1978). Pharmacotherapy. In M. Rutter & E. Schopler (Eds.), *Autism: A reappraisal of concepts and treatment* (pp. 337–355). New York: Plenum.

Cantor, S., Evans, J., Pearce, J., & Pezzot-Pearce, T. (1982). Childhood schizophrenia: Present but not accounted for. *American Journal of Psychiatry, 139,* 758–62.

Cantwell, D., & Baker, L. (1985). Speech and language: Development and disorders. In M. Rutter & L. Hersov (Eds.), *Child and adolescent psychiatry: Modern approaches (2nd ed.) (pp. 526–544).* Oxford: Blackwell Scientific.

Cantwell, D., Baker, L., Rutter, M., Mawhood, L. (in press). *Comparative follow-up study of infantile autism and developmental receptive dysphasia. Journal of Autism and Developmental Disorders.*

Caparulo, B. K., Cohen, D. J., Young, G., Katz, J. D., Shaywitz, S. E., Shaywitz, B. A., & Rothman, S. L. (1981). Computed tomographic brain scanning in children with developmental neuro-psychiatric disorders. *Journal of the American Academy of Child Psychiatry, 20,* 338–57.

Chess, S., Fernandez, P., & Korn, S. (1978). Behavioral consequences of congenital rubella. *Journal of Pediatrics, 93,* 699–703.

Chess, S., Korn, S. J., & Fernandez, P. E. (1971). *Psychiatric disorders of children with congenital rubella.* New York: Brunner/Mazel.

Chick, J., Waterhouse, L., & Wolff, S. (1979). Psychological construing in schizoid children grown up. *British Journal of Psychiatry, 135,* 425–30.

Coleman, P. D., Romano, J., Lapham, L., & Simon, W. (1985). Cell counts in cerbral cortex of an autistic patient. *Journal of Autism and Developmental Disorders, 15,* 245–56.

Corbett, J. A. (1976). Medical management. In L. Wing (Ed.), *Early childhood autism: Clinical, educational and social aspects* (2nd ed.). Oxford: Pergamon.

Corbett, J., Harris, R., Taylor, E., & Trimble, M. (1977). Progressive disintegrative psychosis of childhood. *Journal of Child Psychology and Psychiatry, 18,* 211–29.

Creak, M. (1963). Childhood psychosis: A review of 100 cases. *British Journal of Psychiatry, 109,* 84–9.

Curtiss, S. (1977). *Genie: A psycholinguistic study of a modern-day "Wild Child."* London: Academic.

Damasio, H., Maurer, R. G., Damasio, A. R., & Chui, H. C. (1980). Computerized tomographic scan findings in patients with autistic behavior. *Archives of Neurology, 37,* 504–10.

Darby, J. K. (1976). Neuropathologic aspects of psychosis in childhood. *Journal of Autism and Childhood Schizophrenia, 6,* 339–52.

Dawson, G. (1983). Lateralized brain function in autism: Evidence from the Halstead-Reitan neuropsychological battery. *Journal of Autism and Developmental Disorders, 13,* 369–86.

De Sanctis, S. (1906). On some varieties of dementia praecox. *Riv. Sper. Freniatr., 32,* 141–65. (Translated and reprinted in J. G. Howells (Ed.), *Modern perspectives in international child psychiatry.* Edinburgh: Oliver & Boyd, 1969.)

Deykin, E. Y., & MacMahon, D. (1979). The incidence of seizures among children with autistic symptoms. *American Journal of Psychiatry, 136,* 1310–12.

Deykin, E. Y., & MacMahon, B. (1980). Pregnancy, delivery and neonatal complications among autistic children. *American Journal of Diseases of Children 134,* 860–4.

Eggers, C. (1978). Course and prognosis of childhood schizophrenia. *Journal of Autism and Childhood Schizophrenia, 8,* 21–36.

Eisenberg, L. (1956). The autistic child in adolescence. *American Journal of Psychiatry, 112,* 607–12.

Eisenberg, L. (1972). The classification of childhood psychosis reconsidered. *Journal of Autism and Childhood Schizophrenia. 2,* 338–42.

Evans-Jones, L. G., & Rosenbloom, L. (1978). Disintegrative psychosis in childhood. *Developmental Medicine and Child Neurology, 20,* 462–70.

Fein, D., Skoff, B., & Mirsky, A. F. (1981). Clinical correlates of brainstem dysfunction in autistic children. *Journal of Autism and Developmental Disorders, 11,* 303–16.

Ferrari, M., & Matthews, W. S. (1983). Self-recognition deficits in autism: Syndrome-specific or general developmental delay? *Journal of Autism and Developmental Disorders, 13,* 317–24.

Finegan, J., & Quadrington, B. (1979). Pre-, peri-, and neonatal factors and infantile autism. *Journal of Child Psychology and Psychiatry, 20,* 119–28.

Folstein, S., & Rutter, M. (1988). Autism: familial aggregation and genetic implications. *Journal of Autism and Developmental Disorders. 18,* 3–30.

Folstein, S., & Rutter, M. (1977). Infantile autism: A genetic study of 21 twin pairs. *Journal of Child Psychology and Psychiatry, 18,* 297–321.

Freeman, B. J., Ritvo, E. R., Guthrie, D., Schroth, P., & Ball, J. (1978). The Behavior Observation Scale for Autism: Initial methodology, data analysis, and preliminary findings on 89 children. *Journal of the American Academy of Child Psychiatry, 17,* 576–88.

Freeman, B. J., Ritvo, E. R., & Schroth, P. C. (1984). Behavior assessment of the syndrome of autism: Behavior Observation System. *Journal of the American Academy of Child Psychiatry, 23,* 588–94.

Frith, U. (1971). Spontaneous patterns produced by autistic, normal and subnormal children. In M. Rutter (Ed.), *Infantile autism: Concepts, characteristics and treatment* (pp. 113–131).

Fyffe, C., & Prior, M. R. (1978). Evidence of language recoding in autistic children: A reexamination. *British Journal of Psychiatry, 69,* 393–403.

Geller, E., Ritvo, E. R., Freeman, B. J., & Yuwiler, A. (1982). Preliminary observations of the effect of fenfluramine on blood serotonin and symptoms in three autistic boys. *New England Journal of Medicine, 307,* 165–9.

Gillberg, C. (1983). Identical triplets with infantile autism and the fragile-X syndrome. *British Journal of Psychiatry, 143,* 256–60.

Gillberg, C., & Forsell, C. (1984). Childhood psychosis and neurofibromatosis—More than a coincidence? *Journal of Autism and Developmental Disorders, 14* 1–8.

Gillberg, C., & Gillberg, I. C. (1983). Infantile autism: A total population study of nonoptimal, pre-, peri-, and neonatal conditions. *Journal of Autism and Developmental Disorders, 13,* 153–66.

Gillberg, C., & Schaumann, H. (1981). Infantile autism and puberty. *Journal of Autism and Developmental Disorders, 11,* 365–71.

Gillberg, C., & Svendsen, P. (1983). Childhood psychosis and computed tomographic brain scan findings. *Journal of Autism and Developmental Disorders, 13,* 19–32.

Goldfine, P. E., McPherson, P. M., Heath, G. A., Hardesty, V. A., Beauregard, L. J., & Gordon, S. (1985). Association of fragile X syndrome with autism. *American Journal of Psychiatry, 142,* 108–10.

Green, W. H., Campbell, M., Hardesty, A. S.. Grega, D. M., Padron-Gayol, M., Shell, J., & Erlenmeyer-Kimling, L. (1984). A comparison of schizphrenic and autistic children. *Journal of the American Academy of Child Psychiatry, 23,* 399–409.

Hagberg, B., Aicardi, J., Dias, K., & Ramos, O. (1983). A progressive syndrome of autism, dementia, ataxia, and loss of purposeful hand use in girls: Rett's syndrome: Report of 35 cases. *Annals of Neurology, 14,* 471–9.

Heller, T. (1930). About dementia infantilis. (Reprinted in J. G. Howells (Ed.), *Modern perspectives in international child psychiatry.* Edinburgh: Oliver & Boyd, 1969.)

Hemsley, R., Howlin, P., Berger, M., Hersov, L., Holbrook, D., Rutter, M., & Yule, W. (1978). Training autistic children in a family context. In M. Rutter & E. Schopler (Eds.), *Autism: A reappraisal of concepts and treatment* (pp. 378–411). New York: Plenum.

Hermelin, B., & O'Connor, N. (1970). *Psychological experiments with autistic children.* Oxford: Pergamon.

Herold, S., Frackowiak, R. S. J., Rutter, M., & Howlin, P. (1985). Regional cerebral blood flow, oxygen and glucose metabolism in young autistic adults. *Journal Cerebral Blood Flow and Metabolism 5,* Suppl 1, S189–190.

Hobson, R. P. (1983). The autistic child's recognition of age-related features of people, animals and things. *British Journal of Developmental Psychology, 4,* 343–52.

Hobson, R. P. (1987). The autistic child's recognition of age- and sex-related characteristics of people. *Journal of Autism and Developmental Disorders, 17,* 63–80.

Howells, J. G., & Guirguis, W. R. (1984). Childhood schizophrenia 20 years later. *Archives of General Psychiatry, 41,* 123–8.

Howlin, P., & Rutter, M. (1987). *Treatment of Autistic Children.* Chichester: Wiley.

James, A. L., & Barry, R. J. (1980). A review of psychophysiology in early onset psychosis. *Schizophrenia Bulletin, 6,* 506–25.

James, A. L., & Barry, R. J. (1983). Developmental effects in the cerebral lateralization of autistic, retarded, and normal children. *Journal of Autism and Developmental Disorders, 13,* 43–56.

Kanner, L. (1943). Autistic disturbances of affective contact. *Nervous Child, 2,* 217–30.

Kanner, L. (1973). *Childhood psychosis: Initial studies and new insights.* Washington, D.C.: Winston.

Kolvin, I. (1971). Psychoses in childhood—A comparative study. In M. Rutter (Ed.), *Infantile autism: Concepts, characteristics and treatment* (pp. 7–26). London: Churchill Livingstone.

Kolvin, I. (1974). Research into childhood psychoses: A crosscultural comparison and commentary. *International Journal of Mental Health, 2,* 194–212.

Krug, D. A., Arick, J. R., & Almond, P. J. (1980). Behavior checklist for identifying severely handicapped individuals with high levels of autistic behavior. *Journal of Child Psychology and Psychiatry, 21,* 221–9.

Kydd, R. R., & Werry, J. S. (1982). Schizophrenia in children under 16 years. *Journal of Autism and Developmental Disorders, 12,* 343–58.

Largo, R. H., & Schinzel, A. (1985). Developmental and behavioural disturbances in 13 boys with fragile X syndrome. *European Journal of Pediatrics, 143*, 269–75.

Levitas, A., Hagerman, R. J., Braden, M., Rimland, B., McBog, P., & Matteus, I. (1983). Autism and fragile X syndrome. *Journal of Developmental and Behavioral Pediatrics, 3*, 151–8.

Lord, C., Schopler, E., & Revick, D. (1982). Sex differences in autism. *Journal of Autism and Developmental Disorders, 12*, 317–30.

Lotter. V. (1974). Factors related to outcome in autistic children. *Journal of Autism and Childhood Schizophrenia, 4*, 263–77.

Makita, K. (1974). What is this thing called childhood schizophrenia? *International Journal of Mental Health, 2*, 179–93.

Malamud, N. (1959). Heller's disease and childhood schizophrenia. *American Journal of Psychiatry, 116*, 215–18.

Maudsley, H. (1867). *The physiology and pathology of the mind.* London: Macmillan.

Mrazek, D., & Mrazek, P. (1985). Child maltreatment. In M. Rutter & L. Hersov (Eds.), *Child and adolescent psychiatry: Modern approaches* (2nd ed., pp. 698–719). Oxford: Blackwell Scientific.

Novic, J., Luchins, D. J., & Perline, R. (1984). Facial affect recognition in schizophrenia: Is there a differential deficit? *British Journal of Psychiatry, 144*, 533–7.

Novick, B., Kurtzberg, D., & Vaughn, H. G. (1979). An electrophysiologic indication of defective informate storage in childhood autism. *Psychiatric Research, 1*, 101–98.

Ornitz, E. M. (1978). Neurophysiologic studies. In M. Rutter & E. Schopler (Eds.), *Autism: A reappraisal of concepts and treatment* (pp. 117–39). New York: Plenum.

Parks, S. L. (1983). The assessment of autistic children: A selective review of available instruments. *Journal of Autism and Developmental Disorders, 13*, 255–67.

Paul, R., & Cohen, D. J. (1984). Outcomes of severe disorders of language acquisition. *Journal of Autism and Developmental Disorders, 14*, 405–22.

Paul, R., Cohen, D. J., & Caparulo, B. K. (1983). A longitudinal study of patients with severe developmental disorders of language learning. *Journal of the American Academy of Child Psychiatry, 22*, 252–34.

Petty, L., Ornitz, E. M., Michelman, J. D., & Zimmerman, E. G. (1984). Autistic children who become schizophrenic. *Archives of General Psychiatry, 41*, 129–35.

Prior, M. R., Tress, B., Hoffman, W. L., & Boldt, D. (1984). Computed tomographic study of children with classic autism. *Archives of Neurology, 41*, 482–84.

Pueschel, S. M., Herman, R., & Groden, G. (1985). Brief report: Screening children with autism for fragile-X syndrome and phenylketonuria. *Journal of Autism and Developmental Disorders, 15*, 335–8.

Richardson, S. A., Koller, H., Katz, M., & McLaren, J. (1980). Seizures and epilepsy in a mentally retarded population over the first 22 years of life. *Applied Research in Mental Retardation. 1*, 123–38.

Riikonen, R., & Amnell, G. (1981). Psychiatric disorders in children with earlier infantile spasms. *Developmental Medicine and Child Neurology, 23*, 747–760.

Rimland, B. (1971). The differentiation of childhood psychoses: An analysis of checklists for 2,218 psychotic children. *Journal of Autism and Childhood Schizophrenia, 1*, 161–74.

Rimland, B. (1984). Diagnostic checklist form E2: A reply to Parks. *Journal of Autism and Developmental Disorders, 14*, 343–5.

Ritvo, E. R., Freeman, B. J., Geller, E., & Yuwiler, A. (1983). Effects of fenfluramine on 14 outpatients with the syndrome of autism. *Journal of the American Academy of Child Psychiatry, 22*, 549–58.

Ritvo, E. R., Freeman, B. J., Mason-Brothers, A., Mo, A., & Ritvo, A. M. (1985). Concordance for the syndrome of autism in 40 pairs of afflicted twins. *American Journal of Psychiatry, 142*. 74–7.

Ritvo, E. R., Spence, M. A., Freeman, B. J., Mason-Brothers, A., Mo, A., & Marazita, M. L. (1985). Evidence for autosomal recessive inheritance in 46 families with multiple incidences of autism. *American Journal of Psychiatry, 142*, 187–91.

Rosenbloom, S., Campbell, M., George, A. E., Kircheff, I., Taleporos, E., Anderson, L., Reuben, R.

N., & Korein, J. (1984). High resolution CT scanning in infantile autism: A quantitative approach. *Journal of the American Academy of Child Psychiatry, 23.* 72–7.

Rosenblum, S. M., Arick, J. R., Krug, D. A., Stubbs, E. G., Young, N. B., & Pelson, R. O. (1980). Auditory brainstem-evoked responses in autistic children. *Journal of Autism and Developmental Disorders, 10,* 215–26.

Rumsey, J. M., Duara, R., Grady, C., Rapoport, J. L., Margolin, R. A., Rapoport, S. I., & Cutler, N. R. (1985). Brain metabolism in autism: Resting cerebral glucose utilization as measured with positron emission tomography (PET). *Archives of General Psychiatry, 15.* 448–57.

Rumsey, J., Schwartz, M., Creasey, H., Dwana, R., Rapoport, J. L., Rapoport, S. I., & Cutler, N. R. (1983). *Quantitative CT-scan findings in autism.* Unpublished manuscript, American Psychological Association, Arnheim, California, August 26–30.

Ruttenberg, B. A., Dratman, M. L., Fraknoi, J., & Wenar, C. (1966). An instrument for evaluating autistic children. *Journal of the American Academy of Child Psychiatry, 5,* 453–78.

Rutter, M. (1970). Autistic children: Infancy to adulthood. *Seminars in Psychiatry, 2,* 435–50.

Rutter, M. (1972). Childhood schizophrenia reconsidered. *Journal of Autism and Childhood Schizophrenia, 2,* 315–37.

Rutter, M. (1974). The development of infantile autism. *Psychological Medicine, 4,* 147–63.

Rutter, M. (1978). Diagnosis and definition of childhood autism. *Journal of Autism and Childhood Schizophrenia, 8.* 139–61.

Rutter, M. (1979). Language, cognition and autism. In R. Katzman (Ed.), *Congenital and acquired cognitive disorders.* New York: Raven.

Rutter. M. (1981). *Maternal deprivation reassessed.* Harmondsworth, Middlesex: Penguin.

Rutter, M. (1983). Cognitive deficits in the pathogenesis of autism. *Journal of Child Psychology and Psychiatry, 24,* 513–31.

Rutter, M. (1984). Infantile autism. In D. Shaffer, A. Erhardt, & L. Greenhill (Eds.), *A clinician's guide to child psychiatry* (pp. 48–78). New York: Free Press.

Rutter, M. (1985a). Infantile autism and other pervasive developmental disorders. In M. Rutter & L. Hersov (Eds.), *Child and adolescent psychiatry: Modern approaches* (2nd ed., pp. 545–64). Oxford: Blackwell Scientific.

Rutter, M. (1985b). The treatment of autistic children. *Journal of Child Psychology and Psychiatry, 26,* 193–214.

Rutter, M., & Garmezy, N. (1983). Developmental psychopathology. In E. M. Hetherington (Ed.), *Socialization, personality, and social development, Vol. 4, Mussen's handbook of child psychology* (4th ed., pp. 775–911). New York: Wiley.

Rutter, M., & Gould, M. (1985). Classification. In M. Rutter & L. Hersov (Eds.), *Child and adolescent psychiatry: Modern approaches* (2nd ed., pp. 304–21). Oxford: Blackwell Scientific.

Schopler, E. (1978). Diagnosis and definition of autism. *Journal of Autism and Childhood Schizophrenia, 8,* 167–9.

Schopler, E. (1983). New developments in the definition and diagnosis of autism. In B. B. Lahey & A. E. Kazdin (Eds.), *Advances in clinical child psychology* (Vol. 6, pp. 93–127). New York: Plenum.

Schopler, E., Mesibov, G., & Baker, A. (1982). Evaluation of treatment for autistic children and their parents. *Journal of the American Academy of Child Psychiatry, 21,* 262–7.

Schopler, E., Reichler, R. J., DeVellis, R. F., & Daly, K. (1980). Toward objective classification of childhood autism: Childhood Autism Rating Scale (CARS). *Journal of Autism and Developmental Disorders, 10,* 91–103.

Schopler, E., Reichler, R. J., & Renner, B. R. (1985). *Childhood Autism Rating Scale (CARS).* New York: Irvington.

Schopler, E., & Rutter, M. (1978). Subgroups vary with selection purpose. In M. Rutter & E. Schopler (Eds.), *Autism: A reappraisal of concepts and treatment* (pp. 507–17). New York: Plenum.

Scott, D. W. (1985). Asperger's syndrome and non-verbal communications: A pilot study. *Psychological Medicine, 15,* 683–8.

Skoff, B. F., Mirsky, A. F., & Turner, D. (1980). Prolonged brain-stem transmission time in autism. *Psychiatric Research, 2,* 157–66.

Skuse, D. (1984). Extreme deprivation in early childhood: I. Diverse outcomes for three siblings from an extraordinary family. *Journal of Child Psychology and Psychiatry, 26,* 523–41.

Spence, M. A., Ritvo, E. R., Marazita, M. L., Funderburk, S. J., Sparkes, R. S., A Freeman, B. J. (1985). Gene mapping studies with the syndrome of autism. *Behavior Genetics, 15,* 1–13.

Spiker, D., & Ricks, M. (1984). Developmental relationships in self-recognition: A study of 52 autistic children. *Child Development, 55,* 214–25.

Taft, L. T., & Cohen, H. J. (1971). Hypsarrhythmia and infantile autism: A clinical report. *Journal of Autism and Childhood Schizophrenia. 1,* 327–36.

Tanguay, P. E. (1984). Toward a new classification of serious psychopathology in children. *Journal of the American Academy of Child Psychiatry, 23,* 373–84.

Torrey, E. F., Hersh, S. P., & McCabe, K. D. (1975). Early childhood psychosis and bleeding during pregnancy. *Journal of Autism and Childhood Schizophrenia, 5,* 287–97.

Tinbergen, N., & Tinbergen, E. A. (1983). *"Autistic children": New hope for a cure.* London: Allen & Unwin.

Tsai, L., Stewart, M. A., & August, G. (1981). Implication of sex differences in the familial transmission of infantile autism. *Journal of Autism and Developmental Disorders, 11,* 165–73.

Venter, P. A., Hof, J. O., Coetzee, D. J., Van der Walt, C., & Retief, A. E. (1984). No marker (X) syndrome in autistic children. *Human Genetics, 67,* 107.

Walker, Bettes, B., & McGuire, M. (1984). Recognition and identification of facial stimuli by schizophrenics and patients with affective disorder. *British Journal of Clinical Psychology, 23,* 37–44.

Watson, M. S., Leckman, J. F., Annex, B., Breg, W. R., Boles, D., Volkmar, F. R., Cohen, D. J., & Carter, C. (1984). Fragile X in a survey of 75 autistic males. *New England Journal of Medicine, 310,* 1462.

Williams, R. S., Hauser, S. L., Purpura, D., Delong, R., & Swisher, C. N. (1980). Autism and mental retardation: Neuropathological studies performed in four retarded persons with autistic behavior. *Archives of Neurology, 37,* 749–53.

Wing, L. (1981). Language, social and cognitive impairments in autism and severe mental retardation. *Journal of Autism and Developmental Disorders, 11,* 31–44.

Wing. L., & Gould, J. (1978). Systematic recording of behaviors and skills of retarded and psychotic children. *Journal of Autism and Childhood Schizophrenia. 8,* 79–97.

Wing, L., & Gould, J. (1979). Severe impairments of social interaction and associated abnormalities in children: Epidemiology and classification. *Journal of Autism and Developmental Disorders, 9,* 11–30.

Wolff, S., & Barlow, A. (1979). Schizoid personality in childhood. A comparative study of schizoid, autistic and normal children. *Journal of Child Psychology and Psychiatry, 20,* 19–46.

Wolff, S., & Chick, J. (1980). Schizoid personality in childhood: A controlled follow-up study. *Psychological Medicine, 10,* 85–100.

World Health Organization (1978). International classification of diseases. Geneva: Author.

Yule, W. (1978). Research methodology: What are the "correct controls"? In M. Rutter & E. Schopler (Eds.), *Autism: A reappraisal of concepts and treatment* (pp. 155–62). New York: Plenum.

3

Public Policy and Its Impact on Children with Autism

JAMES J. GALLAGHER

INTRODUCTION

Most professionals who serve children and their families are busy at their tasks of treatment, teaching, or research and rarely take time to think of public policy as it relates to their work. We are only dimly aware of actions taken in far-away legislative halls or courts that often affect us and our ability to do our tasks well and to serve our clients effectively. Just as the child, when asked where milk comes from, may answer, "The refrigerator," we, when asked where our jobs come from, may answer, "The hospital or the university," without pursuing further why the university decided to use one of its precious positions to focus on our area of specialty.

Politics, to many persons, has a vaguely unsavory aroma to it—an activity to be kept far away lest it corrupt us. Actually, politics is the art by which scarce resources in our society are allocated to almost unlimited needs. Public policy actions allocate those resources and, in certain ways, establish the rules or boundaries by which the resources can be used. For those professionals whose interests extend beyond their own patient load to encompass the entire category of autistic children, we need an understanding of how policy decisions are made and how they can be influenced in the future to better achieve our treatment and research goals.

This chapter explores briefly the forces influencing the establishment of relevant public policy for autistic children, the effect that such policy has on our professional work once it has been implemented, and future needs for new policy initiatives.

FORCES INFLUENCING POLICY ESTABLISHMENT

All those working with children with handicaps have benefited enormously through a legislative cornucopia that has been in operation over the last quarter of a century. How did that greatly increased flow of legislation come about, and who was responsible? Although it

JAMES J. GALLAGHER • Frank Porter Graham Child Development Center, The University of North Carolina at Chapel Hill, Chapel Hill, North Carolina 27599-8040.

is fair to say that professional pleas for more resources for handicapped children have been made by individuals, and by some organizations, the powerful initial thrust came, and still comes, from organized parent groups desperately seeking help for their children. Professionals have often been overimpressed with the importance of their own work (who cannot see the obvious value of what I am doing?) and consequently do not, by themselves, represent an active force for reallocating those scarce resources.

Parents and Policy

The role of parents in the setting of public policy for children with developmental disabilities has been crucial to both the design and implementation of policy (Turnbull & Turnbull, 1986). Occasionally, one parent is so frustrated with the experiences undergone while seeking help for his or her child but is aware of how the decision-making system worked, and has made things happen. One such example is described by Wiegerink & Pelosi (1979, p. 12):

> I went to the governor and told him that I had been to every one of the agencies and none of them could help me. They all agreed that I had a problem, they all felt sorry for me and wished they could help; but they all referred me to someone else. Within a couple of weeks they had established a task force to look into the problem of autism and this is how our first public school program got started.

However, it is rare that one person can have such impact. Most of the significant advocacy efforts that have influenced public policy have come through the sustained work of organizations such as the National Association for Retarded Citizens, the National Society for Autistic Children, United Cerebral Palsy, and many similar groups (Boggs, 1985). What the leaders of these organizations found out as they contacted decision-makers was that once the issue of service to handicapped children was brought into the public spotlight, few political figures would wish to run on a platform of saving money by denying the handicapped individual a fair chance to ''make it'' in this society. To the contrary, many legislators took great pride in being the champions of the cause of the child with handicaps, and not a few of them had children in, or close to, their own family that brought such problems home in a personal way. Another important discovery was that if the case of needed resources were argued for all handicapped children, rather than only those with a specific diagnostic entity (e.g., deafness, autism, learning disabilities), the accumulation of supporting agencies and organizations that would be supportive would become powerful in the legislative halls.

The legislative cornucopia (Table I) that came from the Congress in the 1960s and 1970s include authorizations for research, personnel training, demonstration, technical assistance, dissemination, and finally, large sums of money for service delivery, over a billion dollars a year to local school systems, through the P.L. 94-142, the Education for All Handicapped Children Act (Martin, 1985). While there has been follow-up legislative authorization during the 1980s, the innovative thrust in education for the handicapped probably was at its peak in the era of 1965–1975.

Parent advocates can make not only legislative policy but can keep unfavorable executive department actions in the implementation of that policy from taking place. When the Reagan administration wished to modify the regulations for administering programs for handicapped children in ways that the parent groups believed would be highly detrimental, the Congress and the Executive Branch were buried under an avalanche of thousands of letters, telephone calls, and telegrams urging the legislators to stop this action. This im-

Table I. Highlights of Federal Education Policy for Handicapped Children: 1958–1975

Public Law No.	Purpose
P.L. 85-926 (1958)	Grants for teaching in the education of handicapped children, related to education of the mentally retarded
P.L. 88-164 (1963) (Title III)	Authorization of funds for research and demonstration projects in education of the handicapped
P.L. 89-10 (1965)	Elementary and Secondary Education Act: Title III authorized assistance to handicapped children in state-operated and state-supported private day and residential schools
P.L. 89-313	Amendments of P.L. 89-10: grants to state educational agencies for the education of handicapped children in state-supported insitutions
P.L. 90-170 (1967)	Amendments to P.L. 88-164: funds for personnel training to care for the mentally retarded and the inclusion of individuals with neurologic conditions related to mental retardation
P.L. 90-247 (1968)	Amendments of P.L. 89-10: provided Regional Resource Centers for the improvement of education of handicapped children
P.L. 90-538 (1968)	Handicapped Children's Early Education Assistance Act: grants for the development and implementation of experimental programs in early education for the handicapped, from birth to age 6
P.L. 91-230 (1969)	Amendments of P.L. 89-10: Title VI consolidated into one act the previous enactments relating to handicapped children—Education of the handicapped
P.L. 92-424 (1972)	Economic Opportunity Amendments: required that not less than 10% of Head Start enrollment opportunities be available for handicapped children
P.L. 93-380 (1974)	Amended and expanded Education of the Handicapped Act in response to right to education mandates: required states to establish goal of providing full educational opportunity for all handicapped children, ages 0–21
P.L. 94-142 (1975)	Education for All Handicapped Children Act: required states to provide a free appropriate education for all handicapped children between the ages of 3–18 within the state no later than Sept. 1, 1978
P.L. 94-142 Section 619	Amendment to P.L. 94-142 to enhance the expansion of services to preschool handicapped children (aged 3–5) through provision of Preschool Incentive grants

pressive display of interest in public policy is still discussed by congressional staff members, and this advocacy effort resulted in the rescinding of that plan (Weicker, 1985).

The parent organizations have learned an important lesson in democracy, namely, that a small, but well-organized group can often get well-defined wishes cared for in the public arena. There is another message, though, that may not be so evident to the parents. They have been truly successful because the large mass of citizenry is in essential sympathy with their cause. Most citizens have a "there, but for the grace of God, go I" feeling, and there is genuine empathy for the difficulties that these families face and, consequently, a willingness to help, from the public purse, those children who, through no fault of their own, have special problems. There is a fundamental value at work that colors much public policy. Most citizens favor a policy of vertical equity, the unequal treatment of unequals, in order to make them more equal. Children who are poor or handicapped benefit from that value.

Courts and Public Policy

Another major source of policy decisions that have, by and large, aided the delivery of services to handicapped children has been the courts. Over a 20-year period, a series of judicial decisions have established a variety of rights that can serve to guarantee the child with handicapping conditions the opportunity to profit from professional services and community resources. In this domain, too, the parent groups have been active. It is generally agreed that the *Brown v. Board of Education* court decision, which was at the heart of the civil rights for minorities fight during the 1950s and 1960s, was an important precursor to the series of decisions on the rights of handicapped children. But it was the organized parents movement that brought these issues to the attention of the courts.

The right to treatment: This was one significant decision (*Wyatt v. Stickney, 1972*) that forbade the state to institutionalize, or otherwise deprive an individual of liberty, without providing appropriate treatment for the conditions for which he was institutionalized.

The right to education: This right was established in cases that claimed that the mentally retarded and all handicapped children are entitled to a free public education as guaranteed to all children in various state constitutions (*PARC V. Pennsylvania, 1972; Mills v. Board of Education in District of Columbia, 1972*).

The right to avoid discriminatory classification: This right was established to prevent minority children from being classified as handicapped on the basis of tests or instruments that might be invalid for them (*Larry P. v. Riles; Diana v. State Board of Education*).

These decisions were, in part, contradicted by another decision that affirmed the usefulness of tests in the diagnosis of mental retardation (*PASE v. Hannon et al., 1980*).

These court decisions resulted in a much expanded set of services for handicapped children and placed parents of handicapped children in the position of asking for their *rights*, rather than asking for a "favor" from local school districts to provide some appropriate educational services for their child. One recent decision that had tended to temper this set of decisions (*Hendrick Hudson School District v. Rowley, 1982*) determined that the school system did not have the responsibility to provide the "maximum" education for the child, but only sufficient support services to permit the handicapped child to "benefit educationally" from that experience.

The courts will more than likely continue to be a shaper of policy for children with handicapping conditions in the near future. An excellent summary of these court cases may be found in Sage and Burrello (1986) and in Turnbull and Turnbull (1986).

POLICY INFLUENCES ON THE PROFESSIONAL

The large increase in resources emerging from these legislative and court decisions does not come without a price, however, and that price is the rules and regulations that accompany the resources and places limits on what the professional can do. Legislators sometimes speak scornfully of professionals who apparently want the money to be "left on the stump at midnight," or, in other words, want to receive the money with no strings or conditions. That is not the way it is in public policy, nor would we want our tax money to be handed out with no obligations or accountability to farmers, defense contractors, business executives, or others who also seek governmental resources. So, our task is to try to see to it that the inevitable rules that accompany our resources are professionally appropriate.

Eligibility

One of the clear impacts that recent legislation has had has been to change the way we diagnose autistic children. In much of the education legislation, autism is not mentioned specifically as one of the diagnostic categories included in the class of children named handicapped, so the issue has been, "Do autistic children belong?", and, if they belong, under what subtitle are they incorporated? Originally, a decision was made that they fall under the "seriously emotionally disburbed." Currently, however, they are included under "other health impaired."

Such decisions are not mere playing with words. They have major impact on many other professional decisions. The most serious one would be a denial of eligibility for assistance in the first place. Also, if the autistic child is included, what about the "autistic-like" child, that child who shows an unmistakable resemblance to the language and social problems of the autistic child, but at a considerably milder level of severity? What can happen in situations like this is well illustrated by the following example.

Policy and Prevalence

What would we think of the following situation? Suppose that in 1963 a new disease was discovered—a disease that we will call *guny*. Now *guny* had obviously been present before 1963 but had been confused with other similar disorders, so this discovery was an attempt to sort *guny* out from the other conditions and provide differential treatment for the children with the "disease." Originally, the prevalence of such a disease in our society was perhaps thought to be less than one percent of children of any given age, but *guny* has grown into epidemic proportions, increasing by the year. It will affect more than 4.5% or 4 to 5 of every 100 children in the United States in 1987. Should we not say that we have been struck by an enormous epidemic?

Well, we *have* been hit by a major epidemic, only it is not called *guny,* but *learning disabilities.* Children with learning disabilities make up more than 4.5% of school enrollment in the United States, and there is every reason to believe that the number will get larger unless something is done to control it (U.S. Department of Education, 1985). What is this disorder that seems to defeat the very best efforts of the professionals who have identified it and are presumably busily treating it? It appears to be getting worse despite all our attention.

It is highly unlikely that we have been inundated by a new virus bringing on learning problems in children. What we have been struck with are legislative definitions that provide an opportunity for school administrators to obtain additional resources to help them cope with their problem children. Since learning disabilities is one of the categories under P.L. 94-142, which mandates educational services for all handicapped children, then the more children who are identified as *learning disabled,* the more services obtained. The definition of *learning disabilities* is long and complex, but essentially it boils down to a problem the child has in learning or processing information. It seems to be reflected in less than expected school performance. Since professionals have shown an inability to distinguish this condition from other educational problems, by intensity or duration, it is possible to bring more and more cases under the category itself (Kirk & Gallagher, 1986).

Does anyone doubt that the concept of autistic children could be extended to communication disorder children, or children with autistic-like symptoms, and that the category for "autism" would then magically increase in epidemic fashion similar to that of learning disabilities? It is not the nature of the children that would have changed, but the nature of the service system designed to provide help for them and the political system that allocated resources for that help.

Labeling

Why do we label children in the first place? One of the chronic problems involving the classification of exceptional children is the variety of purposes for which such classification takes place. Gallagher (1976) pointed out three major uses of labeling:

1. A means for beginning a classification, diagnosis, and treatment sequence peculiarly designed to counteract certain identifiable negative conditions
2. The basis for further research that will give more insight into the etiology, prevention, and possible treatment applications of such conditions in the future
3. A means for calling public attention to a specific problem in order to obtain additional resources through special legislation and funding

It would indeed be a surprise if the clinical purposes noted in point 1, the etiological purposes noted in point 2, and the political purposes noted in point 3 were equally met by one set of identification procedures. The professional difficulties in classification now being experienced are due, in large measure, to a failure to recognize which purpose is being forwarded at any given time.

Schopler (1983) points out a similar confusion over purposes in the diagnosing of autism,

1. The first, and perhaps most important, basis for naming a syndrome occurs when the cause of the condition is known and can be distinguished from the cause of other conditions. The sorting out of these children becomes more difficult because of the developing continua that may exist with related conditions (Shea & Mesibov, 1985; Batshaw & Perret, 1986).
2. A second meaningful classification basis is the availability of a specific treatment for one definable group of children but not another.
3. When we have neither a specific cause nor a unique treatment, we can still use behavioral description, as in a symptom cluster (pp. 110–111).

There is no escaping the general proposition that when resources are made available for some children, but not others, there is a rush to include more and more children in that special category. There is also a predictable reaction on the part of those who established the policy in the first place who now wish to put tighter eligibility standards on, often to the dismay of the professionals, in order to be sure the money is reaching only the intended target group of children.

Program Quality

One of the other uses of policy beyond establishing the simple level of eligibility is to create an environment in which program quality can be enhanced. This can be done legislatively through the specific authorization and budget support for those support system elements that create the base for program excellence—research, development, leadership training, demonstration, program evaluation, and dissemination. Support for these elements encourages an environment of knowledge seeking and sharing that is at the heart of a healthy profession.

Another way that program goals and quality can be set through policy initiative is to write specific procedures and expectations into the legislation itself. Perhaps the most aggressive legislation in that style has been P.L. 94-142—The Education for All Handicapped Children Act.

In addition to providing large sums of money for the education of handicapped children, P.L. 94-142 laid down six key principles that have had major impact on the service delivery models and the professionals who execute them:

1. *Zero reject.* All children with handicaps are to be provided with a free and appropriate education. There is no local option not to provide services.
2. *Nondiscriminatory evaluation.* Each student must receive a full individual examination before being placed in special education, with tests appropriate to the child's cultural background.
3. *Individualized Education Programs (IEP).* An IEP must be written for every handicapped student who is receiving special education. Goals, procedures, time boundaries, and methods of evaluation are to be specified.
4. *Least restrictive environment.* As much as possible, children who are handicapped must be educated with children who are not handicapped. This does not mean that all handicapped children are to be *mainstreamed,* i.e., placed in the regular classroom. It means that they are taken away from the regular setting only so that beneficial treatment or education may be carried out.
5. *Due process.* These procedures allow parents to call a hearing when they do not agree with the school on the program for their child, to obtain an individual examination by an outside examiner, and take other steps to guarantee the parents' rights.
6. *Parental participation.* Parents are to participate in the development of the program for their child, have access to their child's educational records, and in other ways be an important member of the team helping the child (Kirk & Gallagher, 1986).

These provisions clearly increase the potential of the parent to play a role in their child's educational programming. The *least restrictive environment* provision makes it less likely that an autistic child will be separated off into a separate school program or institution, although it does not necessarily guarantee placement in a regular class. The IEP planning might well conclude that a setting beyond the regular class may be necessary to maximize the child's educational experience.

Essentially, these policies place the burden on the school to demonstrate that they have a special educational program, that this program has been designed cooperatively with parents, and that the child will be incorporated as much as possible into the regular school program. Such policy provisions change the professionals' behavior as well. They now must spend much time on developing IEPs. They must pay attention to parental participation, and concern themselves with due process. None of these changes is free from pain or frustration and is a fine example of the requirements that often accompany increased resources for our professional work.

Paradoxically, the multitude of treatments currently available for children with autism, from megavitamins to psychotherapy, with many variations in between, merely strengthen the belief of many persons that none of the treatments is terribly effective. However, the availability and advocacy for many differing treatments may mean something else. It may mean that different treatments are necessary for different children. Therefore, the proper research or evaluation question is not, "Does treatment X work with autistic children" but rather, "With what children, with which characteristics, under what environmental conditions, does treatment X work?" We must face the fact that respected professionals are putting forth these various treatments. Unless we believe that they are hallucinating, then they must have seen their "treatment" work with someone. The proper question then is, who does it work with and under what set of conditions?

Can policy really have anything to say on such a delicate and complex question as this, where unpredictable and idosyncratic interactions seem to control results? Policy has been considered useful only for the relatively crude distribution of resources designed to cope with a rather large generic problem. But policy can have an important effect on program quality by providing additional sums of money for research and evaluation so that careful and detailed data are collected on a wide array of patients undergoing differing treatments under reasonably controlled conditions. In this way, the relative usefulness of various treatments can be gradually discovered.

Support Services for Quality

The parental pressure is almost always directed to obtaining more services for children and families. It takes special attention by professionals to get additional resources for research, personnel training, or evaluation, all of which are essential support services for quality programs, but which are often overlooked in the press of immediate service delivery problems.

Another contribution to program quality is the development of professional standards of conduct—ethical standards that are applied to the professional community. This is a particularly pertinent point in cases involving children with autism, since many different disciplines are involved, and particularly because some treatments are being employed that force us to draw a fine line between aversive therapy, for example, and downright cruelty to children.

The open door is one of the most important safeguards to the threatened mistreatment of children. Therefore, a policy that allows a parent access to treatment programs, at any time, can forestall some ugly things happening when staff become totally frustrated at their own ability to control or manage a screaming and nonresponsive child. It is, or should be, part of the right of parents, along with the due process rights embedded in P.L. 94-142. Schopler (1986) has pointed out that professionals who have had their state license taken away for questionable practices can merely move to another state and set up business again, which calls for some type of federal licensing to reduce the likelihood of patient abuse.

Program Continuity

One of the clear goals of public policy beyond eligibility and program quality, is to try to draw links between various programs and legislative initiatives that have been developed at different times and for different purposes. This dispersed legislation has resulted in a patchwork quilt of assistance that may or may not carry the child and family over important transition points in the life of the child with handicapping conditions. For example, there has been legislation proposed that would bring services to preschool children but would stop at age 5 or, at most, age 8. Other legislature applies to children with handicaps as long as they are in school. Yet other legislation and policies provide for rehabilitative services after the child is out of school but limited help while the child is still in school. We should specifically investigate the array of current policies to see whether they answer the following questions:

1. Are these services available at the earliest point in life when the child and family are in need of them?
2. Do the services support the child and family during the transition from preschool services to public school services?
3. Are services equally available to the child and family in the child's secondary school years as in the elementary school?
4. Are services available to aid the difficult transition from the world of school to the world of work?

There is a traditional lack of communication between professionals responsible for one particular segment of the life span (e.g., preschool) to another group responsible for another phase (e.g., school). A review of existing policies, as well as how they may ease these transitions for parents with handicapped children, seems called for (Haskins & Gallagher, 1981).

FUTURE POLICY NEEDS

This chapter has so far delineated eligibility, program quality, and program continuity as areas of special policy concern. If we are to build constructively on what now exists for the future, we will need to cope with some of the existing limitations and frustrations.

Eligibility

These are two ways to improve the problems created by eligibility requirements. One would be to sharpen the differential diagnosis between handicapping conditions and between handicapped and nonhandicapped children.

Hobbs (1974, 1975) organized a major review of the labeling issue involving more than 90 scientists and provided a major state-of-the-art statement on the labeling of children. One of his recommendations was "The Secretary of Health, Education and Welfare should contract with appropriate institutions or agencies to develop a comprehensive diagnostic and classification system for handicapped, disadvantaged, and delinquent chilren (p. 234)."

Another, different, strategy to cope with labeling is to make such labels unnecessary to receive services. Under this strategy, support services would be provided for all children needing assistance. This would do away with the necessity for eligibility requirements that eat up an inordinate amount of professional resources in classification and diagnostic procedures that are essentially unrelated to treatment.

One current trend in legislation for children with handicapping conditions is to not specify the specific diagnostic categories but to include a more generic statement of eligibility on the basis of some problem conditions. For example, P.L. 99-457, which reauthorizes the discretionary parts of the Education for the Handicapped Act, has the following definition for "handicapped infants and toddlers (Federal Register 10/8/86, p. 1146):

1. The term handicapped infants and toddlers means individuals from birth to age 2, inclusive, who need early intervention services because they: A. Are experiencing developmental delays as measured by appropriate diagnostic instruments and pro-

cedures in one or more of the following areas; cognitive development, physical development, language and speech development, psychosocial development or self help skills; or B. Have a diagnosed physical or mental condition which has a high probability of resulting in developmental delay.

Such general conditions can easily be met by children who would fit the American Psychiatric Association (DSM-III) category of early *infantile autism* (1980):

1. Lack of responsiveness to other people
2. Gross deficits in language development and peculiar speech patterns such as delayed echolalia
3. Bizarre responses to various aspects of the environment such as resistance to change and peculiar attachment to animate or inanimate objects

All these symptoms develop during first 30 months of life.

Another of the Hobbs's recommendations, now more than a decade old (Hobbs, 1975, p. 265) would propose a flat sum of money calculated on a percentage basis from the regular school budget that would allow for special services to all children in need in the school, thereby avoiding the current "head count" method of reimbursement:

Funds for the support of public school programs for children in need of special assistance should be provided on the basis of a flat percentage of the total appropriation (federal, state, and local) for all children. As a general guideline, a 15% funding formula is recommended. The extra funds should be added to appropriations for all children, not taken away from them.

Future Program Quality

The special future policy concern in regard to program quality would focus more on budget than on authorization. There are probably sufficient laws on the books now for the spport of research, training, and demonstration. The question is whether they are adequately funded in comparison with the service funds being given or as compared with established needs.

One policy consideration might be to tie these support services to the service funds provided in such laws as P.L. 94-142. As the service funds increase, the support services of research and training would go up a proportional amount. There is a good reason why such a provision should be considered. When budget cutbacks are made, it is the research and leadership training areas that often get cut the worst. They have a very small and generally inactive constitutency who rarely scream and protest budget reductions. In contrast, any attempt to cut direct service funds to handicapped children and their families will predictably bring an avalanche of negative mail and telegrams through well-organized lobbying groups. It is not hard to see why funds for "support" services needed for program quality fall further and further behind the service funds and will continue to do so, unless some specific actions are taken such as those suggested earlier.

Program Continuity in the Future

One of the major policy considerations for the immediate future is the failure of existing programs to extend our major life transition periods so that services can be continuous, since it would be the expectation that many persons with moderate to severe cases of autism would need some form of professional assistance over their life span (Coudroglou, 1984). Kyne (1980) pointed out that there is no agency responsible to continue education as a community-based service over age 21. Money is available for institution care, but there is no community support. A situation that runs directly counter to the philosophy embodied in P.L. 94-142, the Education for All Handicapped Children Act, stresses the importance of placing the student in the *least restrictive environment*.

What may be needed first is a careful policy analysis of existing legislation and regulations to see where the service and support system gaps are. Kyne has given one example, but there are surely others.

THE NEED FOR POLICY ADVOCACY

We tend to draw upon analogies as we try to understand a field in which we have not been previously well versed, such as political advocacy and policy. Unfortunately, some of the most common of our images come from athletics, and such images do not serve us well in this instance. In an athletic contest, there is a conflict that has a beginning, a middle, and an end. Someone wins and someone loses, and we go home looking forward to the next encounter.

In the field of public policy, however, the "ball game" is never over. It just keeps going on from one year to another. If one pauses too long to celebrate a temporary triumph, one may find the triumph to be all too temporary indeed. If this year we have passed some needed legislation, then next year, and for all the years after that, there will be appropriations to worry about, regulations to watch out for, and amendments to be wary of.

We are aware that "constant vigilence is the price of freedom." It is also the price for ensuring continued proper services and resources for the handicapped. This does not mean that every professional must man the battlements in the state capital, or in Washington. It does mean that professional groups and organizations need to do so and they deserve our active support.

There is nothing more certain than that tomorrow someone else with a plan to improve the city, the state, the nation, or the planet—or at least the fortunes of their own group—will have ideas of how to allocate differently those scare resources of our society. Their ideas will not likely include our interests but may even have designs on those scarce resources that we have been using.

As Senator Weicker from Connecticut (1985) once said, "It is the task of parents and professionals who care for handicapped children to speak for those who cannot speak for themselves." If that task is left to others, or to fate, the resources and policy initiatives we have become used to may well be eroded or directed to other perceived societal needs.

REFERENCES

American Psychiatric Association. (1980). *Diagnostic and statistical manual of mental disorders* (3rd ed.). Washington, D.C.: American Psychiatric Association.

Batshaw, M., & Perret, Y. (1986). *Children with handicaps: A medical primer* (2nd ed.). Boston: Paul H. Brookes.

Boggs, E. (1985). The future of legislative advocacy for exceptional children. In J. Gallagher & B. Weiner (Eds.), *Alternative futures in special education*. Reston, VA: Council for Exceptional Children.

Coudroglou, A. (1984). Disability: The view from social policy. *Rehabilitation Literature, 45*(11–12), 358–61.

Gallagher, J. (1976). The sacred and profane uses of labeling. *Mental Retardation 141*(6), 3–7.

Haskins, R., & Gallagher, J. (Eds.) (1981). *Models of policy analysis.* Norwood, NJ: Ablex.

Hobbs, N. (1975). *The futures of children.* San Francisco, CA: Jossey-Bass.

Ishii, T. and Takahashi, O. (1983). The epidemiology of autistic children in Toyota, Japan: Prevalence. *Japanese Journal of Child and Adolescent Psychiatry, 24*(5), 311–21.

Kirk, S., & Gallagher, J. (1986). *Educating Exceptional Children,* 5th ed. Boston: Houghton-Miffin.

Kyne, J. (1980). The evolving parent-professional relationship. In B. Wilcox & A. Thompson (Eds.), *Cultural issues in educating autistic children and youth* (pp. 234–24). Washington, D.C.: U.S. Department of Education, Office of Special Education, Division of Innovation and Development.

Martin, E. (1985). Public policy and special education: An unfinished agenda. In J. Gallagher & B. Weiner (Eds.), *Alternative futures in special education.* Reston, VA: Council for Exceptional Children.

National Society for Autistic Children. (1978). Definition of the syndrome of autism. *Journal of Autism and Childhood Schizophrenia, 8*(2), 162–7.

Pizzo, P. (1983). *Parent to parent.* Boston: Beacon Press.

Sage, D. and Burrello, L. (1986). *Policy and management in special education.* Englewood Cliffs, NJ: Prentice Hall.

Schopler, E. (1983). New developments in the definition and diagnosis of autism. In B. B. Lahey & A. E. Kazdin (Eds.), *Advances in clinical child psychology, Vol. 6,* (pp. 93–127).

Schopler, E. (1985). Editorial: Treatment abuse and its reduction. *Journal of Autism and Developmental Disabilities, 16*(2).

Shea, V., & Mesibov, G. (1985). Brief report: The relationship of learning disabilities and higher level autism. *Journal of Autism and Developmental Disorders, 15*(4), 42535.

Turnbull, A., & Turnbull, H. (1986). *Families, professionals and exceptionality: A special partnership.* Columbus, OH: Mental Publishing Co.

Weicker, L. (1985). Sonny and public policy. In H. Turnbull and A. Turnbull (Eds.), *People speak out: Then and now* (pp. 281–287). Columbus, OH: Merrill.

Wiegerink, R., & Pelosi, J. (1979). *Development disabilities: The DD movement.* Baltimore: Paul H. Brookes.

4

Diagnostic Classification for the Clinician

JOHN S. WERRY

INTRODUCTION

This book is about autism—its diagnosis and assessment. Diagnosis means many things, from simply assigning a name or label, to a statement of all aspects relevant to the management of a case. As the title of this chapter suggests, it addresses only the issue of diagnosis in its narrowest sense: the affixing of a label or name which groups together all children with the disorder and states in what way they all resemble each other and can be differentiated from both normal and other types of exceptional children. Furthermore, this chapter is concerned only with the principles and problems of diagnosis in general as a preparation for Part II of this book, which discusses at length the various diagnostic approaches to autism itself. However, to keep this review as germane as possible, the term *autism* is used to illustrate several major points.

First, we look at classification in general; then ask why we should try to classify disorders such as autism, what characterizes a good classification, and how to ensure that the diagnosis made is the right one, look at the types of diagnostic systems available to the clinician and the current popular classification systems; and, finally examine how to choose a system to suit one's own purposes. Throughout, the discussion is kept simple and nontechnical and focuses on clinical concerns.

Classificatory systems are variously known as taxonomies or nosologies, and there is an area of science devoted to their study as phenomena in their own right. Much of this study has been within clinical psychology, perhaps because, unlike clinical medicine, by the time of its origin, there were well-developed concepts and analytic tools by which to study nosology. Strange to say, clinical medicine has been little touched by this area of sicence, yet medicine serves as the touchstone by which classifications in psychopathology are judged. The spectacular successes of modern medicine should not allow us to be mesmerized into believing that there are not still serious root problems in medical diagnosis that extend well beyond our ignorance of the etiology and treatment of major killers like cancer or cardiovascular disease. These root problems are mirrored and magnified in the area of psychiatric disorders such as autism.

JOHN S. WERRY • Department of Psychiatry, School of Medicine, University of Auckland, P.B., Auckland, New Zealand.

WHY CLASSIFY?

There is considerable resistance to classification in psychiatry and abnormal psychology and therefore it is important that it be explained and demystified. Classifying is integral to human activity and no day goes by in which the average human being does not attempt to regularize, codifying, interpret, or try to understand existence by adumbrating daily events from the singular or unusual, to the domain of the familiar. People, weather, politics, economics, and similar day-to-day experiences are all put into groups on the basis of similarities to past experiences or to what we know—so much so that it can be said that there is something about the human brain that makes classification inevitable. It is our way of trying to understand and learn from experience. Without classification, everything that happens to us would be unique and we could not prepare for the future in any way. Scientific classification then, is only an extension of this essential human process and differs only in that it is subject to a set of rules aimed primarily at combating error and self-deception.

Resistance to classification by clinicians is occasioned by a number of factors. Some believe that human beings are unique and that any attempt to classify them is demeaning, prejudicial, stereotyping, and so on. Others object because these classifications are seen as medical in origin and concept and therefore to be resisted by non medical professionals. However, the largest resistance probably comes from the fact that clinicians simply do not find current classifications very useful in their day-to-day work.

There are many good reasons for classifying. These are detailed in the section to follow outlining the characteristics of a good classification. In the end, the most important reason for classifying is that it is essential to the capturing of experience and its application to succeeding cases. Even those who are most opposed to classification actually do classify in that they look at each new case in the light of their previous cases and attempt to find in what way they resembles previous ones so that treatment may be applied in a systematic way. In short, there can be no real argument against classifying, only arguments against particular attempts to do so.

Classification has served humankind spectacularly well—it is where all science begins—noting similarities that permit some kind of grouping. This in turn can lead to hypothesis about the nature of these similarities. Then, through formal testing of these hypotheses, rejection or refinement of the classification can occur. It would be most unwise then, to turn ones back on human history and not operate from the assumption that classification is as likely to be servicable to the needs of clinicians as it has to other areas of human endeavor.

Clinical classifications have distinct purposes, but it is important to bear in mind that there are at least three different types of classification germane to this field (Feinstein, 1967): (1) etiologic/pathologic, (2) treatment/prognostic, and (3) patient management. In medicine, it is easy to separate these three processes because they embrace different classes of phenomena, but in psychiatry all the phenomena are often of a like type (psychological), resulting in confusion. As Feinstein pointed out, much of what is called the "art" of medicine (mostly processes 1 and 2) is probably really unstudied science and can only be called "art" by default because it has not yet been examined in a proper, scientific way. We should all remember that Freud developed psychoanalysis primarily as a tool in his search for a "science of the mind" and, while we may argue about the wisdom of his starting with such difficult unobservables, we ought to respect his aim and maintain his faith that this can be done in the end. Without this faith, we are like a ship without a rudder at the mercy of whatever current wind of fashion is blowing, tossed this way and that, never proceeding systematically in the direction of better patient care or profiting from the paths traversed by others and ourselves.

CHARACTERISTICS OF A GOOD CLASSIFICATION

Some General Values

Having argued that as clinicians we need classification to guide us, we shall now look at the hallmarks of a good diagnosis:

1. It should tell us how to treat—ideally not just how to treat particular symptoms such as gaze avoidance, or disorders such as autism, but the autistic child, which is a much more complex business involving families, schools and so on.
2. It should enable us to tell patients and/or caretakers what the outlook over the next few years and in adulthood is, both with and without treatment.
3. It should tell what the cause or causes are. For example, it is now widely accepted that autism is probably a brain disorder which may have many different causes.
4. Knowing what the diagnosis is, we should then know what commonly associated problems we ought to look out for. For example, epilepsy is one disorder that has a higher than expected association with autism (Coleman & Gillberg, 1985) even though, obviously, most epileptics do not have autism.
5. When we talk to each other about autism it should be clear exactly what we are discussing so that we all recall to mind the same kind of child or person. This is most important in research; otherwise, the findings of one researcher have no relevence to those of others.
6. It should tell us how to prevent the disorder. For example, it is known that there is some link between rubella in pregnancy, prenatal accidents and brain damage in general and autism (Coleman & Gillberg, 1985; Prior & Werry 1986) (see Chapter 7). Thus, rubella vaccination programs and better prenatal care should reduce the frequency of autism, though, since these do not explain all cases of autism, such reduction could not be absolute.
7. While there are social disadvantages to labeling (e.g., a child labeled as autistic may be treated by schools as more handicapped than he or she really is), the very fact that we know what we are dealing with should have a beneficial effect in its own right for patient, family, ecosystem. and clinician alike, which *in toto* should work to the benefit of the patient. Nothing is more frustrating to those working or living with handicapped children than the feeling that no one really knows what is wrong or that there has never been a child with problems like this before. The application of a label such as autism, allows profitless speculation and uncertainty to be put aside and for all then to focus their efforts on management. Parents can then read about the disorder, join parent support groups, and so on.

Put in somewhat more technical language, a good classification should have the following uses: (1) therapeutic, (2) prognostic, (3) etiologic/pathologic, (4) symptomatologic, (5) communicative/heuristic, (6) preventitive, and (7) explanatory.

Obviously, there are vew disorders in psychiatry and, surprisingly, in general medicine that fulfill all these criteria. For example, few medical diagnoses enable the doctor to proceed with complete confidence to program the total management of the patient or to predict or understand all the symptomatology. However, while the diagnosis of autism does tell us a great deal, regrettably, what is of prime interest to clinicians and parents alike—definitively effective treatment and a clearly defined cause—are not among them.

Evaluating the Diagnosis

Moving now from the uses of a diagnosis, let us look at some of the technical properties that, the scientific study of classifications tells us, must be present before we can hope to achieve the usefulness that we seek. These have been detailed elsewhere (e.g., Quay, 1986; Rutter & Shaffer, 1980; Werry, 1976). A knowledge of these properties should prevent wasting much time and effort clinically and in research on useless or invalid taxonomies. Regrettably, such an orderly progression of first testing and then promulgating it is seldom observed. For example, Kanner proposed the diagnosis of autism in 1943; after a slow start, it was then enthusiastically and promiscuously applied to every developmentally deviant group, to the point where Kanner himself became exasperated. The problem was that while Kanner defined a new syndrome, he did not specify clearly enough, what were the necessary and sufficient signs and symptoms or most critically, how they were to be accurately define and measured (Prior & Werry, 1986).

The steps by which a diagnosis should be evaluated, are no different from those which have been rigorously developed for construction of psychological tests as follows:

Reliability

The diagnosis must show agreement between different diagnosers, different places and at different times (if the condition is stable, as autism is), so that any given child can be seen by different clinicians and in different cities and at different times and always receive the same diagnosis. To achieve reliability, the defining characteristics must be as operationally defined and observable as possible, and it is here that most classifications that include autism have failed to measure up. Despite the conspicuous improvements detailed later in this book (see Chapter 9), our fundamental ignorance of the nature of autism, the crudity of measures of behavior, and their remoteness from the brain dysfunctions involved, we necessarily still lack the kind of exactitude that can be achieved, say for the definition of hypertension. However, the history of medicine tells us that, even with crude clinical methods we can get near enough to define a disorder that will serve as a useful and solid starting point. The physician to whom modern medicine owes much of its start (after the Greeks) was the seventeenth century Englishman, Thomas Sydenham, who insisted that it was possible to define diseases by clusters of signs and symptoms carefully observed in the patients themselves and then verified by watching outcome. Sydenham's definition of scarlet fever, for example, is still almost as valid today as it ever was, although now it can be verified quickly by bacteriologic and immunologic tests and terminated dramatically with antibiotics.

In short, we should not be discouraged by the inexactitude of our methods—we do not seek 100% reliability in diagnosis, anything superior to chance is actually a start, since it shows that we are on the way to having a sturdy diagnosis. The important thing is that we must check the reliability before we promulgate diagnoses. That is exactly what happened with the Dianostic and Statistical Manual (3rd ed.) of the American Psychiatric Association (DSM-III) and to a lesser extent with the children's section of the International Classification of Diseases (9th ed.) of the World Health Organization (ICD9) (Quay, 1986).

Covariation

The second property, according to Quay (1986), is covariation of the elements. The defining characteristics (i.e., signs and symptoms) should always be found together, or nearly so, or in certain threshold levels of combinations.

Discriminability

Discriminability is probably the most neglected property of all. The criteria for autism must not only tell what is autism, but also what it is not. We all know—and parents even better—that some professionals diagnose autism widely and some narrowly, so that an autistic child may receive a bewildering variety of, and even quite contradictory, diagnoses ranging from mental retardation to maternal deprivation. This is due to lack of discriminability of these different diagnoses especially when loosely applied.

Further examples of this common problem can be seen in "hyperactivity" and suicide. Studies have shown that with careful diagnosis, there is no major difficulty in discriminating hyperactive from normal children, but there is from those with conduct disorder because of serious overlapping in defining characteristics of the two disorders (Werry, Reeves & Elkind, 1986). One more example, suicide, will suffice to make this most important point about discriminability. A recent study (Shafii, Carrigan, Whittinghill & Derrick, 1985) compared the characteristics of children who had committed suicide with those of a matched group of normal children. About one half the dead children had threatened to kill themselves. It was concluded that clinicians must take threats of suicide very seriously, since they could well portend suicide. However, the same study showed that about 10% of the normal children had also threatened to kill themselves. The annual suicide rate in this age group is about 2 in 20,000. Thus for every child who threatens suicide and then does it, about 2000 will threaten and not do it. Thus, threats of suicide lacks discriminitive power and, on their own, are useless in trying to diagnose suicidal risk. This is a good example of why we must test the discriminability of our diagnoses using proper procedures, since logic suggests that threatening suicide should be a useful clinical predictor, but science shows us that it is not.

Validity

This is the property of being able to confirm the diagnosis by means independent of those by which the diagnosis was made. While there are a number of such external factors by which to do this confirmation, the critical ones for us as clinicians are to be able to define the cause, to choose the right treatment, and accurately to predict outcome. Many diagnoses, psychiatric and, surprisingly, medical too, fail most or all of these criteria. It is obvious that a diagnosis that lacks this critical kind of validity is not going to be of much use clinically.

Since this review is primarily for clinicians, it is not necessary to go into all the details of how these properties are to be checked, suffice it to say that the procedures and the statistical methods of analysis are well established. Most of us are not researchers, nor do we fully understand these procedures and this in turn makes us neglectful, suspicious or misunderstanding of them and of those who would apply them to what we do. This is not helped by the arrogance and clinical naivete often shown by researchers. As clinicians, we should bear in mind that in the end, science is all about objective truth and that the primary motivation for researching diagnosis is to help us do a better job with our patients. If we are not prepared to participate in this process it is our patients who will suffer finally, since they will be denied the attempt to pool our wisdom and build on each other's experience.

HOW TO ACHIEVE A GOOD DIAGNOSIS

A classification system rests inevitably on the data by which it is assembled. Put another way, on the history taking and examinations carried out to determine the signs and symptoms of disorder. No classification however good, can succeed, if its data base is shoddy. Since such features as reliability rest on objectivity and operationalization of necessary and sufficient criteria, it follows that those criteria must be derived from accurate observations of signs and symptoms. This seems to lead automatically and inexorably to the conclusion that unless history taking and examination procedures are standardized and abnormal features always defined, elicited, and measured in exactly the same way, there is unlikely to be a reliable or valid diagnosis. Medical history taking is roughly standardized and the crucial verifying organ-imaging and laboratory tests are rather more so. Furthermore, many of the critical signs and symptoms are quite self-evident, so that errors of detection and measurement are often quite low. As a result, medicine has lagged behind other areas in the use of ways of ensuring reliability.

On the other hand, developers of psychological tests have gone to extraordinary lengths to ensure that data collected is uniform and reliable. It is regrettable, then, that many psychologists who use such tests and seem to have no objection to standardized examination (i.e., data capture) methods in that situation, seem often quite happy with the shapeless interview and examination methods that have come down from medicine through psychiatry. It is probable that the type of interview and the data captured are as likely to be determined by the clinician's preconceptions about the case and what has caused the psychopathology as by any commitment to a need for a standard uniform set of signs and symptoms by which to assess patients. It goes without saying, that any standardized system of interviewing and history-taking has got to yield the maximum amount of useful information in the minimum time. We cannot afford systems of interviewing that are cumbersome, overinclusive, and low on cost–benefit effectiveness. The use of ''gating'' questions and various path-flow systems allows for a compromise between covering the entire field of symptoms and acceptable levels of sampling the key ones, so as to fit the interview to the practicality and constraints of the clinical world. Again, our resistance to such procedures can perhaps be reduced, if we think of this as simply trying to codify what most clinicians do anyway but to pool our experience instead of all going our own way. Several such data capture systems are available or under development at the moment especially for dimensional and medical/categorical systems such as the DSM-III.

CLASSIFICATION OF CLASSIFICATIONS

There are various ways of looking at different types of classifications but the one to be followed here is conceptual or how the classification groups similarities that bind each disorder together and differentiate it from other disorders.

Categorical/Medical/Disease Classifications

Perhaps because psychiatry is an offshoot of medicine, the categorical/medical/disease taxonomy has dominated with autism. The fundamental feature lies in the notion of a disorder or disease that one has or does not have, hence the term categorical. But it is more than just a matter of yes/no dichotomization. Categorical classifications also rely for defining characteristics on signs and symptoms or abnormal features; they presume a single or simple set of underlying causes responsible for the more numerous abnormal defining features (but note that this cause does not need to be physical). There are other assumptions too, such as reasonably uniform response to treatment and so on. The DSM-III and the ICD9 are examples of such classifications. Their strength can be seen in the history of medicine where the careful definition of diseases from the seventeenth to the eighteenth century allowed a quite astonishing rush of discoveries of their causes in the nineteenth century when the critical diagnostic techniques such as bacteriology and microscopic pathology were developed. We are now in a somewhat similar position. Hitherto, methods of examining the brain in life have been crude; apart from a few like the electroencephalograph (EEG), almost exclusively structural and quite insufficient to demonstrate what is wrong in autism and other psychiatric disorders in which any brain disorder is almost certainly functional rather than structural. But exciting new methods such as positron emission tomography (PET) scans promise to change this and help pinpoint exactly what areas of the brain are malfunctioning. As the history of bacteriology shows, when the lesion and even the cause are found, it may require another century or more to find the cure.

By contrast, the weakness of such classifications is easily seen in autism too. As Dr. Wing has shown (see Chapter 7), autism is not only a continuum with all degrees of severity, but the causes are likely to be numerous. As the history of medicine shows, a bad all-embracing classification can sometimes seriously retard progress by premature closure. In the distant future, it is almost certain that autism will be subclassified by cause, some of which will be treatable and others not. However, if one is forced to speculate, autism would seem to be among the small group of psychiatric disorders such as other psychoses, which is most likely to yield to the medical or disease model as the evidence suggesting it is probably due to major brain malfunction is now fairly impressive (Coleman & Gillberg, 1985).

Dimensional Classifications

The assumption of dimensional classification is not one of a clear-cut yes or no categorization, but rather of a continuum or dimension along which every child can be placed somewhere. Height, weight, and IQ are good illustrations of dimensions. Put another way, autism would be seen as a continuum from entirely absent (say 0%) through to the other extreme (100%). Most children would then score 0% and the numbers tail off rapidly to reach only around say 1–2 in 10,000 children with a score of 100% (i.e., the most severe degree of autism possible). This is one half of a normal distribution curve. The point at which the disorder autism is said to exist is then seen to be arbitrary but reflects the clinical reality until it can be defined in some other way than by symptoms (e.g., by etiology). The virtues of such a classification of autism are well-argued in Chapter 7. Most dimensional systems are derived from symptoms commonly seen in clinics and then standardized on total populations. Thus, because autism is rare in the population and even infrequent in clinic patients, dimensional classifications have not been particularly helpful in the diagnosis of autism, but the Rimland checklist could, in theory, be used in this way. Outside autism, there are compelling reasons to believe that much of childhood behavioral difficulties are as well if not better conceptualized as dimensions rather than categories (Quay, 1986). A word of warning: Most normative values for dimensional systems are based on statistical cutoff points such as 2 SD from the mean. Such a concept of abnormality is a clinical nonsense, since there is no *a priori* reason to believe that the frequency of say hyperactivity is necessarily about 2.5% and, in the case of autism, such a figure is clearly false. Cutoff points can only be determined or validated by external criteria such brain patholgy or response to specific treatments.

Process Classifications

The conceptual base in process classifications involves some process, such as systems theory, behavior analysis (stimulus/response/contingency sequences), or outcome, rather than signs and symptoms. For example, an autistic child seen by a behaviorist would not be called autistic but would described in terms of a set of problem behaviors, such as self-mutilation, gaze avoidance, screaming, and rocking. Each problem behavior would then be further subclassified by its eliciting stimuli, setting events, and consequences. Similarly, a family therapist might classify not the child but the family and then in terms of the interpersonal dynamics (e.g., enmeshment). While such classifications are helpful in management, it is hard to see how they have much place in the initial detection of autism, since every child normal or abnormal is subject to such processes. Possible exceptions are developmental classifications, such as the famous but little-used Group for the Advancement of Psychiatry one (Quay, 1986), which classified psychoses by age of onset. However, this classification was never solely developmental but a multidimensional melding of process and medical classification.

Multiaxial Systems

In multiaxial systems, a single diagnosis is eschewed in favor of separate axes that include not only one for the disorder, but also personality, stressors, IQ, and so forth. These classifications represent a significant advance over previous ones in that they recognize that the kind of information needed to deal with patients, transcends just that which defines a disorder. Thus they attempt to diagnose not autism, but the child with autism in all his or her complexity. They are the beginnings of a riposte to Feinstein's criticism (1967) that medicine has ignored everything except an etiologic kind of diagnosis. What axes are needed remains controversial, but it is hard to escape the conclusion that no existing classification has all the axes needed to deal with autism (e.g., IQ in the DSM-III is absent despite its powerful prognostic and treatment value in autism). This type of classification is discussed in more detail in Chapter 8.

Idiographic Approaches

Idiographic approaches are antidiagnostic and claim that each child is unique. Not only is such an attitude anti-intellectual, but it is nonsense, since those who claim to espouse it invariably draw on their past experience, and hence must believe that in some way any particular child resembles others that he or she has seen previously.

POPULAR CLASSIFICATIONS: AN OVERVIEW

Full details of these are given elsewhere in this book. Suffice it to say that no classification has yet demonstrated that it has a premium on truth or utility. For reasons already set out, it seems that multiaxial classifications offer most for comprehensive management. Both of the most popular ones, the ICD9 and DSM-III, are multiaxial (see Chapter 8). There is little doubt that DSM-III has attained a popularity and universality that is exciting to those, like the author, who are accustomed to dissent and sectarianism in child psychopathology, in that it offers, for the first time, a real possibility of a universal language and approach to disorders such as autism. There is little doubt that this popularity is based on the existence of a well-defined set of necessary and sufficient diagnostic critieria for each and every disorder and a manual that summarizes the knowledge about each disorder in convenient form. It has already spawned almost as much research about its properties in 8 years as all previous systems in their entire history. But there are dangers too, as anticipated by Rutter and Shaffer (1980), although perhaps not as serious as they predicted. Feinstein (1967) already noted the disastrous effect on medicine of the premature closure on nosology preceding the nineteenth century. Many of the categories in DSM-III are unreliable or of unknown validity (Quay, 1986). There is also considerable dissatisfaction about the lack of place for psychodynamic and other process aspects of classification and there seems a lack of enthusiasm for some of the axes in clinical practice (Jampala, Sierles & Taylor, 1986). However, the DSM-III is already being fine tuned in DSM-III-R (for revised) and, like the ICD9, will have to be revised for 1989–1990. The ICD9 has not been as successful in child psychiatry as the DSM-III, and other classifications have not found wide audiences. Common sense suggests that we cannot afford competing classifications for child psychiaty let alone autism—we must choose one.

As far as dimensional systems are concerned, none of the most popular, such as those derived from the Child Behavior Checklist (Achenbach, 1980) or the Behavior Problem Checklist (Quay, 1986), is suitable for autism, although they could be helpful to flesh out the total problem profile of the autistic child. Similar remarks can be made about process classifications such as systems theory and behavioral analysis.

WHICH CLASSIFICATION?

The choice of a classification depends on what it is to be used for. As clinicians, we are primarily interested in usefulness in practice and in communicating with colleagues and parents. Choice should be dictated, then, by these considerations. ICD9 and DSM-III have very little difference as far as diagnostic criteria for autism are concerned. However, by being more explicit and by listing a great deal of useful information in crisp and clear form in the manual along with diagnostic criteria, the DSM-III ought to be much more useful to the clinician than the ICD9, provided one is prepared to "live by the book", as it were, and use the manual constantly. This is particularly true for the occasional diagnoser of autism, so that we can strive to talk with one voice and thus avoid confusing and distressing parents unnecessarily.

However, the diagnosis of autism is but a beginning: The management of patient, family, and social environment will call for a wealth of information and knowledge and a set of skills that cannot be captured in any existing diagnostic system. If we bear in mind the sharp limitations of such a diagnostic label, we will be in a better position to appreciate its real usefulness. In any case, we should all be interested in improving our methods of data capture and diagnosis and thus welcome and facilitate the activities of those who have the skills and the will to do so. What is needed is a close partnership between clinician and researcher, so that the result may be greater than the mere sum of the parts contributed by each.

REFERENCES

Achenbach, T. M. (1980). DSM-III in light of empirical research on the classification of child psycho-pathology. *Journal of the American Academy of Child Psychiatry, 19,* 395–412.

Coleman, M., & Gillberg, C. (1985). *The biology of the autistic syndromes.* New York: Praeger.

Feinstein, A. R. (1967). *Clinical judgment.* Baltimore: Williams & Wilkins.

Jampala, V. C., Sierles, F. S., & Taylor, M. A. (1986). Consumers' views of DSM-III: Attitudes and practices of U.S. psychiatrists and 1984 graduating residents. *American Journal of Psychiatry, 143,* 148–53.

Prior, M., & Werry, J. S. (1986). Autism, schizophrenia and allied disorders: The childhood psychoses. In H. C. Quay, & J. S. Werry (Eds.), *Psychopathological disorders of childhood* (3rd ed.). New York: Wiley.

Quay, H. C. (1986). Classification. In H. C. Quay & J. S. Werry (Eds.), *Psychopathological disorders of childhood* (3rd ed.). New York: Wiley.

Rutter, M., & Shaffer, D. (1980). DSM-III: A step forward or a step backward in terms of classification of child psychiatric disorders? *Journal of the American Academy of Child Psychiatry, 19,* 371–94.

Shafii, M., Carrigan, S., Whittinghill, J. R., & Derrick, A. (1985). Psychological autopsy of completed suicide in children and adolescents. *American Journal of Psychiatry, 142,* 1061–64.

Werry, J. S. (1976). Diagnosis. In W. Guy (Ed.), *ECDEU assessment manual.* Rockville, MD: U.S. Department of Health, Education and Welfare. (Publication # ADM 76-338).

Werry, J. S., Reeves, J. C., & Elkind, G. S. (1986). Attention deficit, conduct, oppositional and anxiety disorders in children: A review of research on differentiating characteristics. *Journal of the American Academy of Child & Adolescent Psychiatry, 26,* 144–155.

5

What's in a Name?

MARY AKERLEY

INTRODUCTION

Knowledge, power, control, certainty, identity—all this and more. Names are labels, labels are names. They have scientific uses, social uses, and political uses. Without them, there is no communication.

Try to order a meal without using labels. "I am hungry," you say to the waiter. "Bring me nourishment." That could be anything from a bowl of oatmeal to a seven course banquet, so he will probably ask you to be more specific. "Well," you say, "I want some protein, some carbohydrates, and some vegetables." Now, we are getting somewhere. You have accurately described a meal, but you have not been precise. Serves you right if you get soy beans instead of steak. Your order was the equivalent of a functional definition of a meal. Functional definitions are the trendy alternative to labels in the world of disability. They have their place, but they are not enough because they are not precise. They will only get you soy beans.

Labels can be lifesavers. When one of our children (not the one with autism) was very young, she got hold of a can of charcoal firestarter fluid and helped herself to a drink. When realized what had happened, I grabbed her and the can and rushed to the phone to call the Poison Control Center. Because I had the label right there in front of me, and because the label was precise as to the ingredients, I was able to tell the person at the Center exactly what my daughter had ingested. And because I could do that, the person on the other end could tell me exactly what to do to help her. If we had been working with functional definitions (i.e., "it's the stuff we use to start charcoal fires"), we might have had to guess at what to do, and my daughter might have died before we got to the right guess.

Deceptive labels can be killers. A few years ago, yellow bottles with a lemon on the labels were distributed to homes in my city as a promotion scheme for a new, lemon-scented liquid detergent. The bottle was shaped like a typical detergent bottle, and the label did state that the stuff inside was for washing dishes. Unfortunately, the 2- and 3-year-olds in my town can't read; however, they can all recognize a lemon. Many thought the liquid inside was lemonade, so they drank it. They all got very sick; two of them died.

There's a lesson there. The more a thing resembles something else, the more important it is to label it precisely. Children with autism do resemble children with mental retardation in

MARY AKERLEY • 10609 Glenwild Road, Silver Spring, Maryland 20901.

many ways; they also resemble children who are deaf and children with aphasia. However, if we put the wrong diagnostic label on any of these children, we are going to hurt them. I think that is terribly important, and so do the mothers of the children who drank the lemon detergent.

There are, I admit, dangers—not in the labels themselves, but in the way they are used. We can become too dependent on them, so that they become a substitute for common sense or a way of avoiding doing a hard, sometimes unpleasant, job. There is more to my poisoned daughter story, and it illustrates the point. When I called the Center I was calm and collected. I gave my name, my daughter's age and weight (which I knew could be significant), said she had ingested charcoal firestarter, and read off the active ingredients. I expected an immediate response as to what I should do (the information is on a computer). Instead, I heard, "What is the child's name?" What difference could that possibly make? Surely there is not one antedote for Johns and a different one for Alices!

Wisely, I didn't argue. The bureaucracy moves at its own pace, and refusal to conform simply slows it down, so I answered, "Kathleen." "With a 'C' or a 'K'?" That is label madness. There are times when my daughter's name *is* important; there are even times when the spelling is important, but not when she may be dying. We will need to get it right on the death certificate, but first—please—let's try to save her.

But rightly used, labels are useful, necessary even. They are tools and, like any tool, they must be used for a proper purpose. I can use my hammer to make myself a table or to make myself a widow. If I choose to do the latter it is not the hammer's fault. Assuming the goal is a proper one, the right tool will be the one that gets the user to her goal by the most appropriate means. The label given to a child's disability will—or should—dictate what kinds of help the child gets. Assuming all the necessary services are in place, the right label will get the child to the right program.

And that's what this chapter is all about. Mostly it's about why we need labels in the first place, but with a few directions on how—and how not—to use them. The thesis is a simple one: labeling is not being promoted by this writer as an end in itself; rather, it is offered as a tool, useful only if used as a means to help children with disabilities, their families, and the professionals who work with them.

THE PARENTS' ANSWER (IT'S NOT YOU)

I am here, on these pages, because I am the mother of a son with autism. I would like to tell you how long it took me to find out what was wrong with him. I was not an inexperienced mother when he was born. I have four children; he is the youngest. So I knew something about how babies are supposed to develop. Even before we took him home from the hospital, I knew there was something very different about this child—I didn't know if it was bad or good, but it certainly wasn't like anything I had seen in my other three.

As time went on, it became more apparent that there were developmental problems with this child, and I could not get help. My pediatrician said, "Now, now,—now, now. The other three are very bright; you've finally got a normal one—you don't know what to do with him."

When Ed was 1 year old, the pediatrician died. (I don't really think God was punishing him—he probably would have died anyway.) So we had to find a new pediatrician. This fellow didn't know anything about my style of mothering or about my children's develop-ment. All he could see was that I had this physically beautiful child, absolutely perfect, and I was complaining. He treated me like the psycho he thought he had on his hands. Matters went on in this fashion until Ed had his third birthday and we went for his annual checkup. After the examination, I said to the doctor, "Look, I'm not leaving your office until I get some help. There are other mothers waiting to see you, and they are going to wait a long, long time, because I will sit here until you tell me what to do. If I am wrong, we have only wasted some time; if I am right, we have wasted three years of this child's life."

That convinced him, and then he did a wonderful thing for which I forgave him for everything he had not done in the past: He did not send me to a psychiatrist. He sent me to a neurologist. And that is exactly the right place to start, if you suspect your child has autism. Help from other disciplines can be added as the child develops enough to take advantage of them.

For example, there is no way Ed could have taken advantage of a psychiatrist at that stage in his life. He was totally passive. I didn't even need a playpen; I could put him down, and he would stay put until I moved him.

Happy as I was with this initial referral, life was still not wonderful. The neurologist did as much of an assessment as she could with a subject who wouldn't cooperate. She even had a child psychologist participate in the workup. Then we went back to get the results. After 3 years of world-class anxiety, my husband and I were finally going to find out what was wrong and what to do.

We heard these words; "I've never seen a child like this. I can't tell you what's wrong with him." All the way home, I cried. It seemed it was all up to us. We would have to figure out what to do because no one else knew. "They"—the omniscient, omnipotent authorities—didn't even know what was wrong.

"They," all of "them," did agree that we needed help. That was hardly news. The neurologist did recommend several child therapists; I selected the one closest to our home. My practical basis for the choice proved fortuitous. The therapist was developmentally, not analytically, oriented, and we got a lot done. She even got Ed admitted to an excellent therapeutic nursery school, still without benefit of any diagnosis.

I diagnosed him, from a front-page article in the *Washington Post.* The National Society for Autistic Adults and Children was holding its annual conference in town, and the *Post,* in its news article reporting the event, provided a description of the syndrome. In it I recognized my son.

Dear Reader, if you still disapprove of labels, please reread the last paragraph. The point is, sooner or later, the kid will get the label. Certainly in our case—and I believe in most others'—sooner is better. Had we been told at the beginning that Ed had autism, we would have been sad, terribly so, but we would have been a giant step ahead of sad and frightened.

Imagine yourself in a similar situation. You have a terrible headache, Excedrin 10, so you go to the medicine cabinet and take a double dose of your favorite remedy. Your headache gets better, but just for awhile. Eventually, you decide to see your doctor, who prescribes a drug that, again, works but only temporarily. You go back to the doctor; this time, the doctor runs some tests and tells you the blood vessels on the right side of your head are constricted. You have been given the equivalent of a developmental diagnosis for your child, and it is not enough.

You want to know why those vessels are constricted. Is it a tumor or merely tension? And until you know the why of your headaches, you are going to be a very nervous, frightened, and unhappy person.

Parents of disabled kids also need to know the "why." I don't mean the ultimate, philosophical "why." That is a question for later, perhaps much later. I mean the "why" from the professional's perspective, so that the parent has at least some assurance that the professional can do something to help that child.

Remember, whether we are talking about the headache patient or the parent of a disabled child, we are talking about someone who is frightened. Something awful, truly awful, has happened to that person and, until a measure of control is introduced into the situation, the fear will not go away. The parent is certainly in no position to introduce the control. Unless the parent is, by chance, a pediatrician or psychologist, he or she lacks the requisite knowledge to do so; indeed, the parent is as helpless a victim as the child.

One of the worst fears people have is the fear of the unknown. And, of course, what the parent is dealing with here is an unknown. Not just in this one child, but in the whole family. By the time the parents of a disabled child realize that the home remedies in the medicine cabinet are not working and present themselves for professional help, the entire family has been affected. The other children are very likely angry, sad, resentful and, most assuredly, just as frightened as their parents. No doubt there has also been some finger pointing between Mom and Dad: "It's *your* fault—you've spoiled him!" "*My* fault? You're the one with the funny aunt!"

This cycle of misery is self-perpetuating. It will spin and grow until some detached observer from outside (read: professional) steps in and says "This is what's the matter."

It is important to recognize that, until the child is diagnosed, the parent has another fear: perhaps the child's problem really is his or her fault. I don't mean to suggest here that the parent has read and believed the psychobabble of Freud and Bettleheim; I am discussing what the parent's own common sense will suggest. The parent knows the child will behave as he has been taught, and the parent also knows he (the parent) was the teacher. This child behaves very badly in public (perhaps, like my son, he pitches lemons across the front of the grocery store; perhaps he is content with the ordinary, anti-social indicia of autism such as hand flapping or tantrumming). It therefore follows that the parent (usually mother) has been a bad teacher and thus a bad parent.

Society is all too quick to confirm this misdiagnosis. Ask any parent who has "gone public" with a mentally disabled child, especially one who looks normal, as most children with autism do. That parent has received lots of social feedback in the form of dirty looks, stage whispers about shockingly spoiled children, and sometimes even direct advice ("A good, sharp smack on the bottom is all that child needs!"). All this is devastating to the parent's self-esteem, making her even less able to cope with the basic problem.

It certainly does not help matters that the "bad" behaviors associated with autism are, at least to the uninformed, apparently so easily controllable. The average member of the public cannot really be expected to understand why a mother would permit her child to bang his head on the shoe store floor or why she would not punish him for emptying her purse into the shopping cart.

Once the parent gets professional help, she can distance herself from this social opprobrium but, until she gets it, she cannot. She and her child are a set, a nameless anomaly that is spoiling its community, and it is all her fault. If the child had cerebral palsy or some other visible impairment, the situation would be entirely different. Instead of criticism, the parent would be offered help and perceived with sympathy and even admiration. With undiagnosed autism, the parents must walk alone, with weights on both feet.

Primitive man had the right idea. When he had to deal with something he did not understand, something that frightened him, the first thing he did was to give the thing a name. By doing so, he took the first step in gaining control. The thunder was not so terrifying once it was given the form of a man with the rather silly name of Thor. And recall the Bible story of the Garden of Eden. God gave man dominion over the animals by permitting Adam to name each species.

Parents, too, need to know the name of this thing they fear, this thing that is tormenting their child. You professionals must tell them that. Once you do, no matter how bad the diagnosis, there will be forward progress. The parents may go into a terrible funk, but they will come out of it. They will come out of it because now they can trust you and can believe you have the power to help their child. You knew what was wrong and you were not afraid, for whatever reason (good or bad), to tell them. If you know what ''it'' is, you also know what to do and you will tell them that as well. It will still be a long, hard walk, but you will have taken the weights off their feet.

If you still doubt the wisdom of giving the parents a label for their child's disability, try to understand why. Is it that labels are so final? They need not be. They can be offered differentially, as a place to start, as they often are in a physical medicine. At least you will be getting started. Is it that labels are pejorative and stigmatizing? No, they are neutral. Stigma, like beauty, is in the eye of the beholder. And, since the beholders have already stigmatized this family, the label will not do further harm. Is it that you fear the family is not strong enough to bear the bad news? Then they are certainly not strong enough to continue to bear uncertainty and fear, and the weights on their feet will make them weaker, not stronger. Or, is it that you believe it is best that you retain control of the situation? Surely not, or you would not be reading this book.

Developmental assessment will not do the trick; you cannot offer it as a substitute for a straightforward, honest label. Let me show you why. The mother takes her strangely behaving large-for-his-age 5-year-old to the diagnostician. After many tests, the good doctor offers the following: little Andy has a cognitive age of 12 months, communicates at a 4-month level, and has a social age of 2 months. The mother already knew that or she wouldn't be there. What she wants to know is *why*. To tell her that, you must give her the label. Then you—and she—will be on your way. You both can begin to deal with it.

You will have to give her a lot of help in dealing with it. You will probably even have to explain that there is no pill for what is wrong. But at least tell her, because the need to know what is going on in her child will not go away until you do.

The label also helps the parent understand that it is not the parent's fault, that ''it'' is something external that happened. The parent can deal with that. The label gives the parent something objective on which to focus, something that, at least potentially, can be managed.

There is a caveat. Labels can be effective and helpful only if it is the disability that is labeled and not the child. The child is not a jar of pickles or a bottle of lemon detergent; he is a human being who has something that makes it hard for him to learn. That ''thing'' is what you are labeling. Thus, he has autism, but he is not autistic.

And there are dangers. Certain labels, autism among them, are heard as a death sentence, a condemnation to a life of hopeless uselessness and dependence. When that happens, the professional must explain, perhaps over and over again, what can be done—what has been done—to educate and habilitate such children. Another danger is that the label may engender inflexibility. ''This child has autism. Therefore we must do certain things and we may not do certain other things.'' Clearly, this is nonsense, born of overdependence on the label. Children, all children, even those with disabilities, are developmental creatures, and not all of them develop in exactly the same way. The label is only a starting point; the real guide to the next step is the child himself. Every disabled child is entitled to the same type of creative assessment and programming as is routinely done for a gifted youngster, nothing less.

Finally, be warned. There is abroad in the world a certain perverse type of label snobbery. It is most often seen in parents, but there is no reason to think professionals are immune. In any event, parents with this syndrome need help. Autism may be regarded by some as classier, or at least more acceptable, than mental retardation. Bring them down, but do it gently. And remember, there is no hurry; this is a harmless fault, and it may have some consolation value.

Far worse is its mirror image: the perception that autism is something to be ashamed of. Parents will only feel this way if they have been told, somewhere along the way, that their child's condition is their fault. By now, everyone active in the field knows the obvious effects: the parents feel guilty and/or angry and resentful, and thus require almost as much therapeutic intervention as their child. There are other, less obvious, spillovers. One homely but heartbreaking example will suffice.

I know a young man with autism who, as a young child, subscribed to the belief that everything in the world, even windowsills, was edible. As a result, he and his parents made many trips to the local emergency room. I listened to his mother's stories of these events with great sympathy and with more than a little gratitude that I had been spared this particular misery. Then one day, it was my turn. Ed fell down and cut his ear, a nasty deep gash that required stitches. When we got to the hospital, the emergency room physician attempted to impose the usual protocol: I would remain in the waiting room while Ed was treated. Realizing argument would be futile, I took a different tack (here follows a creative use of the label). In my best I'm-only-thinking-of-you voice, I said, "Doctor, I realize you're busy and haven't had time to read the admitting papers. My son has autism and I really must stay with him." The good doctor wasn't buying it for one minute, so I took the next step. "If you refuse to let me come with him, I cannot be responsible for any damage he may do once he is out of my care." It worked. (I should add here that Ed was never destructive; however, I suspected the doctor would make a negative generalization based on the label "autism," and I was not above taking advantage of his error.)

The next day, I called the mother of the omniverous boy because I thought she would enjoy the story and also because she had expressed her own displeasure with the hospital's policy of separating the injured child from his parents. Now that I knew the secret of how to get through the gauze curtain, I wanted to share it with her. When I finished my narrative, she said, "Oh, Mary, I could never do that." I asked why not. "Because if I said Mark was autistic, they would think I did it. I just say he's retarded."

THE CHILD'S RELIEF (IT'S NOT ME)

Some thought should also be given to labeling from the child's perspective. Some years ago, in connection with the drafting and passage of the federal Education for All Handicapped Children Act, a gentleman by the name of Nicholas Hobbs did a study called "Issues in the Classification of Children." It was about labeling. Unfortunately, not all the people who should have read it did so (it was very thick); but that did not deter them from asserting that Dr. Hobbs unequivocally concluded that labels were bad. He did no such thing; rather, he said many of the things that I have said here, only much more elegantly.

One of the chapters in Hobbs's book is called "Perspectives of the Labeled Child." In it, Hobbs makes a telling observation: labels that describe obvious, visible handicaps (e.g., cerebral palsy, spina bifida) do not carry with them a negative social connotation in the way that labels describing cognitive, social, or emotional handicaps do. The latter are usually pejorative; the former rarely are.

There is no rational reason for this distinction. Both types of labels describe conditions that can be equally devastating developmentally. Why, then, is it an insult to be called retarded, but not to be called crippled? Hobbs suggests that the problem lies not in the label itself, but in the environment, the context in which the label is used. Consider the label "genius," one to which few of us would object. Now imagine someone with that label. He has an IQ of 180, and his hobby is reading obscure historical tomes. His family think he is wonderful, and of course they are right.

But suppose, for reasons we need not trouble ourselves with here, our genius must attend a high school entirely populated by jocks. Everyone except our hero is playing football or leading cheers while he reads his Bulwer Lytton. He is going to be labeled a genius in a pejorative sense. The label has not changed, nor has he. But his environment has. He is now in an environment with different values; now what is different about him is bad rather than good, whereas in his former environment his distinction was a positive one.

So it is not the label that stigmatizes; it is an environment unprepared to accept that which is different. The answer then is not to forgo labels, but rather to change environments. The task is to teach people to regard cognitive and social handicaps no differently from the way they look on purely physical disabilities.

Disabled children have the same needs as their parents. They know there is something wrong with them, and they want to know what it is. I speak from experience. When my son learned the word "autism," he was happy. He had seen the word many times due to our involvement with the National Society for Autistic Adults and Children. When he finally managed to sound it out, something seemed to click. He knew this word related to him. Clearly, his understanding of the concept of autism was, and still is, imperfect; but then so is Eric Schopler's, as good as he is.

Learning the word helped Ed understand himself. Before he had his own label, there had been many times that he had asked me what was wrong with him. His questions seemed to be directed to why he didn't function like other people, especially his siblings. Once he even said to me, "Mommy, I'm broken. Fix me." Those are the words of a child who is aware of his difference and wants help. If I had said to him, "I don't know what's wrong with you," or, even worse, "There's nothing wrong with you," I would have condemned him to that place where I was stuck years before.

When children are told the name of their disability, the limitations inherent in it can also be explained to them. These children will not hate themselves. They will understand, when they cannot make friends easily or cannot learn to read as fast as their peers, that it is not their fault. Rather, it is part of the limitation that they must learn to live with.

If a parent of a child with diabetes refused to explain the disorder to the child, we would be very critical of that parent. Yet I have been severely criticized for discussing Ed's autism with him on the grounds that this candidness would make him feel bad about himself, less human somehow. I believe the reverse is true. I am sharing with Ed my ability, limited as it may be, to control what's wrong with him and to "fix" it as he asked me to, if such be possible. I am also taking the weights off *his* feet.

Before I wrote these words, I asked Ed if he thought it was better to know what was wrong with him than not to know. He was emphatic in saying that it was better to know what he had; he even volunteered, "Then people can help me better."

THE PROFESSIONAL'S TOOL (NOW I CAN GET STARTED)

Last, but certainly not least, there is the perspective of those helpers—the doctors, teachers, psychologists, and therapists who "fix" our broken children. What is the value of labels for them? Suppose that on the first day of school a teacher still does not know what grade or subject she is going to teach. How can she possibly prepare? Special education teachers need advance notice, too. It is only minimally helpful to be told one is going to have a class of children with speech disorders. One still needs to know the "why" of the disorder in order to select the correct intervention. The methods effective for children who are silent because they are deaf are not necessarily the methods of choice for children with aphasia or autism or emotional handicaps.

So professionals need labels, too, at least as guideposts to get them started. Without that much, they will have to rely on trial and error, and our kids don't have time for that. They need help yesterday.

With the advent of mainstreaming, the problem has reached the regular classroom teacher as well. By the time Ed got to senior high school, he was virtually completely mainstreamed. My husband and I went to "Back to School Night" that year with pride that he had come so far along, but with some trepidation too. We were more than a little concerned about how well he was getting along, academically and socially.

The first class was math—"slow" math, to be sure, but real math nonetheless. When we introduced ourselves to the teacher, his pleasure—relief might be a better term—at seeing us there was more of a red flag than a warm welcome. Before he had finished shaking hands with us, he hissed in our ears, "I've got to talk to you!" To appreciate the significance of his behavior, one needs to know the "Back to School Night" ground rules. Any substantive discussion of individual students is strictly prohibited. The purpose of the evening is to acquaint parents with the teachers and the curriculum. The full day's program is presented in brief, and there is simply no time to focus on individual problems. However, Mr. Math was the teacher, so we stayed after class to talk.

He was clearly bamboozled by Ed. "I just don't understand it," he began. "Your son is obviously smart, and this is not hard math. But he is not understanding it, and I don't know why." I was pretty sure I did, and it turned out I was right. No one had ever told this poor fellow what Ed's disability was, yet he was expected to teach him effectively, knowing only that he was a special education student. We gave him a 10-minute crash course in autism and sent him some literature. Apparently that was enough, or perhaps he did some further research on his own. In any event, both he and Ed made it through the course successfully. (Ed got a "B.")

I suppose this is real mainstreaming. Throw the handicapped child into the fast flowing water just as so-called normal youngsters are tossed in. Never mind that the teacher is being thrown into the deep end right along with the students. Unfortunately, the result—easily predictable—is that both will drown.

There is a down side of labeling for professionals. The more precise the label, the harder their job will be. Perhaps all the speech-impaired 9-year-olds in the universe will fit (theoretically) into a single homogeneous class but, once they are separated according to the "why" of the impairment (i.e., once they are labeled), and further divided according to developmental level (also more precise once the "why" is identified), they must have individually designed programs. No more convenient lumping together.

There are some simple rules for using labels. The first is one that doctors already know: Do no harm. The second is: Use labels only for a good purpose. This may sometimes entail using the wrong label. Under the ''labels are tools'' theory, this is fine so long as it gets the child where he needs to go. If the objective is appropriate, the label need not be.

At a very tender age, Ed showed us he understood this principle. I have always believed that humorous sarcasm was a more effective behavior modifier than direct criticism or physical punishment, and I made no exception for Ed. When he failed to control his digestive functions and burped (or worse) audibly, I would say ''Charming!'' He knew full well I was not suggesting he do it again.

One lovely Easter morning, we all went out to brunch after church. The restaurant was crowded. Midway through the meal, the happy chatter of the diners was interrupted by a prolonged crash—a busboy had dropped a full tray of dirty dishes. In the palpable silence that ensued, Ed said, very loudly, ''Charming!'' Clearly what the busboy did was not charming, but who would ever say that was not an appropriate use of an inappropriate label?

So, when the perfect program for a child you know is labeled ''TMR,'' forget that yesterday the child had autism. Today the child has moderate mental retardation and will fit right in. Situational ethics is a valuable survival skill.

Finally, never use a label to dehumanize. When we say ''autistic children'' or ''this child is autistic,'' we are equating the child with the disability, and that is dehumanizing. The child is one who has autism, and that is how the child should be described. Admittedly, the preferred phrasing is awkward to use. It takes longer to say and is much less convenient than the shorthand to which we are accustomed. But I submit to you, it is very awkward to have autism, very inconvenient to have mental retardation. The very least we helpers can do is take a bit of that inconvenience upon ourselves.

II

Diagnostic Issues

6

Classification and Diagnosis of Childhood Autism

FRED R. VOLKMAR and DONALD J. COHEN

INTRODUCTION

The Range of Syndrome Expression: Seeing the Forest for the Trees

Kanner's (1943) description of the autistic syndrome stands as a classic example of the contribution of an individual clinician investigator to psychiatric taxonomy. Despite subsequent modifications, this description has proven remarkably enduring; it stands as a benchmark against which all subsequent attempts to refine the diagnostic concept must be measured. Kanner's description also suggested false leads for research (e.g., parental psychopathology) and colors current conceptions of this disorder almost irrevocably. How might we view these disorders today if Kanner had never published his initial case reports?

The challenge of this thought experiment suggests both the scope of Kanner's vision and the difficulties investigators continue to face. Assume that an interdisciplinary group of investigators, well acquainted with current methods of assessment and diagnosis but unacquainted with the concept of infantile autism, were presented with a sizeable sample of individuals who reflected, in the broadest possible sense, the range of individuals now termed autistic. Assume, in addition, that our hypothetical colleagues were told that this group of individuals exhibited one or more disorders and that their task was to determine the best system for classification.

Probably the most striking initial impression would be of tremendous sample variability. The sample would include some infants and some old men, some eccentric piano tuners with IQs of 110 and some profoundly retarded institutionalized individuals. Some gentle wraithlike 7-year-old might be observed as would be some screeching adolescent who banged his head to the point of skull fracture. A few individuals with idiosyncratic interests in train or bus schedules would be represented as would be many individuals who appeared unable or unwilling to communicate. Our hypothetical team of investigators would probably initially make some simple demographic observations. They would most probably observe a prepon-

FRED R. VOLKMAR and DONALD J. COHEN • Child Study Center, Yale University, New Haven, Connecticut 06510-8009.

derance of boys to girls, some evidence of various medical/neurologic findings and conditions in certain individuals, and an occasional child with an inborn error of metabolism, rubella, or enlarged ventricles on computed tomographic (CT) brain scan, or with nonspecific electroencephalographic (EEG) abnormality. A wide range of performance on standard psychometric tests and difficulties with cognition, communication, relatedness, motility, and perception would be noted. Age differences would be a source of concern. Assessments using behavior checklists and structured interviews would probably demonstrate a vast array of problems, including fears and phobias, poor attention, isolation, aggression, lack of appropriate self-care skills, and immaturity. Biochemical abnormalities (e.g., high peripheral serotonin levels) would be exhibited by some cases, but no single biochemical marker would be observed. In their deliberations, the research team would be forced to grapple with the problems posed by developmental change, intellectual level, differential treatments, associated medical conditions, and the range of outcomes. They would debate all the aspects of "the syndrome" which, at various points in time, have been assumed to be in some sense primary. Probably various statistical approaches (e.g., cluster analysis, correlations) would be employed to examine alternative diagnostic schemes. In the end, however, it is not at all clear that our hypothetical group of investigators would be able to derive a single unitary diagnostic concept encompassing their entire sample. The most skeptical members of the team would probably decide to study a simpler question, arguing that the "trees" comprising this particular sample were too heterogeneous to provide an ecologically valid "forest."

Fortunately, Kanner did publish his initial observations. Our hypothetical situation illustrates both the significance of his capacity to see a thread connecting his cases as well as the tremendous problems posed by the marked heterogeneity of subjects now generally believed to fall under the umbrella of "autism" erected by Kanner. An appreciation of these problems may help clarify the long and controversial history of the concepts surrounding autism and the complications posed for classification schemes.

Historical Background

Kanner was neither the first nor the last investigator to attempt to identify meaningful diagnostic categories among severely impaired children. The interest in childhood, inspired by Locke and Rousseau, led in the nineteenth century to systematic observation of children and a general interest in the role of experience, maturation, and biologic endowment in child development, e.g., early reports of feral children, such as the "wild boy" (Itard, 1801, cited in Lane, 1977). In the mid-1800s Maudsley suggested that children could exhibit "insanity." Most importantly, Kraeplin's description of the syndrome of dementia praecox, or what is now termed schizophrenia, and his organic approach to classification stimulated tremendous interest in the importance of diagnosis and classification in psychiatry. Kraeplin's concept was rapidly extended to children by DeSanctis (1906) and other investigators. At the same time, attempts by educators and psychologists such as Binet helped systematize conceptions of mental subnormality.

Before Kanner's report and for many years subsequently, many clinicians and investigators assumed, largely on the basis of severity, a fundamental continuity between severe psychotic illness in adults (e.g., schizophrenia) and severe psychiatric disturbances in childhood. Despite the attempts of Potter (1933) and others, the term *childhood schizophrenia* became synonymous with childhood psychosis.

Kanner's initial cases did not, in his opinion, fit existing notions of schizophrenia. His cases exhibited disturbances in the first years of life that were characterized by marked disturbances in social relatedness, communication, and unusual environmental responsivity rather than the florid thought disorder and hallucinations typical of adult schizophrenics. Subsequently, various diagnostic concepts, such as autistic psychopathy (Asperger, 1944), atypical personality development (Rank, 1949, 1955), disintegrative psychosis (Evans-Jones & Rosenblum, 1978), and symbiotic psychosis (Mahler, 1952), were also proposed for severe childhood psychiatric disturbance. Controversy regarding the validity and boundaries of these disorders predominated the clinical and research literature for many years. Was Kanner's syndrome merely an early variant of schizophrenia? Were neurobiologic or experiential factors more important for pathogenesis? In what ways were "psychotic" conditions in childhood continuous with the psychoses of adult life? How were the social disabilities of autism to be understood? Research findings of the past four decades have contributed to the resolution of some of these issues.

Kanner's phenomenologic description of infantile autism proved, in general, to be remarkably accurate; yet, as Kanner himself speculated, subsequent research, particularly from longitidunal studies, suggested need for some modification. It became apparent that autism could be observed in association with other conditions, e.g., congenital rubella (Chess, Fernandez & Korn, 1974), was often associated with gross evidence of CNS damage such as seizures (Rutter, 1972), and was typically associated with mental retardation (DeMyer, Hingtgen & Jackson, 1981). Furthermore, the preponderance of available evidence clearly came to support the notion of an underlying organic pathologic process so that it became more reasonable to believe that the child, rather than the parent, was disordered (DeMyer *et al.*, 1981). Various lines of evidence supported the validity of Kanner's concept; children with Kanner's syndrome could be differentiated reliably from children with other disorders on the basis of various features (Rutter & Garmezy, 1983; Dahl, Cohen & Provence, 1986). This chapter summarizes current areas of consensus and controversy in regard to the clinical phenomenology of the disorder. Both alternative diagnostic approaches and existing classification schemes are considered.

CLASSIFICATION

Uses and Purposes of Classification

The ability, and urge, to classify is fundamental. Classifications enable us to make use of information for purposes of explanation, prediction, and communication. The assignment of a label to a phenomenon or set of phenomena provides all of us with a sense of comfort in a changing and unpredictable world. The classification of children and adults with what we now term autism or the "pervasive developmental disorders" has, historically, been the subject of much controversy for various reasons (reviewed by Cohen, Volkmar & Paul, 1986*b*). Classification schemes vary in orientation and purpose and can take several forms (Werry, 1985).

The medical model of classification is oriented around categorical diagnoses, e.g., appendicitis. This approach rests on a substantial historical tradition and assumes the existence of discrete disease entities usually on an organic basis. Commonalities among all cases assigned a given diagnostic label are presumed to outweigh individual differences and provide important implications for prevention, treatment, prognosis, and so forth. This approach need not be theoretically based, e.g., Kanner's syndrome; when based on theory the theory need not be correct, e.g., Down's syndrome.

An alternative approach to classification relies on the assessment of dimensions of function or dysfunction. This approach, more common in nonmedical settings, reduces phenomena to one or more dimensions along which any child can be placed, e.g., short stature or retardation. Common examples of such approaches are exemplified by the use of continuous variables (e.g., weight or hemoglobin), rating scales, or checklists and the use of standardized developmental or intellectual tests and the IQ score. This approach is not incompatible with the medical one, since dimensions can be further reduced to discrete categories, e.g., levels of mental retardation.

The developmental approach to classification considers children in the light of the unfolding of developmental processes (e.g., such as coping skills or capacities for language) and in comparison with others of the same age. This approach is common in dealing with developmental phenomena and, in its most basic sense, focuses on embryologic aspects of development and relates phenotypic expression to underlying processes of gene expression in interaction with the environment.

Finally, the idiographic approach rejects simple labels and focuses on the totality of the individual and the context of his or her problems in "formulating a case" and prescribing a course of treatment. Practically, this approach is the one most commonly used by clinicians in planning and monitoring treatment.

Classification schemes act to synthesize information and facilitate communication in a concise and, hopefully, valid and reliable fashion. Like other human constructions, classification schemes can be abused or ill-used but can also serve an important function (Hobbs, 1975; Rutter & Shaffer, 1980). To further complicate issues of diagnosis and classification, labels assigned can be used for purposes other than those for which they were originally intended. Accordingly, legal, financial, or educational implications of a diagnosis may be important, if sometimes unintended, aspects of the diagnostic process, e.g., when regulations and laws mandate special services for specific diagnostic groups (Schopler, 1983). Advances in nomenclature and classification may take many years before being disseminated into common usage, and the multiplicity of classification schemes can be a source of confusion to parents and professionals alike.

The diagnostic process in child psychiatry (Cohen, 1976) is complicated by these issues as well as those unique to the child. Developmental changes and intellectual level may obscure or illuminate aspects of classification. In the Diagnostic and Statistical Manual (3rd edition) of the American Psychiatric Association DSM-III (APA, 1980), for example, severe or profoundly retarded children cannot, by definition, exhibit attention deficit disorder. This does not mean that such individuals never exhibit severe attentional problems, rather this distinction attempts to achieve greater validity and reliability in diagnosis. Ultimately the usefulness of any classification scheme can be confirmed only be extensive empirical research and demonstrable clinical utility (Rutter, 1978a).

Earlier Diagnostic Systems

Prior to DSM-III, various attempts were made to differentiate autistic and other "psychotic" conditions. Eisenberg and Kanner (1956) emphasized two essential features needed for the diagnosis of autism: extreme aloneness and preoccupation with the preservation of sameness. Other groups, e.g., the British Working Party (Creak, 1961) and the Group for Advancement of Psychiatry (1966), attempted to differentiate autism as well as place it within a broader classification scheme. Only as evidence accumulated regarding the validity and distinctiveness of autism was it included in official diagnostic schemes. Rutter (1978b) provided an important synthesis of Kanner's original description and subsequent research; his description emphasized onset before 30 months and the prominence of social impairments, language deviance, and stereotypy. The National Society for Autistic Children's definition (1978) noted the early onset and social and communicative abnormalities but also included disturbances in rates and/or sequences of development and unusual responses to sensory stimuli. Of these various definitions, that of Rutter (1978b) proved most influential, probably because, like Kanner's original (1943) description, it most closely paralleled clinical experience.

The DSM-III Diagnostic System

Autism was accorded official diagnostic status in DSM-III (APA, 1980), which represents the most recent comprehensive approach to diagnosis of autism and related disorders. In DSM-III, an atheoretical phenomenologic approach that employs explicit, operational diagnostic criteria (Spitzer, Endicott & Robins, 1978) was adopted. It provided for multiaxial classification (Rutter et al., 1975); i.e., it was possible to use different axes to specify associated medical problems, psychosocial stressors, and levels of adaptive functioning as well as psychiatric or developmental diagnosis. In DSM-III, autism is grouped under the broad class of pervasive developmental disorder. Disorders in this general class include infantile autism (IA), childhood-onset pervasive developmental disorder (COPDD), and atypical pervasive developmental disorder (atypical PDD) as well as "residual" IA or COPDD (e.g., once was, but no longer is, autistic as strictly defined). COPDD is a disorder first described in DSM-III without a substantial research foundation. This term is proposed to account for those rare children in whom a severe developmental disorder develops later in childhood, but the criteria proposed for this disorder seem to imply less severe autism (Volkmar, Stier & Cohen, 1985b). Atypical PDD is proposed in the sense of related to the paradigm disorder but "otherwise unclassified," and not in the sense of Rank's (1949) earlier use of the concept of atypical development. All the PDDs are characterized by distortions of multiple psychological functions involving social and linguistic development. Childhood schizophrenia is no longer included as a separate diagnostic category (Cantor, Evans & Pezzot-Pearce, 1982) and individuals with hallucinations, delusions, and so forth, are specifically excluded from the PDD diagnoses reflecting the substantial agreement that autism and schizophrenia are not related (Makita, 1966; Kolvin, 1971; Rutter, 1972).

Several aspects of the DSM-III scheme have proved problematic (Cohen et al., 1986b) (see Chapter 2). Briefly, issues arise in respect to multiaxial placement and diagnosis (Rutter & Schaffer, 1980), diagnostic concepts proposed (Volkmar et al., 1985b), and specification of explicit diagnostic criteria (Volkmar, Cohen & Paul, 1986). Practically criteria may be difficult to apply meaningfully particularly to older or higher functioning autistic individuals (Cohen et al., 1986b). However, on the whole, DSM-III appears to have done a service. It has again focused attention on fundamental features of the phenomenology of these disorders and has suggested studies to futher clarify the nature of the spectrum of pervasive or autistic disorders.

Issues in Classification of Autism and Related Disorders

"Core" Characteristics: What Is Primary?

The attempt, as in DSM-III, to adopt explicit operational criteria for autism immediately raises the question of what features are truly "core" aspects of the disorder. Diagnostic criteria are, in fact, complex syntheses of individual features or symptoms of the disorder; the practical delineation and application of such criteria can prove problematic (Helzer & Coryell, 1983). In its approach to diagnostic criteria for autism, DSM III was heavily influenced by Rutter's (1978b) synthesis of Kanner's description as modified by subsequent experience. DSM-III emphasizes early onset, pervasive social unresponsiveness, language deficits and deviance, and bizarre responses to the environment. Since the intent of DSM-III was to be phenomenologic, atheoretical, and as parsimonious as possible, other aspects of the syndrome or speculations regarding etiology were not included, e.g., perceptual inconstancy (Ornitz & Ritvo, 1968) or disturbances in developmental rates or sequences (NSAC, 1978). Since many different behaviors are exhibited by the range of autistic individuals over the course of development and since many of these behaviors are also exhibited by nonautistic children, the task of arriving at final diagnostic criteria is most complicated.

Another approach has focused on the attempt to statistically determine which symptoms most robustly discriminate autistic and nonautistic youngsters. Using data from the Rimland checklist, Prior, Perry, and Gajzago (1975) found that only three specific behaviors (the desire for sameness, islets of special ability, and skill in manipulation of small objects) discriminated autistic and nonautistic psychotic children. Similarly, Freeman, Schroth, Ritvo, Guthrie, and Wake (1980) conducted a careful study of 67 behaviors in autistic, retarded, and control subjects matched for mental and chronological age and found substantial symptom overlap between groups. The considerable overlap and variability in symptom expression prove problematic in attempts to develop criteria which differentiate diagnostic groups on the basis of exclusive, necessary, and sufficient findings.

It is important to note that criteria included in any diagnostic system need not necessarily be "primary" in an etiologic sense; i.e., they may be primary aspects of syndrome definition but be unrelated to underlying pathophysiologic mechanisms. A skin rash of a particular progress, distribution, and color may define a childhood exanthem unequivocally yet be different from the viral pathogenesis. In the past, investigators focused on one particular feature of the autistic syndrome, i.e., linguistic (Rutter et al., 1971), perceptual (Ornitz & Ritvo, 1968), cognitive (Prior, 1979), or social-affective (Kanner, 1943) as if these were isolated processes. However, communication, social development, and other cognitive skills emerge in an interdependent fashion over the course of the child's development. The search for a single, unitary, pathogenic explanation for autism is further complicated by the association of autism with various other conditions, as well as symptom variability within and between subjects. The final behavioral syndrome we term infantile autism may well be the final common expression of various and unrelated factors; i.e., it is possible that many different insults act through one or more mechansisms to produce the autistic syndrome. As Rutter and Garmezy (1983) have pointed out, it is best to recall that all aspects of the child's development are affected and it is misleading to consider any aspect of development apart from development as a whole.

Developmental Changes: The Age Factor

Changes in the syndrome with age further complicate the specification of diagnostic criteria (DeMyer *et al.*, 1981). The presence of an "age factor" is commonly observed in diagnostic and assessment instruments (Parks, 1983). Attempts to circumvent this problem, by inquiring about or scoring data only about the child's early development, have been employed in various rating scales and checklists. Age effects are noted, however, even when parents are asked to report only on the child's early development (Volkmar *et al.*, 1986*b*), suggesting the importance of a child's developmental change on later parental retrospections. Younger preschool autistic children may seem most profoundly unrelated and noncommunicative (Ornitz, Guthrie & Farley, 1977) but may develop selective, if deviant, attachments as they mature. Communication skills may develop. Similar changes are noted in the expression of stereotyped and other behaviors. Marked changes in adjustment during adolescence are not uncommon, though even the highest functioning child typically remains markedly deviant as an adult (Volkmar & Cohen, 1985). The changes in syndrome expression over development complicate application of diagnostic criteria. The DSM-III criteria, for example, are most applicable to younger and more impaired children (Volkmar *et al.*, 1986) while the provision of a "residual" autism category seems to imply that autistic children "grow out" of autism when, in fact, they almost always continue to have profound difficulties of a social-communicative nature. Practically autistic children become autistic adults and the elaboration of more developmentally appropriate criteria, encompassing the entire age range, is an important area for investigation.

PHENOMENOLOGIC ISSUES AND CLASSIFICATION

Developmental Level

Although Kanner (1943) framed his observation of social deviance within a developmental context, his additional impression that autistic individuals are not retarded proved incorrect. Early efforts to account for poor test performance by poor "testability" or lack of motivation proved incorrect. Although certain peak skills may be exhibited, IQ scores remain relatively stable over time and predict outcome. Probably 75% of autistic individuals function within the retarded range, with more than 50% having IQs less than 55 (Schopler, 1983). In retrospect, Kanner's original cases appear to have been somewhat higher functioning; while the range of IQ has been expanded it remains easiest to make the diagnosis in higher functioning individuals. Developmental level and IQ are strongly associated with the onset of seizure disorder (Rutter, 1972) and with the range of maladaptive behaviors exhibited (Schopler, Reichler, DeVellis & Daly, 1980; Freeman *et al.*, 1980).

The presence of increased frequency of "autistic-like" behaviors (e.g., social withdrawal, stereotypy) in children with subnormal IQs has been widely reported (e.g., Wing & Gould, 1979). This observation raises an important and as yet unanswered question regarding syndrome boundaries. From the point of diagnostic criteria, one goal might be to achieve syndrome homogenity by establishing explicit demarcation points regarding IQ, e.g., much like criteria for ADD in DSM-III. However, while this would increase the ease of definition, it is clear that many autistic children are cognitively very impaired (Schopler, 1983) and the exclusion of the mute, seizure disordered autistic child would be problematic both for service as well as research.

Wing and Gould (1979) in an epidemiologic study noted that severely retarded children commonly exhibited autistic features. The question of a possible increased incidence of autism in the severely retarded remains open. Data from our own center (Fig. 1), based on full-scale IQ scores obtained on a variety of tests, demonstrate a preponderance of lower IQ scores in the sample as a whole. This result differs somewhat from the IQ data reported from the TEAACH sample (Schopler, 1983). While questions of test selection, administration, and so forth, complicate the interpretation of these data, the available information clearly supports the need for criteria applicable to the entire IQ range. As a practical matter, the assessment of autistic individuals should, to the extent possible, include administration of various standardized, normative assessment instruments (Cohen, Paul & Volkmar, 1986a).

Social Dysfunction

Kanner (1943) regarded social deficits and deviance as a primary aspect of autism. While most diagnostic schemes do include such deviance for purposes of syndrome definition, subsequent investigators have tended to regard these deficits as secondary to cognitive or communicative ones (reviewed by Fein, Pennington, Markowitz, Braverman & Waterhouse, 1986). In part, this has reflected an awareness of the changes in relatedness over the course of development (Lotter, 1978) as well as an implicit "cognitive primacy hypothesis" (Cairns, 1979), i.e., that cognitions are primary determinants of social behaviors.

The capacity and predisposition to form social relationships can be traced to the first days of infancy; this capacity appears to be intimately related to communicative and cognitive

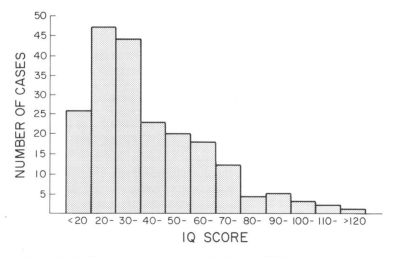

Fig. 1. IQ distribution for 203 autistic individuals, Child Study Center sample.

skills (reviewed by Volkmar, 1986). The course of social development in autism is strikingly different from the norm and differs, as well, from that observed in children reared in institutions, with Down's syndrome, and other problems. For example, the human face, normally the most interesting aspect of the infant's visual environment, holds little interest for the autistic infant; lack of eye contact, poor or absent attachments, and a general lack of social interest are typical (Ornitz *et al.*, 1977). These deficits stand in stark contrast to unusual sensitivities to other aspects of the environment and appear to make the autistic social dysfunction (Cohen *et al.*, 1986*b*) a primary aspect of definition of the disorder. As with other aspects of development, changes in the capacity to form social relations do occur in autism but are typically manifest, even in high-functioning adults, by difficulties with social interaction, pragmatic communication, and the understanding of implicit meanings and emotional nuances, etc. Autistic individuals do not seem to simply be incapable of encoding information regarding social transactions, rather the use of such information seems to be disordered (Rutter & Garmezy, 1983).

Compared with other aspects of development the social ones have been the target of remarkably little systematic study. Wing and Gould's (1979) epidemiologic study suggested that social deficits were notable among the severely retarded. If the autistic social dysfunction is more broadly defined, its incidence, over that of more strictly defined autism, may increase several fold to affect perhaps as many as 1 in 500 children. In light of the IQ information, the incidence of autistic social dysfunction may be as low as 1 in 20,000 children with normal IQ and as high as 1 in 75 with severe or profound mental retardation. If atypical PDD were included, the incidence would be even higher. The study of autistic social dysfunction may provide important information regarding syndrome boundaries, particularly in the severely retarded.

Communication

Compared with social aspects of development, communicative development has been more extensively studied. Communicative (or sometimes only linguistic) criteria are typically encompassed in definitions of the autistic syndrome. The most obvious communication impairment is a lack of speech with about one half of autistic persons remaining mute. The speech of those who do communicate verbally is remarkable in a host of ways (reviewed by Paul, 1986). The study of language characteristics within a broad communicative context has revealed that symptoms such as echolalia can be viewed adaptively, e.g., as attempts to prolong interaction, and earlier impressions of such behaviors as exclusively pathologic must now be revised. Pragmatic deficits are common and communicative competence is strongly associated with outcome (DeMyer *et al.*, 1981). While language problems are common targets for intervention they typically prove resistant to dramatic change. The language and communicative deficits in autism are unique and differ from those seen, for example, in the developmentally language disordered child (Paul, 1986). It is important that diagnostic criteria reflect the broad range of communicative, and not simply linguistic, dysfunctions.

Age of Onset

The distinction, as in DSM-III, between diagnostic groups on the basis of age of onset of the condition rests on a body of research suggesting a bimodal distribution of psychotic illness in childhood (Kolvin, 1971). Some children appear to develop autism after a period of some months or even years of normal development (Harper & Williams, 1975); a few children develop an autstic illness after 30 months of age (Kolvin, 1971; Wing & Gould, 1979; Volkmar et al., 1985b). The practical demarcation of a precise age of onset can, however, be problematic (DeMyer et al., 1981), and most children with developmental problems arising in the first years of life are not autistic. Practically, age of onset might more properly be termed age of recognition and effects of parental sophistication and denial and the generally poor reliability of parental reports (Robbins, 1963) might reasonably be expected to color the age of syndrome recognition. The choice of 30 months, as in DSM-III, is arbitrary and determined, in part, by the attempt to differentiate autism from other disorders, e.g., disintegrative psychosis, which develop after some years of normal development.

Volkmar et al. (1985b) ascertained age of recognition in 103 individuals with well-documented histories of autism. The resulting data are presented in Fig. 2. While most cases exhibited difficulties during the first year of life, five children were reported to have had an onset after 30 months of age. In three of these cases, the onset appeared to result from gross central nervous system (CNS) insult; in the other two cases, parental variables may have colored the report of later onset. The five later-onset cases did not differ from other cases in terms of clinical features apart from age of onset. This result is consistent with those of Wing and Gould (1979) and Kolvin (1971). While autism is clearly an early-onset disorder, it may be more helpful practically to specify behavioral features for diagnostic purposes and include age of onset as an associated rather than a defining feature.

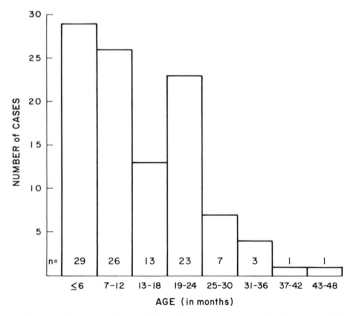

Fig. 2. Age of recognition of autism/childhood-onset pervasive developmental disorder. (Data adapted from Volkmar et al., 1986.)

Other Features

Additional criteria relating to other aspects of the autistic syndrome are variably included in diagnostic schemes. Unusual responses to the environment, resistance to change, and stereotyped or self-injurious behaviors are commonly observed in autistic individuals, although developmental changes are noted in their expression (Freeman *et al.*, 1980). These are commonly included as either primary or associated diagnostic features. Other features of the disorder are less often included in diagnostic schemes. Wing, Gould, Yeates, and Brierly (1977), for example, have emphasized the importance of deficits in symbolic play and imagination in syndrome definition. Play skills, however, are related to attachment, and may be part of the broader symbolic deficit observed (Sigman & Ungerer, 1984). Thus, the specific inclusion of deficits in symbolic play in diagnostic schemes remains a topic for futher study. Similar issues have arisen in regard to disturbances in perception or arousal. Tinbergen and Tinbergen (1972) suggested that high levels of arousal might account for the autistic syndrome; available evidence, however, contradicts this view (Rutter & Garmezy, 1983; Volkmar, Hoder & Cohen, 1985a).

ALTERNATIVE DIAGNOSTIC APPROACHES

Dimensional Approaches to Diagnosis

Although the categorical approach to diagnosis of autism has tended to predominate, various attempts to define dimensions of dysfunction have been made. The dimensional approach is exemplified, for example, by the use of standard normatized assessment instruments such as standard tests of intelligence or communicative competence. The importance of such measures, necessarily grounded within a developmental context, is well established (DeMyer *et al.*, 1981). Some investigators have designed rating scales or checklists for purposes of assessment explicitly for the autistic population (reviewed by Parks, 1983).

Several problems stand in the way of creating and using such instruments. Fundamental questions of validity and reliability have yet to be sufficiently addressed (Parks, 1983). Other problems are posed by issues of design and method. Some instruments focus on parental reports of early development and suffer from attendant issues of reliability (Robbins, 1963). Other instruments are based on teacher report or direct observation and problems of the generalizability of the results over settings and time complicates interpretation. Further problems are posed by the range of syndrome expression. Typically a deviance, as opposed to a developmental (Zigler, 1969) model is employed; i.e., deviant behaviors are sampled or rated and, unlike developmentally based instruments, issues of standardization and comparison prove problematic.

Volkmar and co-workers (1987) reported the use of a well-standardized normative assessment instrument, the revised Vineland Adaptive Behavior Scales (Sparrow, Balla & Cicchetti, 1984) to document social deficits in autism. Fifty-seven consecutive referrals (35 autistic and 22 nonautistic developmentally disabled) subjects constituted the sample. As compared with nonautistic subjects, the autistic group exhibited significantly greater deficits in adaptive social behaviors especially in terms of interpersonal skills. The results are summarized in Table I. The result suggests the utility of a well-standardized normative assess-

Table I. Sample Characteristics and Vineland Age Equivalent Scores:
Mann-Whitney U Tests[a]

| | Autistic | | Nonautistic | | | |
	X̄	SD	X̄	SD	U	p
Age	12.37	7.64	11.14	6.44	318	NSD
IQ	49.03	17.05	58.32	26.98	412	NSD
Mental age	5.24	4.57	5.64	3.60	321	NSD
Communicaton	3.73	3.93	4.71	3.48	277	<0.10
Receptive	3.18	3.91	3.45	1.19	256	<0.04
Expressive	2.91	2.82	4.41	3.70	275	<0.10
Written	4.39	4.52	5.12	3.92	341	NSD
Daily living skills	4.26	2.98	4.62	2.68	333	NSD
Personal	4.45	3.45	4.66	2.81	348	NSD
Domestic	4.91	3.62	4.79	2.61	356	NSD
Community	3.59	3.32	4.31	3.04	308	NSD
Socialization	2.14	1.83	3.85	2.81	224	<0.01
Interpersonal relations	1.59	1.05	3.61	2.73	207	<0.003
Play–leisure time	2.51	3.05	3.55	2.85	263	<0.04
Coping skills	2.71	2.03	4.44	3.03	255	<0.03
Motor	2.38	2.71	4.47	2.74	27	NSD
Composite score	2.38	0.98	3.00	0.87	277	<0.10

[a]Number of cases = 35 autistic, 22 nonautistic developmentally disabled except for motor domain, where autistic N = 12 and nonautistic N = 7. Table adapted, with permission, from Volkmar, Sparrow, Goudreau, Cicchetti, Paul, and Cohen (1987).

ment instrument for documenting autistic social dysfunction. Dimensional approaches to diagnoses are not incompatible with categorical views; dimensional data, if reliable and valid, may provide important insights into syndrome boundaries and areas of continuity and discontinuity across disorders.

Subtypes

Given the heterogeneity in syndrome expression, it is not surprising that attempts have been made to discover subtypes of autism. Such a typology might be based on a host of factors, including age of onset, IQ, associated medical conditions such as seizures, biochemical abnormalities such as elevated peripheral serotonin levels. The DSM-III system subtypes explicitly on age of onset (IA versus COPDD) and implicity on severity, in that criteria for COPDD appear to be less stringent than those for autism (Volkmar et al., 1985b). Various factors mitigate against such attempts. Probably the strongest case for subtyping could be made for IQ (Prior, 1979). Individuals with higher IQ scores have better outcomes, greater communicative competence, and a decreased incidence of seizures. The prepotence of IQ is not unique to autism, but its use in establishing at least two broad subgroups (higher and lower functioning, demarcated by a global IQ of 55) merits some consideration (Cohen et al., 1986a). Biochemical markers for autism have yet to be identified. The association of autism and the fragile X syndrome (Haggerman, McBogg & Haggerman, 1983) in a small subgroup of autistics remains to be firmly established as a useful subgrouping, since most patients with fragile X are not autistic. The presence of organic factors or elevated serotonin levels has not been shown to clearly distinguish behavioral features of the disorder (e.g., Wing & Gould, 1979). Wing and co-workers (Wing & Gould, 1979; Wing & Atwood, 1986) have proposed a typology based on clinical features and interactional style (aloof, passive, or active but odd). Although descriptive, these categories have yet to be shown to have validity and stability. Clearly, the lack of knowledge regarding fundamental mechanisms of pathogenesis limits efforts to subtype.

Other Diagnostic Concepts

While Kanner's diagnostic concept has proved most enduring, alternative concepts have been proposed for disorders with variable degrees of similiarity to autism. Boundaries between disorders, e.g., autism and severe mental retardation and autism and Asperger's syndrome, have become the topic of debate. Generally, the validity of these alternative diagnostic concepts is much less firmly established than strictly defined autism. However, the issues of possible continuities/discontinuities across groups raise important questions for research.

Atypical PDD—Atypical Development

DSM-III includes an atypical PDD category; this term is used in the DSM-III sense of not typical for those children whose disorders resemble autism but who fail to meet full criteria for a specific pervasive developmental disorder. The choice of this term, although consistent throughout DSM-III, is unfortunate, since it suggests the earlier diagnostic concept of atypical personality development (Rank, 1949, 1955) proposed to encompass those children who exhibited unusual sensitivities and responses to the environment but who were not as intellectually impaired as autistic children. Such children may be more common than autistic ones, although they are less frequently studied. The lack of explicit criteria for children with nonautistic but serious and "pervasive" early-onset disorders complicates efforts to study them. The few available studies (e.g., Brown, 1960; Dahl et al., 1986; Sparrow, Rescorla, Provence, Condon, Goudreau & Cicchetti, 1986) suggest that the disorder is persistent over time and exhibit considerable symptomatic overlap with autism (Dahl et al., 1986). The validity of this concept and its relationship to autism and other PDDs remains unclear. Greater specification of "atypical" cases may illustrate aspects of continuity and discontinuity with autism. In particular, the development of more explicit diagnostic criteria for purposes of research (Cohen et al., 1986a) should be helpful in this regard.

Asperger's Syndrome, Schizoid Personality

In 1944, Asperger proposed the autistic psychopathy concept to describe a disorder with many points of similarity to Kanner's autism. Such cases appear less frequently than autism, and attempts to differentiate Asperger's syndrome have focused on the relative later age of onset, relative preservation of linguistic skills, and less prominent signs of CNS dysfunction (Van Krevelen, 1971). However, social-communicative transactions are impaired (Wing, 1981), and the apparent later onset may be a function of higher intellectual level. The concept of schizoid personality disorder (Wolff & Chick, 1980) has also been proposed. In both disorders, problems of empathy, attachment, and social relatedness are prominent, suggesting some similarities to autism. The possibility remains that at least some cases of Asperger's syndrome represent high-functioning autism.

Childhood Schizophrenia

Despite the many years of research on childhood schizophrenia, little is known about this disorder (Tanguay & Asarnow, 1985). The earlier use of this term as a catch-all for every severely disturbed child was based on the incorrect presumption of continuity between adult and childhood psychosis. A substantial body of research (Rutter, 1972) casts considerable doubt on this assumption. If this concept is strictly and explictly defined, children with schizophrenia can be differentiated from autistic children on the basis of such factors as age of onset, clinical features, and family history; in DSM-III, individuals with delusions/hallucinations are excluded from an PDD diagnosis and must satisfy the criteria for schizophrenia. However, the DSM-III criteria for schizophrenia are not particularly developmental in nature, and their applicability to children may prove problematic (Cantor et al., 1982). Petty, Ornitz, Michelman & Zimmerman (1984) have again raised the issue of continuity between autism and schizophrenia in at least some individuals.

Some point of diagnostic similarity between the two concepts is to be expected; Kanner's (1943) choice of Bleuler's (1911) term *autism* suggests some point of similarity to schizophrenia. This semantic similarity need not, of course, imply diagnostic congruence. However, the classification of some individuals may be difficult. For example, the higher-functioning autistic adult may exhibit idiosyncratic interests or unusual experiences bordering on the delusional or hallucinatory. Similarly, many "residual" schizophrenic patients lack interest in social relationships and communication. Careful diagnostic assessment will generally not be diverted by such superficial similarities (Green, Campbell, Hardesty, Grega, Padron-Gayol, Shell & Erlenmeyer-Kimling, 1984). The clear preponderance of evidence suggests that the two disorders are distinctive (Rumsey, Rapoport & Scerry, 1985). It is important to assess carefully the significance of the observation that autistic individuals can become schizophrenic or that some "autistic features" may precede full blown schizophrenia (Petty et al., 1984). Given that about one half of autistic people never talk, it may be difficult to define the presence of schizophrenia in autism. The co-occurrence of the disorders also should not be surprising, since there is no reason to assume that having autism protects an individual from a schizophrenic episode later in life. Having PDD or any other neurobiologic disorder may represent an added risk. The study of associated psychiatric disorders in autism has received comparatively little attention in the research literature and is important for both clinical and research purposes. The use of new structured interview techniques for parents and caregivers and an awareness that autistic people can develop other conditions may help illuminate associations with other forms of psychopathology.

CONSENSUS AND CONTROVERSY

Areas of Agreement

Important areas of consensus regarding the description and validity of the concept of autism have emerged in recent years. Most investigators would now agree that autism is an early-onset disorder characterized by core features such as disturbances of relatedness, communication, and cognition. This disorder appears to differ from other childhood psychiatric disorders in its course, development, and clinical features. On the whole, available evidence suggests that autism does not simply "shade off" into normality. The autistic social dysfunction is of a type quite different from that found in other disorders. Most investigators would agree that the disorder is unrelated to childhood schizophrenia, although boundaries of the disorder would be the topic of debate. The mental retardation of most autistic individuals would be seen by virtually all investigators as a fundamental aspect of the disorder and not as simply "functional" or "secondary." Greatest diagnostic consensus would be achieved for those children who are not severely or profoundly retarded. The importance of using a detailed multiaxial classification scheme and of standard assessment instruments would not entail much debate.

Areas of Controversy

Areas of diagnostic controversy are related to questions of syndrome boundaries and definition. These two aspects of classification are intimately related. The questions of possible continuities of autism among higher-(intellectually) functioning persons (e.g., Asperger's syndrome, atypical PDD) and lower-functioning severely and profoundly retarded individuals remain to be answered. The phenomenologic and etiologic heterogeneity of all the various syndromes proposed is an obstacle for research studies. It is clear that developmental changes may be significant, that autistic infants grow into autistic adults rather than "growing out" of autism, and that diagnostic schemes should encompass the entire life span. The study of syndrome boundaries appears to be of great interest. The diagnostic process may be facilitated by the use of newer dimensional assessment techniques. Diagnostic schemes for purposes of research should not be limited by "official" schemes (e.g., DSM-III). For example, atypical PDD children have rarely been studied. Attempts to provide greater diagnostic specificity for this population have been made (e.g., Cohen *et al.*, 1986); the definition of groups for research purposes need not conform to official diagnostic schemes. This is not to suggest that official diagnostic schemes are unimportant; rather, such schemes should not preclude attempts to provide greater knowledge about areas of controversy. The urge toward a broader diagnostic conception of autism and related disorders should be tempered by a recollection of the misuse of the childhood schizophrenia concept; i.e., diagnostic categories should not be so broad as to be meaningless. Subgroups for specific studies should continue to be selected as is reasonable for the specific research purpose, e.g., only verbal subjects for studies of echolalia, and higher functioning for some attentional studies. When such subgroups are selected, it is important to realize that indeed a subgroup is being studied and that results may or may not generalize to the larger population of autistic persons. The interpretation of research would be facilitated by expanded sample descriptions using any of a variety of means (Cohen *et al.*, 1986).

SUMMARY

Over the past four decades, significant progress in validating Kanner's concept of infantile autism has been achieved. It is clear that the syndrome differs from other severe psychiatric disorders of childhood in clinical features and course. While precise etiologic mechanisms have yet to be identified, it is clear that the preponderance of available evidence suggests the importance of multiple biologic factors acting through one or more mechanisms to produce the autistic syndrome. No aspect of development can be considered primarily disordered in an etiologic sense; however, our understanding of the autistic social dysfunction remains quite limited and appears to be an important area of inquiry. The current resurgence of interest in issues of diagnosis and classification has stimulated considerable research. The study of lower and higher intellectually functioning autistic or autistic-like individuals appears to hold considerable promise in helping to refine diagnostic concepts and criteria. While the validity of other proposed syndromes remains less firmly established, the study of such concepts will help to illuminate aspects of continuity/discontinuity with autism. There is no reason to assume that having autism acts as a specific protective factor against other forms of psychopathology. In moving toward greater diagnostic precision it will be important to balance the need for reasonable conservatism in nomenclature against the need to incorporate newer research findings. The elaboration of more specific, and operational, diagnostic criteria grounded in the phenomenology of the disorder remains an important topic for research.

ACKNOWLEDGMENT. This chapter was supported by the W. T. Grant Foundation, the John Merck Fund, grant MH00418 from the National Institute of Mental Health, grant HD-03008 from the National Institute of Child Health and Human Development, grant 30929 for the Mental Health Clinical Research Center and grant RR00125 for the Children's Clinical Research Center. The support of Leonard Berger is gratefully acknowledged.

REFERENCES

American Psychiatric Association. (1980). *Diagnostic and Statistical Manual* (3rd ed.). Washington, D. C.: American Psychiatric Association.

Asperger, H. (1944) Die "autistichen Psychopathen" im Kindersalter. *Archiv. fur psychiatrie und Nervenkrankheiten, 117,* 76–136.

Bleuler, E. (1950). *Dementia praecox oder Gruppe der Schizophrenien* (J. Zinkin, trans.), New York: International Universities Press. (Originally published 1911.)

Brown, J. (1960). Prognosis from presenting symptoms of preschool children with atypical development. *American Journal of Orthopsychiatry, 30,* 382–90.

Cairns, R. B. (1979). *Social development: The origins and plasticity of interchanges.* San Francisco: W. Freeman.

Cantor, S., Evans, J., & Pezzot-Pearce. (1982). Childhood Schizophrenia: present but not accounted for. *American Journal of Psychiatry, 139,* 758–762.

Chess, S., Fernandez, P., & Korn, S. (1974). Behavioral consequences of congenital rubella, *Journal of Pediatrics, 93,* 699–712.

Cohen, D. J. (1976). The diagnostic process in child psychiatry. *Psychiatric Annals, 6,* 404–16.

Cohen, D. J., Caparulo, B., Gold, J., Waldo, M., Shaywitz, B., Ruttenberg, B., & Rimland, B. (1978). Agreement in diagnosis: clinical assessment and behavior rating scales for pervasively disturbed children. *Journal of the American Academy of Child Psychiatry, 17,* 689–95.

Cohen, D. J., Volkmar, F. R., & Paul, R. (1986*b*). Issues in the classification of pervasive developmental disorders and associated conditions: History and current status of nosology, *Journal of the American Academy of Child Psychiatry, 25,* 158–61.

Cohen, D. J., Paul, R., & Volkmar, F. R. (1986*a*). Issues in the classification of Pervasive Developmental Disorders and associated conditions: Towards DSM IV. *Journal of the American Academy of Child Psychiatry, 25,* 213–20.

Creak, M. (1961). Schizophrenic syndrome in childhood: Progress report of a working party. *Cerebral Palsy Bulletin, 3,* 501–4.

Dahl, K., Cohen, D. J., & Provence, S. (1986). Developmental disorders evaluated in early childhood: Clinical and multivariate approaches to nosology of PDD. *Journal of the American Academy of Child Psychiatry, 25,* 170–80.

DeMyer M. K., Hingtgen J. N., & Jackson R. K. (1981). Infantile autism reviewed: a decade of research. *Schizophrenia Bulletin, 7,* 388–451.

DeSanctis, S. (1906). Sopra alcune varieta della demenza precoce. *Rivista Sperimentale De Feniatria E. Di Medicina Legale, 32,* 141–65.

Eisenberg, L., & Kanner, L. (1956). Early infantile autism 1943–1955. *American Journal of Orthopsychiatry, 26,* 556–66.

Evans-Jones, L. G., & Rosenblum L. (1978). Disintegrative psychosis in childhood. *Developmental Medicine and Child Neurology, 20,* 462–70.

Fein, D., Pennington, B., Markowitz, P., Braverman, M., & Waterhouse, L. (1986). Towards a neuropsychological model of infantile autism: Are the social deficits primary? *Journal of the American Academy of Child Psychiatry, 25,* 198–212.

Freeman, B. J., Schroth, P., Ritvo, E., Guthrie, D., & Wake, L. The Behavior Observation Scale for Autism (BOS): Initial results of factor analyses. *Journal of Autism and Developmental Disorders, 10,* 343–6.

Group for the Advancement of Psychiatry (GAP). (1966). *Psychopathological disorders in Childhood: Theoretical considerations and a proposed classification,* 6, Rep. No. 62, New York: GAP.

Green, W. H., Campbell, M., Hardesty, A. S., Grega, D. M., Padron-Gayol, M. Shell, J., & Erlenmeyer-Kimling, L. (1984). A comparision of schizophrenic and autistic children. *Journal of the American Academy of Child Psychiatry, 23,* 399–409.

Haggerman, R. J., McBogg, P., & Haggerman, P. (1983). The fragile X syndrome: history, diagnosis, and treatment. *Developmental and Behavioral Pediatrics, 4,* 122–30.

Harper, J., & Williams S: (1975). Age and type of onset as critical variables in early infantile autism. *Journal of Autism and Childhood Schizophrenia, 5,* 25–35.

Helzer, J. E., & Coryell, W. (1983). More on DSM III: How consistent are precise criteria. *Biological Psychiatry, 18,* 1201–3.

Hobbs, N. (Ed.) (1975). *Issues in the classification of children* (Vols. 1 and 2). San Francisco: Jossey-Bass.

Kanner, L. (1943). Autistic disturbances of affective contact. *Nervous Child, 2,* 217–50.

Kolvin, I. (1971). Studies in childhood psychoses. I. Diagnostic criteria and classification, *British Journal of Psychiatry, 118,* 381–4.

Lane, J. (1977). *The wild boy of Aveyron.* London: Allen & Unwin.

Lotter, V. (1978). Follow-up studies. In M. Rutter & E. Schopler (Eds.), *Autism: A reappraisal of concepts and treatment,* New York: Plenum.

Mahler, M. (1952). On child psychoses and schizophrenia: Autistic and symbiotic infantile Psychoses, *Psychoanalytic Study of the Child, 7,* 286–305.

Makita, K. (1966). The age of onset of childhood schizophrenia. *Folia Psychiatrica Neurologica Japonica, 20,* 111–21.

National Society for Autistic Children (NSAC). (1978). National Society for Autistic Children definition of the syndrome of autism. *Journal of Autism and Developmental Disorders, 8,* 162–7.

Ornitz, E. M., & Ritvo, E. R. (1968). Perceptual inconstancy in early infantile autism. *Archives of General Psychiatry, 18,* 76–98.

Ornitz, E. M., Guthrie, D., & Farley, A. H. (1977). Early development of autistic children. *Journal of Autism and Childhood Schizophrenia, 7,* 207–29.

Parks, S. L. (1983). The assessment of autistic children: A selective review of available instruments. *Journal of Autism and Developmental Disorder, 13,* 255–67.

Paul, R. (1986). Communication in autism. In D. J. Cohen and A. Donnellan (Eds.), *Handbook of autism.* New York: Wiley.

Petty, L. K., Ornitz, E. M., Michelman, J. D., & Zimmerman, E. G. (1984). Autistic children who become schizophrenic. *Archives of General Psychiatry, 41,* 129–35.

Potter, H. W. (1933). Schizophrenia in children. *American Journal of Psychiatry, 89,* 1253–70.

Prior, M. R. (1979). Cognitive abilities and disabilities in infantile autism: A review. *Journal of Abnormal Child Psychology, 7*, 357–80.

Prior, M., Perry, D., & Gajzago, C. (1975). Kanner's syndrome or early-onset psychosis: A taxonomic analysis of 142 cases. *Journal of Autism and Childhood Schizophrenia, 5*, 71–80.

Rank, B. (1949). Adaptation of the psychoanalytic technique for the treatment of young children with atypical development. *American Journal of Orthopsychiatry, 19*, 130–9.

Rank, B. (1955). Intensive study and treatment of preschool children who show marked personality deviations or "atypical development" and their parents. In G. Caplan (Ed.), *Emotional problems of early childhood*. New York: Basic Books.

Robbins, L. C. (1963). The accuracy of parental recall of aspects of child development and child rearing practices. *Journal of Abnormal and Social Psycholoy, 6*, 261–70.

Rumsey, J. M., Rapoport, J. L., & Scerry, W. R. (1985). Autistic children as adults: psychiatric, social, and behavioral outcomes. *Journal of the American Academy of Child Psychiatry, 24*, 465–73.

Rutter, M. (1970). Autistic children: infancy to adulthood. *Seminars in Psychiatry, 2*, 435–50.

Rutter, M. (1972). Childhood schizophrenia reconsidered. *Journal of Autism and Childhood Schizophrenia, 2*, 315–38.

Rutter, M. (1978a). Diagnostic validity in child psychiatry. *Advances in Biological Psychiatry, 2*, 2–22.

Rutter, M. (1978b). Diagnosis and definition. In M. Rutter & E. Schopler (Eds.), *Autism: A reappraisal of concepts and treatment*. New York: Plenum.

Rutter, M., Bartak, L., & Newman, S. (1971). Autism—a central disorder of cognition and language. In M. Rutter (Ed.), *Infantile autism: Concepts, characteristics and treatment*. London: Churchill Livingstone.

Rutter, M., & Garmezy, N. (1983). Developmental Psychopatholgy. In E. M. Hetherington (Ed.), *Handbook of Child Psychology* (Vol. 4). New York: Wiley.

Rutter, M., & Shaffer, D. (1980). DSM-III: A step forward or back in terms of the classification of child psychiatric disorder? *Journal of the American Academy of Child Psychiatry, 19*, 371–94.

Rutter, M., Shaffer, D., & Shepherd, M. (1975). *A multiaxial classification of child psychiatric disorders*, Geneva: World Health Organization.

Schopler, E. (1983). New developments in the definition and diagnosis of autism. In B. B. Lakey and A. E. Kazdin (Eds.), *Advances in clinical child psychology*, New York: Plenum.

Schopler, E., Reichler, R. J., DeVellis, R. F., & Daly, K. (1980). Toward objective classification of childhood autism: Childhood Autism Rating Scales (CARS) *Journal of Autism and Developmental Disorders, 10*, 91–103.

Sigman, M., & Ungerer, J. (1984). Attachment behaviors in autistic children, *Journal of Autism and Developmental Disorders, 14*, 231–44.

Sparrow, S., Rescorla, L. A., Provence, S., Condon, S., Goudreau, D., & Cicchetti, D. (1986). Follow-up of "atypical" children—a brief report. *Journal of the American Academy of Child Psychiatry, 25*, 181–4.

Sparrow, S., Balla, D., & Cicchetti, D. (1984). *Vineland Adaptive Behavior Scales*. Circle Pines, MN: American Guidance Service.

Spitzer, R. L., Endicott, J. E., & Robins, E. (1978). Research diagnostic criteria, *Archives of General Psychiatry, 35*, 773–82.

Tanguay, P., & Asarnow, R. (1985). Schizophrenia in children. In R. Michaels (Ed.), *Psychiatry*, Philadelphia: J. B. Lippincott.

Tinbergen, E. A., & Tinbergen, N. (1972). Early childhood autism: An ethological approach. *Advances in Ethology, Journal of Comparative Ethology*, Suppl. No. 10. Berlin: Paul Perry.

Van Krevelen, D. A. (1971). Early infantile autism and autistic psychopathy. *Journal of Autism and Childhood Schizophrenia, 1*, 82–6.

Volkmar, F. R. (1986). Social Development. In D. J. Cohen and A. Donnellan (Eds.), *Handbook of Autism*. New York: Wiley.

Volkmar, F. R., & Cohen, D. J. (1985) The experience of infantile autism: A first person account by Tony W. *Journal of Autism and Developmental Disorders, 15*, 47–54.

Volkmar, F., Cohen, D. J., & Paul, R. (1986). An evaluation of DSM-III criteria for infantile autism. *Journal of the American Academy of Child Psychiatry, 25,* 190–7.

Volkmar, F. R., Hoder, E. L., & Cohen, D. J. (1985*a*). Compliance, "negativism," and the effects of treatment structure in autism: A naturalistic, behavioral study. *Journal of Child Psychology and Psychiatry, 26,* 865–77.

Volkmar, F. R., Sparrow, S. A., Goudreau, D., Cicchetti, D. V., Paul, R., & Cohen, D. J. (1987). Social deficits in autism: An operational approach using the Vineland Adaptive Behavior Scales. *Journal of the American Academy of Child Psychiatry, 26,* 156–161.

Volkmar, F. R., Stier, D. M., & Cohen, D. J. (1985*b*). Age of recognition of pervasive developmental disorder. *American Journal of Psychiatry, 142,* 1450–2.

Werry, J. S. (1985). ICD9 and DSM III classification for the clinician. *Journal of Child Psychology and Psychiatry, 26,* 1–6.

Wing, L. (1981). Asperger's syndrome: A clinical account. *Psychological Medicine, 11,* 115–29.

Wing, L., & Atwood, A. (1986). Syndromes of autism and atypical development. In D. J. Cohen and A. Donnellan (Eds.), *Handbook of Autism.* New York: Wiley.

Wing, L., & Gould, J. (1979). Severe impairments of social interaction and associated abnormalities in children: Epidemiology and classification. *Journal of Autism and Developmental Disorders, 9,* 11–30.

Wing, L. Gould, J., Yeates, S. R., & Brierly, L. M. (1977). Symbolic play in severely mentally retarded and autistic children. *Journal of Child Psychology and Psychiatry, 18,* 167–78.

Wolff, S., & Barlow, A. (1979). Schizoid personality in childhood: a comparative study of schizoid, autistic, and normal children. *Journal of Child Psychology and Psychiatry, 20,* 29–46.

Wolff, S., & Chick, J. (1980). Schizoid personality in childhood: A controlled follow-up study. *Psychological Medicine, 10,* 85–100.

Zigler, E. (1969). Developmental versus difference theories of mental retardation and the problem of motivation. *American Journal of Mental Deficiency, 73,* 536–49.

7

The Continuum of Autistic Characteristics

LORNA WING

INTRODUCTION

As a result of the accumulation of findings from biologic, psychological, and clinical research, views of the etiology and nature of childhood autism have evolved and changed since Kanner (1943) published his first description of the syndrome that bears his name. However, disagreements continue concerning the clinical criteria for diagnosis, and the boundaries between autism and other conditions in which there are impairments of skills and abnormalities of behavior.

Knowledge of causes and their physical effects provides the most reliable foundation for diagnostic criteria but, in most psychiatric conditions, including autism, details of etiology and pathology are still unknown. Definitions of autism and related conditions have, perforce, been based on combinations of postulated psychological dysfunctions and manifestations in overt behavior, with all the unreliability this entails.

In this situation, theories, classifications, and labels abound. Kanner believed his syndrome to be a unique and specific condition. Other investigators have taken the opposite view and have grouped autism together with all so-called "childhood psychoses" under some general label, usually childhood schizophrenia (Bender, 1947, 1961; Despert, 1938; Goldfarb, 1970).

Kolvin and colleagues (Kolvin, 1971; Kolvin, Ounsted, Humphrey & McNay, 1971) demonstrated that "psychosis" with early childhood onset could be differentiated from the rare cases, virtually never seen before age 7, with the clinical features of psychoses of adult life. However, these studies did not show whether Kanner's syndrome could be reliably separated from other early childhood psychoses.

Epidemiologic research is particularly useful in identifying the prevalence and the boundaries of clinical phenomena. For such tasks, studies in which complete populations living in specified geographic areas are examined avoid the biases inherent in samples referred to clinics, even if these are district based. The techniques of epidemiology were used in a study in which the relationships among Kanner's syndrome, other childhood psychoses, and mental retardation were examined in a population of children from one area of southeast London (Camberwell) (Wing & Gould, 1979; Wing, 1981*a*). The same children, now adoles-

LORNA WING • MRC Social Psychiatry Unit, Institute of Psychiatry, University of London, London SE5 8AF, England.

cents or adults, are currently being followed up. All adults known to the Camberwell mental retardation services have also been studied (Wing & Hayhurst, 1974), as have 890 adults living in a hospital (institution) for the mentally retarded (Shah, Holmes & Wing, 1982).

The formulation presented in this chapter was based on the results of the work mentioned above in conjunction with recent experimental and clinical work by other workers. It is hypothesized that Kanner's syndrome is part of a continuum or spectrum of autistic disorders. The central problem, which, by definition, is both necessary and sufficient for the diagnosis of a disorder in this continuum, is an intrinsic impairment in development of the ability to engage in reciprocal social interaction, which is fundamentally different from those described in neurotic or conduct disorders. This can occur on its own, but in most cases it is accompanied by impairments of other psychological functions, some much more commonly than others. The manifestations of the social and other problems vary widely in type and severity, and all kinds of combinations of impairments are seen in clinical practice. Some of these combinations have been named as syndromes, but many have not been assigned a separate identity. Thus the term continuum represents a concept of considerable complexity, rather than simply a straight line from severe to mild.

This chapter describes the manifestations of the abnormality of social interaction and of commonly associated impairments of psychological function. The relationship among the various named syndromes, other developmental disorders, and the autistic continuum is discussed. The current standard diagnostic criteria for childhood autism adopted, respectively, by the American Psychiatric Association (1980) and the World Health Organization (1977) are commented on in the light of the above formulation. The clinical implications of the hypothesis are outlined and suggestions made for further research.

COMPONENTS OF THE AUTISTIC CONTINUUM

The ways in which each of the dysfunctions described below can be shown are listed from the most to the least severe. It should be noted that the descriptions are of selected points along a continuum, and all possible intermediate forms may be found in clinical practice.

Impairment of Social Interaction

Interest is growing in the development from birth of the capacity to interact with others, biologically inherent in normal infants. Deficit in this capacity is now recognised as being at the root of the problems of autistic people. Impairment of social interaction can conveniently be divided into three separate, but closely related facets, each of which varies in its overt manifestations, depending on the severity of the dysfunction. They are referred to as the triad of impairments of social interaction—or the triad for short (Gould, 1986; Wing, 1981a, 1982; Wing & Gould, 1979).

Impairment of Social Recognition

Social recognition refers to the ability to recognize that other human beings are the most interesting and potentially rewarding features of the environment. In the normal infant, social recognition is observable during the early weeks of life (Newson & Newson, 1975, 1979; Schaffer, 1974, 1979).

Levels of agreement between two trained observers rating the presence of a problem in this area have been calculated from an ongoing unpublished study of mentally retarded adults, about one third of whom have the triad. There was 92% agreement on the presence of impairment of social recognition. Absence or deficit may be shown in different ways (Wing & Gould, 1979). Levels of agreement for the different manifestations are given below.

1. The most severe form is aloofness and indifference to other people. Those with this degree of impairment tend to ignore or even actively avoid social or physical contact with others. Some children and adults displaying this behavior are aloof and indifferent in all situations. Others make approaches to obtain things they want but return to aloofness once the need is gratified. Some like simple physical contact such as cuddling, tickling, or games of chasing but have no interest in the purely social aspects of the interaction. In children, the social indifference is especially marked toward age peers. (Level of agreement on presence was 95%.)

2. A less marked form is seen in those who do not make social contact spontaneously but who amiably accept approaches and do not resist if others pull them into activities. Some children of this kind are liked by their classmates because they can be used, for example, as babies in a game of mothers and fathers or as patients for doctors and nurses. They remain in their allotted role as long as the others are playing, but they wander off at the end of the game unless redirected by their peers. (Level of agreement on presence was 67%.)

3. Some people with this problem do make active social approaches, but in an odd, one-sided fashion. Their behavior is inappropriate because it is undertaken mainly to indulge some repetitive, idiosyncratic preoccupation. They have no interest in, and no feeling for, the needs and ideas of others. They do not modify their speech or behavior to adapt to others but continue to pursue their own topics or favorite activities, even in the face of active discouragement. Those with little or no speech make intrusive, even embarrassing, physical contacts. (Level of agreement on presence was 82%.)

4. In its mildest and most limited manifestation, seen in adults who were socially impaired as children, but who have made considerable progress, the problem is present in a subtle form that is difficult to describe and recognize on brief acquaintance, but is detectable on longer contact. It is best described as a poverty of grasp of the most subtle rules of social interaction and a lack of perceptiveness towards others. People with this type of impairment give the impression that they have acquired a superficial knowledge of social behavior through intellectual learning rather than through intuition. (No figures for agreement on ratings are available for this type of social interaction.)

Impairment of Social Communication

Impairment in the area of social communication affects the giving and receiving of nonverbal, preverbal, and verbal social signals, the pleasure in conversation, and, at a more sophisticated level, the ability and desire to talk about feelings and exchange ideas. In the normal child, the earliest forms of these activities are seen in the first 2 or 3 months of life when the baby takes part in conversational exchanges by smiles, movements, and noises indicative of enjoyment (Bullowa, 1979; Schaffer, 1974; Trevarthen, 1974) and uses intoned sounds to indicate feelings that can be interpreted by parents (Ricks, 1975, 1979; Ricks & Wing, 1975). The absence of speech, by itself, does not prevent social communication, since nonspoken means can be used effectively by people with speech problems who do not have impairment of social interaction.

The manifestations of impairment vary as follows (Wing & Gould, 1979; Wing, 1981a):

1. There may be absence of any desire to communicate with others.
2. At a less severe level, needs are expressed, but there is no other form of communication.
3. Those with speech may make factual comments, but these are not part of a social exchange and are often irrelevant to the social context.
4. Some older children and adults talk a great deal, but do not engage in true reciprocal conversation. Instead, they ask questions repetitively or deliver lengthy monologues regardless of the content of the conversation, the responses of the listener, or expressions of boredom and desire to leave.

In a study of autistic, normal, and Downs' syndrome subjects, Attwood (1984) found that the autistic children did not use gesture to initiate social interaction or to express feelings; for example, they did not touch someone to give comfort, or encouragement.

Impairment of Social Imagination and Understanding

The problem of impaired social imagination and understanding affects the ability to copy other people's actions with genuine understanding of their meaning and purpose. It interferes with the development of the type of pretend play that involves the imaginative act of putting oneself in the position of another person, real or fictional, and of experiencing their thoughts and feelings, as distinct from empty copying of their actions. It also adversely affects the capacity to estimate what others are likely to know or not to know. What Baron-Cohen, Leslie, and Frith (1985) have called the absence, in autistic people, of any theory that other people have minds, is a striking description of this aspect of the triad. Normal children begin to develop these imaginative social abilities from the second or third year of life (Bretherton, McNew & Beeghley-Smith, 1981; Shantz, 1983). Copying of the mother's facial expressions is observable during the first few months of life (Pawlby, 1977; Trevarthen, 1974).

Impairment of social imagination may be shown as follows (Gould, 1982, 1986; Wing, Gould, Yeates & Brierley, 1977).

1. Copying and pretend play may be entirely absent.
2. Copying of other people's actions may be present, but without real understanding of their meaning and purpose. A child at this level may mechanically copy other children's play actions, such as bathing a doll and putting it to bed, but will not have any spontaneous pretend play. A few children tend to echo automatically other people's gestures with the same lack of comprehension as other children with these problems echo speech.
3. There may be repetitive, stereotyped enacting of a role, such as a television character, an animal, or an inanimate object such as a train, but without variation or empathy.
4. In older and more able people with social impairment there can be recognition that

something goes on in other people's minds, but no understanding of how to guess at or otherwise discover what this may be.

5. Some people with the triad appear to have some ability to recognize other people's feelings, but the capacity exists on an intellectual level without empathic sharing of the emotions.

Repetitive Patterns of Activity

The presence of the triad of impairments of social interaction described above is essential for the diagnosis of a disorder in the autistic continuum. It is typically associated with unusual patterns of self-chosen activities (Wing & Gould, 1979; Gould, 1982). The manifestations of these activities vary widely, but their range is always, in different degrees, limited, and there is a marked tendency for them to be repetitive and stereotyped in form. Although characteristically occurring with the triad, repetitive behavior is not, on its own, diagnostic of the autistic continuum because it can be seen in young normal children, and in severely retarded children, even if they do not exhibit the triad. However, in neither of these groups does it dominate the whole spontaneous activity pattern as it does in those with impairment of social interaction.

The many different types of repetitive behavior can be approximately grouped as follows:

1. In those who have profound cognitive as well as social impairment there may be virtually no spontaneous activity, but an insistence on adopting the same bodily posture, often in the same place in the room or on the same chair. They may strongly resist any attempts to involve them in occupation or recreation. They may show small bodily movements, such as teeth grinding or clenching and unclenching of the fists.
2. Some display simple bodily stereotypies, such as rocking, finger flicking, aimless pacing, or fascination with simple sensory stimuli.
3. More complex bodily movements may be seen, or absorption in complex stimuli such as a particular piece of music, or repetitive manipulation or arrangement of objects, or intense attachment to particular objects, such as pebbles, bits of plastic, and empty detergent packets, which may be amassed in large quantities.
4. The repetitive behavior may take the form of insisting on carrying out particular sequences of actions, such as a bed time ritual, always following the same route to familiar places, or drawing or making models of the same types of objects, which, once finished, may be ignored or destroyed.
5. At the highest level, the problems are manifested in verbal or intellectual forms, such as absorption in particular books which are constantly reread, or in amassing facts on subjects such as railway time tables, astrophysics, the characteristics of British mammals, the genealogy of royalty. The list of possible subjects for these circumscribed interests is endless, but the peculiar intensity with which they are pursued is common to all.

Other Psychological Functions

There is a marked tendency for various other psychological functions to be affected together with the triad.

Language

The pragmatic aspects of language, i.e., the comprehension and use of language within a social context, rather than the understanding of its literal meaning, are always impaired in disorders in the autistic continuum (Baltaxe, 1977; Cromer, 1981; Frith, 1982; Tager-Flusberg, 1981). In the most able people, the manifestations of this problem may be subtle, for example, showing lack of awareness of other people's responses to conversational topics, and the need for turn-taking in social interchanges.

The formal aspects of communication, i.e., the mechanics of language, including vocabulary, syntax, and semantics, are delayed and deviant in development in most, but not all people with autistic disorders. Comprehension and use of language (spoken, manually signed, and written) may be completely absent or retarded in development to varying degrees. Such delay is not distinguishable from that in other conditions causing language backwardness (Frith, 1982), but certain abnormalities are characteristic of the autistic continuum, although not always present. These include immediate and delayed echolalia, idiosyncratic use of words and phrases, and confusion over words, such as pronouns and prepositions, that shift in meaning with the speaker and the situation (Fay & Schuler, 1980; Kanner, 1949; Schopler & Mesibov, 1985; Ricks & Wing, 1975). Discrepancies between levels of comprehension and use of language are common. Most often comprehension is better than use, but the opposite may also be found in some persons. Sooner or later, some people with the triad develop fully adequate vocabulary and grammar but, even among these, speech tends to be repetitive, long winded, devoid of idiomatic expressions, and filled with long words where short ones would suffice.

A few of the autistic children and adults who remain mute develop the ability to communicate in writing by hand or on a typewriter, or by using some electronic device (see, e.g., Schawlow & Schawlow, 1985). Others learn a manual sign system. In the cases the present author has knowledge of, the communications have the characteristics of repetitiveness and lack of social empathy found in autistic speech.

Play needing social empathy is always affected. Pretend play with objects, which many workers regard as the outward sign of the first stages of development of inner symbolic language, is often but by no means always absent. Some children with the triad do develop this type of play, although it is limited and repetitive in form (Gould, 1982, 1986). They may use toy animals or dolls in such play but, if so, these playthings tend to be treated as objects and not as if they were alive. Some try to involve other children, but only as robotlike assistants, and not for the pleasure of their company. This kind of activity should be distinguished from truly social imaginative play. Also, the use of one object to represent another, such as pretending that a stick is a gun, is especially unusual in children with the triad (Baron-Cohen, 1985).

The nonverbal accompaniments of normal speech, including facial expression, eye contact, bodily posture, gesture, and miming, are almost always affected, but the way in which this problem is shown varies from complete absence at one end of the scale to an inappropriate use of large and random gestures and an intense fixed stare at the other. Attwood's (1984) findings concerning absence of gestures expressing sympathy and interpersonal empathy have already been mentioned, though this author found that the autistic children he studied did use instrumental deictic (indicative) gestures on the occasions when they interacted with others. They did not use gesture to describe objects or properties of objects, unlike the normal and Downs' syndrome subjects in the study. Peculiar vocal intonation or difficulty with controlling the volume of sound is almost but not completely universal.

Motor Coordination

On intuitive grounds, abnormalities of language do not appear to be surprising in association with the triad of impairments. Less apparently predictable is the frequent observation of peculiarities of motor coordination affecting posture, gait and complex skilled movements (DeMyer, 1976; Damasio & Maurer, 1978).

These peculiarities are difficult to predict and define, because there can be any mixture of motor skills and deficiencies. Some children are late in walking and are clumsy and awkward in large movements. They tend to be nervous of activities requiring climbing and balancing. Others are swift and agile in movement and undertake breathtaking feats such as jumping around on window ledges and walking along roof ridges. Fine finger dexterity is equally variable, and degree of skill in this area is not predictable from that in large movements. A child may be able to operate the controls of a record player and unerringly place the needle on one specific spot on the record but may be unable to kick a football. Operations requiring combinations of different movements, such as turning a door handle and pulling the door at the same time, pose particular difficulties for some children.

Postures of the hands, with fingers hyperextended, are common. By the time of adolescence, even those most agile as children tend to show oddities in gait and posture. These include walking without arm swinging, odd disjointed puppetlike movements, and standing with head bowed and elbows flexed.

Responses to Sensory Stimuli

Those with the triad may respond with indifference, fascination or distress to sensory input in any modality (Coleman & Gillberg, 1985; Kanner, 1943; Ornitz, 1974; Rutter, 1966). Ignoring sounds; oversensitivity to sounds; indifference to heat, cold, and pain; fascination with shiny objects, things that spin, and self-spinning; and dislike of a gentle touch, despite enjoying being tickled and swung round appear to be particularly common examples, although there is great individual variation. In the present author's experience, corroborated by the Camberwell study, these problems are most characteristic of young children with the triad and of those who are severely handicapped. They are not essential diagnostic criteria for the triad as they may not be observed in the more able people, especially those within the normal range of intelligence.

Cognitive Skills

Most people with the triad are mentally retarded, and all or most of their cognitive skills are impaired to varying degrees. In the Camberwell study of the children below the age of 15, overall intelligence was estimated using both language and non-language-dependent tests; 3% of all those with the triad were within the normal range (IQ 70+), 14% were mildly retarded (IQ 50–69), 42% were severely retarded (IQ 20–49), and 41% were profoundly retarded (IQ <20). Almost one half of the last group were nonmobile (Wing 1981a). But the psychological functions that do not require social perception and language for their performance, such as visuospatial and mathematical skills, are usually, but by no means always, less affected than sociability and language (DeMyer, 1976; Lockyer & Rutter, 1969; Wing & Gould, 1979). In a small minority of cases, there can be above-average, even superior, levels of ability in one or more of these areas, sometimes referred to as islets of ability. Some have musical skills, such as absolute pitch, accurate recognition or reproduction of tunes, and the ability to play a musical instrument or even to compose music. Unusually good rote memory seems to underlie some of these special skills, such as knowledge of routes or timetables or the amassing of facts on specific subjects, although O'Connor and Hermelin's work (1984) suggests that calendar calculators use rule-based strategies as well as memory. Recall of information outside the areas of special interest often seems to be impaired (Boucher, 1981). Parents commonly report that their children cannot answer appropriately when asked, for example, what they had for dinner at school that day, even if they have more than adequate vocabulary and grammar for this task. This may, however, result from a failure to understand the meaning of the question rather than a failure of memory.

In the above descriptions, the assumption has been made that for each psychological function, the different manifestations of impairments form a sequence along a continuum of severity. In some cases, the idea of a related sequence seems reasonable, e.g., the increasing complexity of the forms of stereotyped repetitive activities. In other cases, for example, the scale of social recognition, which varies from indifference to others at one end, to active but odd one-sided approaches at the other, the relationship between the points along the sequence is less obvious. The hypothesis that they are on a continuum derives from observations showing that children can change from one point on the scale to another with increasing age and in different environments (Lord, 1984).

Many other elements may be present (DeMyer, 1979; Rutter, 1970; Wing, 1980). These include poor attention span, overactivity, high levels of anxiety, and disturbances of behavior such as aggression, self-injury, destructiveness, and temper tantrums. There may be abnormalities of fluid or food intake or sleeping patterns; physical handicaps, including epileptic fits, visual or hearing impairments, or cerebral palsy; and superimposed psychiatric conditions, such as depression, especially in adolescence or adult life (Wing, 1981b). Episodic catatonic phenomena may be seen in adolescents, sometimes in response to stressful situations. However, these features are variable in occurrence and are not specific to the autistic continuum, so they are not included among the essential diagnostic criteria. Finally, it should be emphasized that individual temperament and personality have an important effect on behavior and outcome.

PATTERNS OF IMPAIRMENTS AND SKILLS

The epidemiologic studies mentioned above, as well as other clinical evidence, show that psychological impairments in autism and related conditions can vary in severity independently of each other. Also, any combination may be found, apart from certain obvious constraints, such as the impossibility of verbal stereotypies occurring in someone who is mute. Sometimes there are extreme contrasts, as in the case of Nadia, who was socially aloof and severely retarded on intelligence tests but who, from around 3 years of age, could draw with remarkable photographic realism (Selfe, 1977). Similar discrepancies were seen in another autistic artist and in the twins who did arithmetic calculations, described by Sacks (1985). One possible reason that individual profiles of psychological functions in people with the triad may be so uneven is the apparent lack or poverty of mechanisms that normally facilitate integration of the various specific areas of skills. Psychological and clinical studies (Bartak, Rutter & Cox, 1975; Frith & Snowling, 1983; Gould, 1986) have shown that autistic persons and others with the triad have difficulty in comprehending the wider meaning of their experiences and fail to place items of knowledge into context. People who do not have the triad build up a complex interconnecting network of associations between concepts. By contrast, those with the triad, if they associate concepts at all, do so in straight and narrow lines with few or no cross-connections. This would appear to be causally associated with the repetitive, limited, apparently meaningless patterns of activities that characterize people with disorders in the autistic continuum. The lack of ability to integrate different areas of skill into a coherent framework and the consequent concentration on very limited interests may in turn exacerbate the inherent tendency for some aspects of cognitive function to develop to a higher level than others. Whether the poverty of associations is the cause or the effect of the social impairments or whether there is some other type of relationship is unknown. In practice, the important point is that the relative independence between levels of impairment of different psychological functions results in a wide variety of possible profiles.

Patterns in a Population of Children

The findings of the ongoing epidemiologic study of 95 Camberwell children with disorders in the autistic continuum, identified from among a total population of 35,000 under age 15 at the end of 1970 (Wing & Gould, 1979; Wing, 1981), suggested that, while any combination of impairments might be observed in individuals, some regularities could be detected. However, there were exceptions to every rule.

First, the picture before age 7 years will be discussed. Those children who were aloof and indifferent to others at this stage of their development comprised the largest single group, 58 in all. Most were severely or profoundly mentally retarded and included 16 who did not achieve independent mobility. Most had no comprehension or use of language and no pretend play of any kind, and almost all, when young, had simple stereotypies and abnormal responses to sensory stimuli. There was a strong tendency for social aloofness to be associated with severe or profound handicaps. Nevertheless, 17 of the 58 had elaborate repetitive routines as well as simple stereotypies, which qualified them for the diagnosis of Kanner's syndrome using the two criteria specified by Kanner and Eisenberg (1956); that is, profound lack of affective contact with others and elaborate stereotypies.

Seven out of this group of 17 had visuospatial intelligence in the mildly retarded or normal range, together with special musical, visuospatial, or rote memory skills. They demonstrated the five criteria Kanner listed in his early publications on the syndrome (1943, 1949): (1) profound lack of affective contact; (2) anxious desire for the preservation of sameness; (3) fascination with objects that are handled with skill; (4) mutism or language that does not serve interpersonal communication; and (5) good cognitive potential shown by feats of memory, or skills on performance tests, especially the Seguin form board. Kanner was unaware that a high score in such areas could be associated with a low level of general cognitive ability.

The study included 21 children who, before age 7, were passive in social interaction, and who were all able to walk independently. Fifteen, i.e., about two thirds, were in the mildly retarded or normal IQ range, had useful practical and self-care skills, and had some language. All of these comparatively able children displayed repetitive behavior, but this tended to be of an organized elaborate kind. Some copied other children's pretend play with dolls and other toys or played repetitively with such materials. However, the remaining six passive children functioned as severely retarded, with few or no skills, no play, and little or no language and had simple stereotypies.

Those who, before age 7, were active but odd in social interaction numbered 16 in all. They were all fully mobile. Nine had IQs in the mildly retarded or normal range or had useful practical and self-care skills and at least some language. These children had markedly repetitive speech and repetitive play, including copying the actions of characters from television or books. In some children in this group, the use of speech was at a higher level than comprehension and the verbal IQ on the Wechsler test was higher than the performance IQ. But the remaining seven of the active but odd group were severely retarded with few or no skills and little or no speech. These children made inappropriate physical approaches to others and had limited repetitive patterns of activity.

The age of onset was reported to be after 30 months in four children, being 32, 36, 40, and 60 months respectively. The first three were aloof, two of these showing Kanner's two criteria, and the last was odd. In the first three cases, the abnormalities followed encephalitis; theoretically, the diagnoses could have been Heller's syndrome (described by Hulse, 1954), or disintegrative psychosis (World Health Organization, 1977), or childhood-onset pervasive developmental disorder (American Psychiatric Association, 1980), but the clinical picture of the children did not differ from that of others in the same subgroups. The fourth child with later reported onset fitted Asperger's description of his syndrome and was almost certainly abnormal before 60 months, but his parents were unaware that his development was deviant.

Changes with Age

Follow-up evaluation of the teenage years of the 89 subjects (out of the original 95) who were still alive and in England showed that none became normally sociable and most remained in the groups to which they were assigned in early childhood. However, some changes were recorded in 20 children (22% of those followed up). Nineteen of these had visuospatial intelligence in the mildly retarded or normal range, six had been aloof, 12 passive, and two odd. Fourteen of those who changed tended to engage in more social contact with increasing age, but six children resembled Kanner's descriptions more closely in their teens than as young children, five of them, previously passive or odd, because they became more socially withdrawn and developed more complex repetitive routines, and one, who had always been aloof, because he also developed complex routines. Seven of those with more social approaches by their teens developed the features described by Asperger (1944) as characteristic of his syndrome. Three of these children had had classic Kanner's syndrome, three were passive, and one was odd. The criteria Asperger listed for his syndrome are lack of empathy and naive inappropriate one-sided social interaction; little or no ability to form friendships; long-winded repetitive speech; poor nonverbal communication; circumscribed interests in subjects such as timetables, archeology, and astronomy, but without real understanding of the facts amassed; ill-coordinated movements; and, overall, a marked lack of common sense. Asperger also found specific learning disabilities affecting reading or arithmetic in many of his group. In a previous paper, it was noted that six of the Camberwell children had Asperger's syndrome (Wing, 1981b). Since then, the characteristic features have become more obvious in a seventh child. In fact, all the teenagers with IQs of 50 or above who were passive or who were active but odd in social interaction had at least some of the features of Asperger's syndrome, although only seven had the full picture. This diagnostic category was not applied when the children were below 7 years of age, because they were too young for the circumscribed interests, difficulty in making friendships, and long-winded repetitive speech to be clearly manifested.

Some of those with active but odd social interaction and repetitive speech possibly fitted Mahler's (1952) symbiotic psychosis. Some who were aloof and mobile and with marked motor stereotypies might have been diagnosed as Earl's (1943) primitive catatonic psychosis of idiocy, but the published descriptions are not precise enough for certainty.

There is no doubt that the clinical pictures in the active but odd children with speech would be classified by some workers as childhood schizophrenia, and their repetitive enacting of characters from fiction or animals might be referred to as delusional. The changes in the clinical picture over time, as described here, support the view that the active but odd group are more appropriately placed within the autistic continuum (see also Wing, 1981b).

The Camberwell study illustrates some of the dilemmas in classification. Many children showed features of Kanner's autism, and the other named syndromes, but few precisely fitted any of the descriptions. As might be expected, the longer the list of criteria for any group, the smaller the numbers of people who could be included. The reasons for the problems can be summarized as follows:

1. Since each of the items making up the profiles lies on a continuum, arbitrary cut-off points have to be specified where no sharp dividing lines exist.
2. There is considerable overlap between the criteria for the so-called syndromes, and many children have features of more than one at the same time; the more criteria specified, the more overlap that is found, but the fewer subjects fit the full picture.
3. In some children, especially those who are less severely handicapped and less aloof, behavior varies with the environment they are in, although the impairments are always present.
4. Children, mainly those who are more able (including those with Kanner's syndrome in early years), can move from one syndrome to another as they grow up. A few become more markedly aloof as they grow older. More often, aloofness lessens, and passivity or oddness take its place. A small minority improve so much they become apparently normal, with only minor traces of the characteristic abnormalities, although there can be marked problems with intimate social relationships.
5. The degree to which the different impairments are manifested varies from extremely severe to very mild, and each shades into near normality.

Taking all these factors into account, it is not difficult to see why some children could be classified under more than one named syndrome, and others not classified at all, especially if their behavioral patterns in different places and at different times are taken into account.

RELATIONSHIP TO OTHER DEVELOPMENTAL DISORDERS

The foregoing discussion has focused on developmental impairment of social interaction as the central issue, with problems affecting other skills viewed as associated abnormalities. It is legitimate to ask why social interaction should be regarded as the key variable. If degree of impairment of each of the functions considered can vary independently of the others, why not place any of them in the centre of the stage? The answer is that, in principle, there is no reason why this should not be done, and that, for some variables, it has been done, though not in a systematic fashion. Developmental receptive and expressive disorders of language have been intensively studied, and associations with poor motor coordination and with impairments of social interaction have been noted (Paul & Cohen, 1984; Paul, Cohen & Caparulo, 1983). Developmental clumsiness and visuospatial disorders have been examined in their own right and, again, associations with other impairments, including that of social interaction, have been commented on (Rourke, Young, Strang & Russell, 1986). If, in one specified geographic area, several epidemiologic studies were to be carried out simultaneously, one to identify all those with the triad of social impairments, others for developmental receptive language disorders, poor reading comprehension, motor clumsiness, and so on, then, depending on the total count of problems, some children would appear in all or most of the surveys, some in a few and some in only one.

Disagreements over diagnosis are particularly likely to occur concerning children with the triad who are of borderline or normal intelligence, since the autistic features may be present in less obvious forms. It is quite possible, for example, for such a child to be viewed by some as being impaired in social interaction, by others as having a developmental language impairment or as having a disorder of the ''pragmatic'' aspects of language (Rapin & Allen, 1983), and by yet others as a clumsy child. Provided that full investigation has confirmed that all these separate features are present, each of these diagnoses contributes information but tells only part of the story.

Schopler (1985) called attention to the overlap with learning disability of higher level autism and Asperger's syndrome. Examples of differing viewpoints on what appear to be similar problems can be found in the literature. Working in the field of behavioral neurology, Weintraub and Mesulam (1983) described 14 adults in whom (as pointed out by Denckla, 1983) the clinical picture resembled Asperger's syndrome, although there was no mention of circumscribed interests or other repetitive activities. Weintraub and Mesulam classified the problems as developmental learning disabilities of the right hemisphere. Rourke *et al.* (1986) examined and followed up a group of children with a cluster of arithmetic disabilities, poor visuomotor skills, and marked social abnormalities, which he referred to as central processing difficulties. These resembled the problems of the children classified in the present paper as active but odd, with repetitive speech. A linguist (McTear, 1985*a,b*) gave a detailed account of the speech of a child with marked impairment of conversational interaction, which the author termed pragmatic disorder. Similarly, Blank, Gessner and Esposito (1979) described a child with marked discrepancy between the conceptual and the social–interpersonal aspects of verbal behavior. The style of communication in both cases appeared to be the same as that found in people in the autistic continuum. Writing about a man he had studied over many years, Luria (1969) the famous Russian psychologist, concentrated on the bizarre hypertrophy of memory and on the literal interpretations of words, but there are hints throughout the account of a pattern of behavior that might now be considered to be within the more able end of the autistic continuum. Yet another point of view comes from the field of psychiatry. Wolff and colleagues (Wolff & Barlow, 1979; Wolff & Chick, 1980) classified a group of adolescents as schizoid personality, many if not all of whom have the syndrome described by Asperger. It would be beneficial both to the affected children and adults and to their families if workers in child development, neurology, and psychiatry were able to take a broad view of the subject and understand how the different approaches overlap and complement each other. Nevertheless, beyond all the other problems that may also be present, the triad of impairments of social interaction of the kind described here has such serious implications for the individual and his family that it must be recognized, whatever other handicaps are present.

HOW SPECIFIC ARE THE NAMED SYNDROMES?

Given that there is a tendency for some patterns to occur more often than others, even though there are no absolute divisions between them, it is appropriate to speculate on the reasons for this clustering. It seems unlikely that the patterns are related to gross aetiology. Any of the named or unnamed syndromes can be associated with a history of conditions likely to affect brain function, such as tuberose sclerosis, maternal rubella, perinatal trauma, encephalitis, or infantile spasms (Chess, 1971; Chess, Korn & Fernandez, 1971; Coleman & Gillberg, 1985; Wing & Gould, 1979). It appears likely that genetic factors are important in some cases (Folstein & Rutter, 1977). Recent reports point to an association with the fragile X chromosome (Gillberg, 1983; Mergash, Szymanski & Gerard, 1982), but it is by no means clear how specific this is to any one group within the range of those with the triad. The Camberwell epidemiologic study showed that evidence from the history or the present state suggestive of possible gross brain damage tends to be associated most often with social aloofness and severe general retardation, rather than with any particular named syndrome (Wing & Gould, 1979; Wing, 1981a).

A more likely hypothesis is that a particular area of the brain is concerned with the potential for social recognition, communication, and imagination and that the triad occurs when any pathologic process leads to its dysfunction. In this formulation, the triad is seen as primary, and not as a result of other impairments such as language disorders. It could, in theory at least, occur as the only problem, but much more often would be part of more widespread pathology. It appears that the brain areas organizing the development of language, nonverbal communication, and aspects of motor coordination are especially likely to be involved when the area responsible for social interaction is affected. Visuospatial and rote memory skills can also be impaired but are more likely to be spared than language and motor abilities. The tendency for clustering of particular impairments could perhaps be related to anatomic proximity of the relevant brain areas or to functional association, perhaps because of the biochemical mechanisms involved. When the triad occurs in almost pure form in people of borderline or normal intelligence, presumably the pathology must be precisely located and therefore limited in its effects.

There is no conclusive evidence concerning the specificity, whether defined by cause, or by brain area, or function affected, of any of the named syndromes within the range of the triad. However, it is very likely that advances in neuropathology will eventually allow subgroups to be defined reliably (Fein, Pennington, Markowitz, Braverman & Waterhouse, 1986; Fein, Skoff & Mirsky, 1981; Fein, Waterhouse, Lucci & Snyder, 1985). The profiles that have received particular attention are comparatively rare but have, in common, marked discrepancies in psychological functions, with high levels of performance in some areas contrasting with poor performance in others. These are so different from the usual picture, found in most normal people, of a moderately even level of skill in all areas, that they appear mysterious and fascinating to the lay public and to clinicians. By contrast, the single most common profile within the autistic continuum found in the Camberwell study was that seen in 24 children. It comprised social aloofness, severe or profound retardation, with no areas of better skills, apart from independent mobility, and with only simple (not complex) repetitive routines. The age-specific prevalence of this subgroup was 6.9 per 10,000 compared with 4.9 for Kanner's syndrome defined on two criteria and 2.0 defined on five criteria. It was the most stable clinical picture over time and place but has never been named as a syndrome. People with such problems have, on the whole, like the nonmobile group with the triad, been cared for by the services for the severely mentally retarded and have not come to the attention of psychiatrists, psychologists, neurologists, or linguists.

CLINICAL IMPLICATIONS

All aspects of development are important for the eventual achievement of independence in adult life, but social interaction has a special significance. Chronic impairment of this ability, however subtle, has a major effect on a child's ability to learn the rules of social life and to make use of any other skills he or she may have. This is true, whatever the person's level of intelligence and however helpful the upbringing and environment. Its presence militates against personal contentment, even in the tiny minority who have high academic achievements. It also has important implications for education, management, and treatment, regardless of IQ or the presence of other types of handicaps (Howlin & Rutter, 1987; Schopler, Reichler & Lansing, 1979a,b). The problems and needs are common to all forms of the triad and not just to the named syndromes. In clinical and educational practice, it is recognition of the triad that is crucial, and not the diagnosis of "specific" syndromes within the autistic continuum.

Children with the triad present particular problems to teachers, because of their severe behavioral and learning difficulties. Some are educated in specialist schools, but in all countries in which these are available they cater only for a small minority of affected children. Most have to be fitted into schools for other handicapped or for normal children. In such schools, those who are socially impaired stand out as different from and more difficult to help than the rest. Recognition of the nature of their disabilities and a full explanation are helpful to teachers. When they understand the reasons for the child's perplexing behavior, they can make use of the special techniques of education that have been developed for autistic children, insofar as pressures of time and the demands of others in the class allow. The principles underlying such techniques, suitably tailored to the individual child, are relevant across the whole IQ range, from profound retardation to superior ability. They are also relevant regardless of any other handicaps that may be present. Thus, a deaf child who is also autistic needs education based primarily on methods developed for autism, with secondary modifications to take account of the deafness, and similarly for other associated physical or psychological problems.

Parents, like teachers, are greatly helped if the presence of the triad, whether in severe, moderate, or mild form, is recognized early in the child's life. They need to know that the child is autistic or has a condition related to autism. This provides them with a reference group of other parents and helps relieve the feeling of isolation produced by having a child with a comparatively uncommon form of handicap. A diagnosis also gives them access to national and local voluntary societies for autistic people and to agencies providing specialist information and advice, including reading material. Many parents have never had the comfort of such sources of help because their children do not show the picture of typical Kanner's autism, although they do have the triad of impairments and need the same kind of education and management as the classically autistic child. There are also implications for prognosis. If the triad is present, prediction of outcome must be guarded. Those in the autistic continuum are likely to do less well than their IQ peers who do not have social impairment (Shah, 1985; Wing, 1981).

STANDARDIZED DIAGNOSTIC SYSTEMS

Identification of the presence of disorders in the autistic continuum has major implications for the individual and the family. Diagnostic practices are heavily influenced by the widely accepted standardized systems, so their adequacy is of considerable importance for both theory and practice.

The World Health Organization's *International Classification of Diseases* (9th edition) (ICD9) (WHO, 1977) and the American Psychiatric Association's *Diagnostic and Classification Manual* (3rd edition) (DSM-III) (APA, 1980) each contain systems for classifying autism and related conditions.

The ICD9 classification has the general heading, Psychoses with Origin Specific to Childhood. The ICD9 subgroups cover (1) typical autism, with onset up to 30 months (299.0 infantile autism); (2) a condition including social interaction impairment and stereotyped behavior beginning after a few years of normal development (299.1 disintegrative psychosis); (3) atypical autism, especially the form seen in severely retarded children (299.8 other); and (4) a remainder category (299.9 unspecified). This classification is a major advance on ICD8 that simply mentioned autism under *schizophrenia,* but it can now be seen to be unsatisfactory. *Psychosis* is an ill-defined term that should be replaced by a heading that indicates the developmental impairments underlying autistic and related behavioral patterns.

The description of typical autism is reasonably clear, but it would be difficult to fit the other clinical phenomena associated with the triad into the remaining categories. The higher-functioning groups, including the one described by Asperger, would be particularly difficult to classify. A further problem is the use of the age of onset as a defining criterion for *infantile autism* and for so-called *disintegrative psychosis.* Children are seen at clinics at varying times after the appearance of behavioral abnormalities, sometimes years later, and age of onset is notoriously difficult to establish. There is no statement in the literature clearly specifying the clinical differences between autistic or autistic-like behavior present from birth or reportedly following a period of normal development. Until there is a method of establishing age of onset reliably, or rules for distinguishing autism and disintegrative psychosis on clinical or other grounds, it would appear best to diagnose and subclassify on currently available clinical criteria alone and to note reported age of onset separately.

The DSM-III system refers to *pervasive developmental disorder,* which is a considerable improvement on *psychosis,* but can be criticized on the grounds that many people with autism and similar conditions have better skills in some areas than others, so the term *Pervasive* is not entirely appropriate. It was presumably chosen because of the great importance and pervasive impact of the impairment of social interaction, but it can easily be misunderstood.

Again, the DSM-III system emphasizes age of onset, listing (1) infantile autism (299.0) with age of onset before 30 months, and (2) childhood-onset pervasive developmental disorder (299.9) with onset after 30 months but before age 12 years. The distribution of behavioral items between these two categories is particularly odd, since each seems to have been assigned one half of the features described in detailed accounts of typical autism, and it is not clear how or why they have been divided in this way. Thus, immediate and delayed echolalia are mentioned only under infantile autism, and abnormal movements such as tiptoe walking only under childhood-onset disorder, although both are found in those with infantile onset. There is also a remainding category (3) atypical pervasive developmental disorder (299.8).

As with the ICD, DSM-III presents problems in finding suitable categories for many people with the triad, especially the most and the least severely handicapped.

However, DSM-III-Revised (APA,1987) does cover the full range of social impairment under the general heading of Pervasive Developmental Disorder. Only two categories, namely Autistic Disorder, and Pervasive Developmental Disorder Not Otherwise Specified, are used. Age of onset is coded on a digit separate from the clinical condition.

Standardized diagnostic systems have to balance uneasily between representing views generally accepted at the time of formulation, and permitting scope for research leading to new ideas on classification. In the present state of knowledge, there is much to be said for having a general category that includes all those with the triad, with subcategories based on the two factors that are demonstrably related to current needs for education and other services, and to eventual prognosis, i.e., level of intelligence (Rutter, 1970) and quality of social interaction (aloof, passive, and odd) (Shah, 1985; Wing, 1981). Perhaps such a pragmatic scheme is too far removed from received wisdom to be acceptable. A possible compromise would be to define "typical Kanner's autism", and "other," and to subdivide each of these into mildly, moderately and severely handicapped depending upon levels of intelligence. In clinical practice, some system of naming is needed that will differentiate the more able from the more handicapped, since many parents find it difficult to accept a diagnosis that places a child of normal or superior intelligence in the same category as one who is severely or profoundly retarded.

A really comprehensive and helpful system of classification would be one that included all types of developmental disorders of psychological function and the ways in which they influence each other. However, this requires further progress in understanding the relationships between patterns of cognitive, language, and social skills and overt behavior.

FUTURE RESEARCH

The issues discussed in this chapter pose many questions that cannot yet be answered. Detailed studies of the clinical phenomena would help to clarify the relationships among the different manifestations of the triad. Population-based studies, including long-term follow-up, would be of particular value. This would permit an examination of the borderlines between social impairment and other developmental disorders of psychological functions and also between mild social impairment and eccentric normality. Some variations in the clinical picture may prove to be related to etiologic factors. The comparison of impairment of social interaction dating from early childhood with the loss of social skills following severe psychiatric illness in adult life would also be of interest. Devising psychological and psychophysiologic techniques to explore the same problems would be of special value, since they would permit more standardization of method than is possible with clinical observation.

The development of standardized measures of quality of social interaction would greatly facilitate work in this field. The major problem would be to create methods of assessment that could be adapted for subjects of any level of age and IQ.

Kanner believed the fundamental problem in autism to be a "profound lack of affective contact with others." The ideas expressed in this chapter represent a return to this view, but with modifications and elaborations based on research carried out since Kanner's original papers. It is now generally agreed that the cause is brain dysfunction and has nothing to do with the parents' methods of childrearing or the child's early experiences. However, there is a division of opinion as to whether the social impairment is primarily an abnormality of the brain areas concerned with social and affective behavior (Fein et al., 1986; Hermelin & O'Connor, 1985) or is based on lack of certain specific cognitive skills needed to interpret and respond to social situations (Baron-Cohen, 1985; Baron-Cohen et al., 1985, 1986). Data can be found to support either of these views (Shah & Wing, 1986). The important task is to identify the brain mechanisms responsible for empathic social interaction, regardless of whether this ability should be termed emotional or cognitive, or a combination of both. So far, investigations by brain scans or at post mortem have revealed no specific pathology, but the techniques available are still relatively crude. It is to be hoped that advances in the methodology of examining the brain during life will eventually provide the answers.

REFERENCES

American Psychiatric Association. (3rd ed., 1980). *Diagnostic and statistical manual of mental disorders*. Washington, DC.: American Psychiatric Association.

American Psychiatric Association. (3rd ed. rev., 1987). *Diagnostic and statistical manual of mental disorders*. Washington, DC.: American Psychiatric Association.

Asperger, H. (1944). Die autistischen psychopathen im kindersalter. *Archiv fur Psychiatrie und Nervenkrankheiten, 117,* 76–136.

Attwood, A. (1984). *The gestures of autistic children*. Unpublished doctoral thesis, University of London.

Baltaxe, C. A. M. (1977). Pragmatic deficits in the language of autistic adolescents. *Journal of Paediatric Psychology, 2,* 176–80.

Baron-Cohen, S. (1985). *Social cognition and pretend play in autism*. Unpublished doctoral thesis, University of London.

Baron-Cohen, S., Leslie, A. M., & Frith, U. (1985). Does the autistic child have a ''theory of mind''? *Cognition, 21,* 37–46.

Baron-Cohen, S., Leslie, A. M., & Frith, U. (1986). Mechanical, behavioural and intentional understanding of picture stories in autistic children. *British Journal of Developmental Psychology, 4,* 113–25.

Bartak, L., Rutter, M., & Cox, A. (1975). A comparative study of infantile autism and specific developmental receptive language disorder. I. The children. *British Journal of Psychiatry, 126,* 127–45.

Bartak, L., Rutter, M., & Cox, A. (1977). A comparative study of infantile autism and specific developmental speech disorders. III. Discriminant function analysis. *Journal of Autism and Childhood Schizophrenia, 6,* 297–302.

Bender, L. (1947). Childhood schizophrenia: A clinical study of 100 schizophrenic children. *American Journal of Orthopsychiatry, 17,* 40–56.

Bender, L. (1961). The brain and child behaviour, *Archives of General Psychiatry, 4,* 531–47.

Blank, M., Gessner, M., & Esposito, A. (1979). Language without communication: a case study. *Journal of Child Language, 6,* 329–52.

Boucher, J. (1981). Memory for recent events in autistic children. *Journal of Autism and Developmental Disorders, 11,* 293–302.

Bretherton, I., McNew, S., & Beeghley-Smith, M. (1981). Early person knowledge as expressed in gestural and verbal communication: When do infants acquire a ''theory of mind''? In M. E. Lamb & L. R. Sherrod (Eds.), *Infant social cognition.* Hillsdale, NJ: Erlbaum.

Bullowa, M. (Ed.) (1979). *Before speech: the beginning of interpersonal communication.* London: Cambridge University Press.

Chess, S. (1971). Autism in children with congenital rubella. *Journal of Autism and Childhood Schizophrenia, 1,* 33–47.

Chess, S. (1977). Follow-up report on autism in congenital rubella. *Journal of Autism and Childhood Schizophrenia, 7,* 69–81.

Chess, S., Korn, S. J., & Fernandez, P. B. (1971). *Psychiatric disorders of children with congenital rubella.* New York: Brunner/Mazel.

Coleman, M. & Gillberg, C. (1985). *The biology of the autistic syndromes.* New York: Praeger.

Cromer, R. F. (1981). Developmental language disorders: Cognitive processes, semantics pragmatics, phonology, and syntax. *Journal of Autism and Developmental Disorders, 11*(1), 57–73.

Damasio, A. R., & Maurer, E. G. (1978). A neurological model for childhood autism. *Archives of Neurology, 35,* 777–86.

DeMyer, M. (1976). Motor, perceptual–motor and intellectual disabilities of autistic children. In L. Wing (Ed.), *Early childhood autism* (2nd ed.). Oxford: Pergamon.

DeMyer, M. (1979). *Parents and children in autism,* Washington, D. C.: Winston.

Denckla, M. (1983). The neuro-psychology of social-emotional learning disabilities. *Archives of Neurology, 40,* 461–3.

Despert, J. C. (1938). Schizophrenia in children. *Psychiatric Quarterly, 12,* 366–71.

Earl, C. J. C. (1943). The primitive catatonic psychosis of idiocy. *British Journal of Medical Psychology, 14,* 230–53.

Fay, W., & Schuler, A. L. (1980). *Emerging language in autistic children.* Baltimore: University Park Press.

Fein, D., Pennington, B., Markowitz, P., Braverman, M., & Waterhouse, L. (1986). Toward a neuropsychological model of autism: Are the social deficits primary? *Journal of the American Academy of Child Psychiatry, 25,* 198–212.

Fein, D., Skoff, B., & Mirsky, A. F. (1981). Clinical correlates of brain-stem dysfunction in autistic children. *Journal of Autism and Developmental Disorders, 11,* 303–15.

Fein, D., Waterhouse, L., Lucci, D., & Snyder, D. (1985). Cognitive subtypes in developmentally disabled children; a pilot study. *Journal of Autism and Developmental Disorders, 15,* 77–96.

Folstein, S., & Rutter, M. (1977). Infantile autism: A genetic study of 21 twin pairs. *Journal of Child Psychology and Psychiatry, 18,* 297–322.

Frith, U. (1982). Psychological abnormalities in early childhood psychoses. In J. K. Wing & L. Wing (Eds.), *Handbook of psychiatry* (Vol. 3). Cambridge: Cambridge University Press.

Frith, U., & Snowling, M. (1983). Reading for meaning and reading for sound in autistic and dyslexic children. *British Journal of Developmental Psychology, 1,* 329–42.

Gillberg, C. (1983). Identical triplets with infantile autism and the Fragile X syndrome. *British Journal of Psychiatry, 143,* 256–60.

Goldfarb, W. (1974). *Growth and change of schizophrenic children.* New York: Wiley.

Gould, J. (1982). *Social communication and imagination in children with cognitive and language impairments.* Unpublished doctoral thesis, University of London.

Gould, J. (1986). The Lowe & Costello Symbolic Play Test in socially impaired children. *Journal of Autism and Developmental Disorder, 16,* 199–213.

Hermelin, B., & O'Connor, N. (1985). Logico-affective states and non-verbal language. In E. Schopler & G. Mesibov (Eds.), *Communication problems in autism.* New York: Plenum.

Hobson, R. P. (1986). The autistic child's appraisal of expressions of emotion. *Journal of Child Psychology and Psychiatry, 27,* 321–42.

Howlin, P., & Rutter, M. (1987). *Treatment of autistic children.* Chichester: Wiley.

Hulse, W. C. (1954). Dementia infantilis. *Journal of Nervous and Mental Diseases, 119,* 471–7.

Kanner, L. (1943). Autistic disturbances of affective contact. *Nervous Child, 2,* 27–250.

Kanner, L. (1946). Irrelevant and metaphorical language in early childhood autism. *American Journal of Psychiatry, 103,* 242–6.

Kanner, L. (1949). Problems of nosology and psychodynamics in early childhood autism. *American Journal of Orthopsychiatry, 19,* 416–26.

Kanner, L., & Eisenberg, L. (1956). Early infantile autism 1943–1955. *American Journal of Orthopsychiatry, 26,* 55–65.

Kolvin, I. (1971). Studies in the childhood psychoses. I. Diagnostic criteria and classification. *British Journal of Psychiatry, 118,* 381–4.

Kolvin, I., Ounsted, C., Humphrey, M., & McNay, A. (1971). II. The Phenomenology of Childhood psychoses. *British Journal of Psychiatry, 118,* 385–95.

Lockyer, L., & Rutter, M. (1969). A five to fifteen year follow-up study of infantile psychosis. III. Psychological aspects. *British Journal of Psychiatry, 115,* 865–82.

Lord, C. (1984). The development of peer relations in children with autism. In F. J. Morrison, C. Lord, & D. P. Keating (Eds.), *Advances in applied developmental psychology.* New York: Academic.

Luria, A. R. (1969). *The mind of a mnemonist.* London: Jonathan Cape.

McTear, M. F. (1985). Pragmatic disorders: A question of direction. *British Journal of Disorders of Communication, 20,* 119–27.

McTear, M. F. (1985). Pragmatic disorders: A case study of conversational disability. *British Journal of Disorders of Communication, 20,* 129–42.

Mahler, M. S. (1952). On child psychoses and schizophrenia: autistic and symbiotic infantile psychoses. *Psychoanalytic Study of the Child, 7,* 286–305.

Mergash, D. L., Szymanski, L., & Gerald, P. (1982). Infantile autism associated with fragile X syndrome. *Journal of Autism and Developmental Disorders, 12,* 295–301.

Newson, J., & Newson, E. (1975). Intersubjectivity and the transmission of culture: On the social origins of symbolic functioning. *Bulletin of the British Psychological Society, 28,* 437–46.

Ornitz, E. M. (1974). The modulation of sensory input and motor input in autistic children. *Journal of Autism & Childhood Schizophrenia, 4,* 197–216.

O'Connor, N., & Hermelin, B. (1984). Idiot savant calendrical calculators: Maths or memory? *Psychological Medicine, 14,* 801–6.

Paul, R., & Cohen, D. J. (1984). Outcomes of severe disorders of language acquisition. *Journal of Autism and Developmental Disorders, 14,* 405–22.

Paul, R., Cohen, D. J., & Caparulo, B. K. (1983). A longitudinal study of patients with severe developmental disorders of language learning. *Journal of the American Academy of Child Psychiatry, 22,* 525–34.

Pawlby, S. (1977). Imitative interaction. In H. R. Schaffer (Ed.), *Studies in mother-infant interaction* New York: Academic.

Rapin, I., & Allen, D. A. Developmental language disorders: Nosologic considerations. In U. Kirk (Ed.), *Neuropsychology of language, reading, and spelling.* New York: Academic Press.

Ricks, D. M. (1975). Vocal communication in pre-verbal normal and autistic children. In N. O'Connor (Ed.), *Language, cognitive deficits and retardation.* London: Butterworths.

Ricks, D. M. (1979). Making sense of experience to make sensible sounds. In M. Bullowa (Ed.), *Before Speech: The beginning of interpersonal communication.* Cambridge: Cambridge University Press.

Ricks, D. M., & Wing, L. (1975). Language, communication, and the use of symbols in normal and autistic children. *Journal of Autism and Childhood Schizophrenia, 5,* 191–221.

Rourke, B. P., Young, G. C., Strang, J. D., & Russell, D. L. (1986). Adult outcomes of central processing deficiencies in childhood. In I. Grant, and K. M. Adams (Eds.), *Neuropsychological assessment of neuropsychiatric disorders.* Oxford: Oxford University Press.

Rutter, M. (1966). Behavioural and cognitive characteristics. In J. K. Wing (Ed.), *Early childhood autism.* Oxford: Pergamon.

Rutter, M. (1970). Autistic children: Infancy to adulthood. *Seminars in Psychiatry, 2,* 435–50.

Rutter, M. (1972). Psychiatric causes of language retardation. In M. Rutter and J. A. M. Marten (Eds.), *The child with delayed speech,* London: Heinemann.

Sacks, O. (1985). *The man who mistook his wife for a hat.* London: Duckworth.

Schaffer, H. R. (1974). Early social behaviour and the study of reciprocity. *Bulletin of the British Psychological Society, 27,* 209–16.

Schaffer, H. R. (1979). Acquiring the concept of the dialogue. In M. H. Bornstein and W. Kessen (Eds.), *Psychological development from infancy: image to intention.* Hillsdale, NJ: Erlbaum.

Schaffer, H. R., Collis, G. M., & Parsons, G. (1977). *Vocal interchange and visual regard in verbal and pre-verbal children.* London: Academic.

Schawlow, A. T., & Schawlow, A. L. (1985). Our son: the endless search for help. In M. P. Brady and P. L. Gunter (Eds.), *Integrating moderately and severely handicapped learners.* Springfield, IL: Charles C Thomas.

Schopler, E. (1985). Editorial: Convergence of learning disability, higher level autism and Asperger's syndrome. *Journal of Autism and Developmental Disorders, 15,* 359–60.

Schopler, E., & Mesibov, G. B. (1985). *Communication problems in autism.* New York: Plenum.

Schopler, E., Reichler, R. J., & Lansing, M. (1979a). *Individualized assessment and treatment for autistic and developmentally disabled children. Vol. 1. Psychoeducational profile.* Baltimore: University Press.

Schopler, E., Reichler, R. J., & Lansing, M. (1979b). *Individualized assessment and treatment for autistic and developmentally disabled children. Vol. 2. Teaching strategies for parents and professionals.* Baltimore: University Press.

Selfe, L. (1977). *Nadia: A case of extraordinary drawing ability in an autistic child.* London: Academic.

Shah, A. (1985). Impairment of social interaction in autism and mental retardation: A 12 year follow up study. Paper given at the *7th World Congress of the International Association for the Scientific Study of Mental Deficiency.* New Delhi.

Shah, A., & Wing, L. (1986). Cognitive impairments affecting social behaviour in autism. In E. Schopler & G. Mesibov (Eds.), *Social behavior problems in autism.* New York: Plenum.

Shah, A., Holmes, N., & Wing, L. (1982). Prevalence of autism and related conditions in adults in a mental handicap hospital. *Applied Research in Mental Retardation, 1982, 3,* 303–17.

Shantz, C. U. (1985). Social cognition. In J. H. Flavell and E. M. Markman (Eds.), *Cognitive development: handbook of child psychology* (Vol. 3). New York: Wiley.

Spitzer, R. (Chairman) (1985). *Draft of DSM-III-Revised in development.* Washington, D.C.: American Psychiatric Association.

Tager-Flusberg, H. (1981). Sentence comprehension in autistic children. *Applied Psycholinguistics, 2,* 5–24.

Trevarthen, C. (1974). Conversations with a two-month old. *New Scientist, 62,* 230–5.

Weintraub, S., & Mesulam, M. M. Developmental learning disabilities of the right hemisphere. *Archives of Neurology, 40,* 463–8.

Wing, L. (1980). *Autistic children: A guide for parents.* London: Constable.

Wing, L. (1981). Cognitive and social skills associated with outcome in childhood autism and related conditions. Paper given at the *25th Anniversary of the Children's Clinic, Department of Neuropsychiatry, Kyoto University Hospital.* Kyoto.

Wing, L. (1981a). Language, social and cognitive impairments in autism and severe mental retardation. *Journal of Autism and Developmental Disorders, 11,* 31–44.

Wing, L. (1981b). Asperger's syndrome: A clinical account. *Psychological Medicine, 11,* 115–29.

Wing, L. (1982). Development of concepts, classification and relationship to mental retardation. In J. K. Wing & L. Wing (Eds.), *Psychoses of uncertain aetiology: Handbook of psychiatry* (Vol. 3). Cambridge: Cambridge University Press.

Wing, L., & Gould, J. (1979). Severe impairments of social interaction and associated abnormalities in children: Epidemiology and classification. *Journal of Autism and Developmental Disorders, 9,* 11–29.

Wing, L., Gould, J., Yeates, S. R., & Brierley, L. M. (1977). Symbolic play in severely mentally retarded and in autistic children. *Journal of Child Psychology and Psychiatry. 18,* 167–78.

Wing, L., & Hayhurst, M. (1973). A study of mentally retarded adults in Camberwell. In D. J. Hall., N. C. Robertson, & R. J. Eason (Eds.), *Proceedings of the Conference on Psychiatric Case Registers, University of Aberdeen, March 1973.* London: D.H.S.S. Statistical and Research Series No. 7, Her Majesty's Stationery Office.

Wolff, S., & Barlow, A. (1977). Schizoid personality in childhood: A comparative study of schizoid, autistic and normal children. *Journal of Child Psychology and Psychiatry, 20,* 29–46.

Wolff, S., & Chick, J. (1980). Schizoid personality in childhood: A controlled follow-up study. *Psychological Medicine, 10,* 85–100.

World Health Organization. (1977). *Manual of the international statistical classification of diseases, injuries and causes of death* (9th rev. Vol. 1). Geneva: World Health Organization.

8

Multiaxial Diagnostic Approaches

DENNIS P. CANTWELL and LORIAN BAKER

INTRODUCTION

This chapter deals with diagnostic approaches in child psychiatry. The chapter begins with a discussion of why diagnostic classification is desirable and a summary of the basic principles of such classification. The goals and requirements of a classification system are outlined, and four types of classification systems (categorical, dimensional, uniaxial, and multiaxial) are explained. The type of multiaxial classification system used in DSM-III is explained, and two case histories of autistic children are provided to illustrate how such an approach is superior to a uniaxial system. Finally, some of the unresolved issues having to do with the DSM-III classification system are presented, and the relevance of these issues to the diagnosis and classification of autism is noted.

RATIONALE FOR CLASSIFICATION

Purposes and Principles of Classification in Child Psychiatry

The most significant purpose of a diagnostic classification system is to facilitate professional communication. This communication is enhanced by the use of a diagnostic classification system both with regard to individual practitioners communicating about a specific patient and with regard to the broader communication that occurs in the field through professional journals and meetings.

By referring to a particular diagnostic label rather than listing all the features that constitute a disorder, professional communication is considerably expedited. Furthermore, the use of a system of common terminology facilitates research by means of the uniform identification of patients and permits comparison of research studies from different facilities. In this way, a diagnostic system can allow for the prediction of the natural course of a condition and the identification of commonly associated features that are important in management.

This point is well illustrated by the specific syndrome of autism. Kanner (1958) argued

DENNIS P. CANTWELL and LORIAN BAKER • Neuropsychiatric Institute, University of California at Los Angeles, Los Angeles, California 90024.

in his early work that it was crucial from the standpoint of treatment to differentiate autistic children not only from mentally retarded children, but also from other types of psychotic children. At the time of the delineation of the syndrome by Kanner (1943), little was known about the natural outcome or response to treatment of the disorder. However, although there is still considerable controversy about the disorder, much is now known about its long-term effects (DeMyer, Hingtgen & Jackson, 1981).

The basic principles of classification of childhood psychopathology have been discussed fully in a previous publication (Cantwell, 1980). However, it is necessary to reiterate briefly some of the basic principles as they apply to diagnosis and classification of childhood psychopathology in general, and in particular to the classification of autism and pervasive developmental disorders. First, it is currently accepted that any successful psychiatric classification system will be based on facts rather than on theoretical concepts.

Second, etiology has generally not turned out to be a fruitful way of classifying childhood psychopathology. Many disorders of childhood and adolescence that present with the same phenomenologic picture may have developed on the basis of different etiologic factors in different children. Since there are major differences in thinking about the etiology of various disorders, etiology could not form the basis of a system to be used for communication between individuals with different theoretical orientations.

For example, with regard to the syndrome of autism, it was formerly believed that autism developed on some type of psychosocial basis. It is now clear that most autistic children have some form of brain damage or brain dysfunction that can be demonstrated. Nevertheless, no specific, unique, agent, mechanism, or correlate has been discovered to produce autism. Nonetheless, although professionals from different theoretical backgrounds may disagree about how autism develops, they can agree on the presence of the diagnosis of autism in a particular child.

Goals of a Classification System

A good child psychiatric classification system will provide adequate differentiation between different disorders and between disordered children and normal children. A good system will also provide adequate coverage of patients who present with different types of disorders. No child psychiatric classification system is ideal. An ideal system would ensure that every child who presents for evaluation will meet the criteria of one and only one disorder within that particular classification system. This is not realistic. We know that at least 25% of psychiatrically ill adults receive a diagnosis of ''undiagnosed mental disorder'' if strict diagnostic criteria are used (Goodwin & Guze, 1979).

In addition to adequate coverage, an ideal classification system would also provide adequate differentiation between the various diagnostic conditions described in the system. It is important not only to provide categories that permit adequate differentiation of disordered children from normal children, but also adequate differentiation of children with different types of psychiatric disorders from each other.

Specifically, with regard to autism, the classification system should allow not only differentiation of autistic children from normal children but also of autistic children from children with schizophrenia, children with developmental language disorders, children who suffer severe psychosocial and environmental deprivation, children with mental retardation, children with severe significant hearing problems and others that may be confused with autism. Furthermore, it would be most useful to be able to classify children who do not meet clear clinical criteria for autism but who are clearly psychiatrically disordered and have a disorder that is somewhat similar to autism in one or more of the basic core symptom areas. It was this type of child that the childhood-onset pervasive developmental disorder diagnosis was attempting to categorize in DSM-III.

It is also important that a classification system for childhood psychopathology be able to distinguish children with these disorders at various ages. Children are still developing organisms, and it is not realistic to expect that their phenomenologic symptom pattern will remain clearly the same in infancy, preschool, early grade school, late grade school, early adolescence, mid-adolescence, late adolescence, early adult life, and so forth. Classification systems of childhood psychopathology have the added problem of defining normality versus abnormality for different ages and different developmental levels. Thus, a developmental framework in any classification system of childhood psychopathology is crucial.

Two necessary features of a diagnostic classification system are: (1) that it can be used reliably, and (2) that the disorders it describes have some degree of validity. Reliability refers to the extent to which the users of a classification system can agree on its usage when applied to specific cases.

There are multiple sources of unreliability in the diagnosis of childhood psychopathology (Spitzer & Williams, 1980). These include some combination of information variance (when clinicians have different sources of information), observation and interpretation variance (when clinicians differ in their interpretations of the same information), and criterion variance (when there are differences in the criteria that clinicians use to summarize data into diagnoses). Among these types of unreliability, a classification system can only affect criterion variance by delineating specific diagnostic criteria that must be present for the disorder to be diagnosed.

Deciding which criteria are right leads to the question of validity. Autism is one disorder that has a good degree of face validity and descriptive validity. It has face validity in that a number of clinicians agree that a disorder exists with a clinical picture generally similar to that which was originally described by Leo Kanner. Also, autism is characterized by symptoms, particularly the social relatedness symptoms, that are not commonly seen in persons with no mental disorder or in individuals with other types of mental disorders. Thus, autism among all child psychiatric disorders has a good degree of descriptive validity. Autism also has a good degree of predictive validity among child psychiatric disorders. (Ways of fully validating disorders in any classification system are discussed below in the comparison of categorical and dimensional systems.)

TYPES OF CLASSIFICATION SYSTEMS

Defining Disorders by Categorical or Dimensional Methods

Categorical Approaches

Two general approaches to the categorization of symptoms into a diagnostic classification system are (1) the categorical approach, and (2) the dimensional approach. Categorical systems have formed the basis of most of the "official" classification systems of psychiatric disorder both for adults and for children. This includes the current International Classification of Diseases (ICD), its predecessors, and the current DSM-III and its predecessors.

The categorical approach owes much to the medical model. The implication is that children who present with a particular clinical picture differ not only from normals but also from children with other clinical pictures in ways other than their clinical picture, including outcome, etiology, and treatment response. In developing criteria for a categorical diagnostic system, workers must first form a clinical concept for which there is some degree of face validity. Then, attempts are made to increase the descriptive validity of the category by narrowing the definition so as to discriminate persons with the disorder.

This process can be seen with regard to the syndrome of infantile autism. Leo Kanner originally described 11 children who presented with a rather unique clinical picture he referred to as infantile autism. Later clinicians used and refined that prototype model to decide whether particular children met Kanner's criteria for infantile autism.

On a larger scale, the development of a categorical classification system for a number of psychiatric disorders was pioneered by the Washington University group in St. Louis. Their work, which became known as the "Feighner criteria" (Feighner et al., 1972) presented criteria for the diagnosis of a limited number of psychiatric disorders that had been validated in a five stage scheme: (1) clinical description, (2) delimitation from other disorders, (3) laboratory studies, (4) family studies, and (5) follow-up studies.

This approach has been modified and expanded by a number of researchers, including Cantwell (1975); Spitzer, Endicott, and Robins (1978); and Klerman (1983). Cantwell (1975) modified the original Washington University five phase scheme for the validation of psychiatric disorders for particular use with disorders of childhood. His six-stage scheme for validation of categorical diagnoses in childhood psychiatry included (1) clinical picture, (2) physical and neurologic factors, (3) laboratory studies, (4) family studies, (5) follow-up studies, and (6) treatment studies.

Klerman (1983) outlined an approach for validation of categorical diagnoses that expanded on the Washington University scheme. Once one established criteria for a particular syndrome such as infantile autism and collected reliable clinical data, the first step would be the demonstration of internal validity. This essentially means that the consistency of the symptoms that comprise the essential diagnostic criteria for this syndrome can be demonstrated, usually by correlational statistical methods. The second step would be the external validation of the clinical syndrome using as external validating criteria (1) epidemiologic data, (2) family aggregation data, (3) biologic laboratory studies, (4) correlation with psychosocial factors, (5) natural history studies, and (6) response to treatment studies.

Such approaches to establishing the diagnostic criteria for categorical classification systems are far more sophisticated than the early attempt by Kanner to define infantile autism. Although the original description of infantile autism began with a clinical description and a delimitation from other disorders, there was no attempt to demonstrate validity using biologic laboratory data, natural history studies, or other data. Nonetheless, later in life, Kanner did follow up his original group. He also suggested initially that there may be a particular type of family situation associated with the clinical description of autism.

Currently, of all child psychiatric disorders, autism is one of the best studied and best validated both along internal validation lines and external validation lines as outlined above. Space precludes a complete discussion of this issue.

Dimensional Approaches

A second approach to categorizing symptoms into a diagnostic classification system is the dimensional approach. This involves the derivation of diagnostic categories by various mathematical procedures. The use of the dimensional approach grew out of the recognition that child psychopathology is characterized by "an immense variety of behaviors, most of which are displayed to some extent by most children" (Achenbach, 1980). It was hoped that the application of mathematical procedures would result in the emergence of new diagnostic categories that had not been detected by clinical practice.

The use of the dimensional approach begins with quantifying of behaviors and examining the tendency of specific items of behavior to occur together. Once correlations among individual items of behavior are computed, groups of items that regularly co-occur together can be detected by multivariate statistical analyses of the correlations.

The simplest example of this approach is the factor analysis in which factors are established consisting of groups of items. An item (usually a symptom) can load on one or more factors, and the loading will range from -1.0 to $+1.0$. The loading of an item on a factor shows how strongly the item correlates with a dimension defined by a particular factor. Thus, for example, items like: "can't relate to people," "treats people the same as objects," "ritualistic–compulsive behavior," "deviant or delayed language" may load on an "autism factor" but may also load on other factors. The higher the correlation of an individual item with a particular factor, the greater the loading on that particular factor.

Factor analysis, however, only classifies types of behavior and does not classify individuals in the way that categorical classification systems do. In order to classify individuals using a dimensional approach, cluster analysis is used. Cluster analysis forms groups of individuals that are mutually exclusive in that each individual is a member of only one cluster. This poses potential problems for those individuals with borderline types of disorders or overlapping syndromes (who would receive two separate diagnoses such as infantile autism and attention deficit disorder in a categorical system).

A second problem with the dimensional approach has to do with the validity of the classifications it makes. Although the dimensional approach was conceived as a highly objective method, in fact there is considerable arbitrariness in the selection of items to input into the model and in the selection of which mathematical criteria to use to execute the model. As a result, the syndromes created using this type of approach often cannot be cross-validated in other samples. Review of dimensional classifications of psychiatric disorders reveals that there are several syndromes that occur repeatedly and cut across all studies (called broadband syndromes).

There are, however, a large number of syndromes that have been repeatedly diagnosed by categorical systems and are well-studied but that do not turn up in these dimensional statistical studies. One such condition is infantile autism.

Autism is a relatively rare condition. Thus, unless any patient sample or broad-based epidemiologic sample is extremely large, it is not likely that many autistic children will be included. When no autistic subjects are included in the sample used to determine multivariate-based syndromes, no autistic factor can emerge from the initial data analysis. By extension, no autistic syndrome can emerge when mathematical techniques of cluster analysis are applied. Thus, autism and related behavioral clusters have rarely turned up in large scale epidemiologic studies using multivariate statistical techniques.

Multiaxial versus Uniaxial Classification Systems

The above discussion regarding dimensional and categorical approaches to the classification of psychiatric syndromes centered on observable symptomatology. However, other aspects of syndromes also are relevant to their classification. Such aspects include medical factors (physical disorders, neurologic symptoms, data from laboratory studies), psychosocial factors (family data, demographic information) and assessment factors (natural history, functioning and/or impairment in various areas, and treatment data).

One way to capture these aspects in a psychiatric classification system is to use a multidimensional or multiaxial system in which various domains or axes are classified separately. (To avoid confusion with the dimensional approaches described above, we use the term multiaxial to refer to this type of multidimensionality.) Within such a multiaxial scheme, classifications on the different axes could be either categorical or dimensional.

There are conceptual and pragmatic reasons why having a multiaxial system is potentially richer than having a uniaxial diagnostic system. Conceptually, having different domains that should be coded each time one evaluates a patient offers the potential for a much richer description of an individual child in terms of factors such as family factors, other psychosocial factors, intelligence, presence or absence of developmental disorders, all of which may predict outcome and response to treatment better than any particular single diagnosis could. For research purposes, the coding of multiple domains may permit recognition of associations between particular disorders and environmental or biologic factors that have hitherto been unrealized. Pragmatically, the coding of multiple domains may prevent overlooking important issues that are present in a particular clinical patient.

The use of a multiaxial classification system may be particularly desirable when dealing with children because of the variety of disciplines involved in helping children. When childhood problems first manifest themselves, the most appropriate source of help is not always clear. This is particularly true for a pervasive disorder such as autism where functioning is likely to be impaired in cognitive, linguistic, social, emotional, educational, and behavioral domains. Children presenting with such a disorder might, with almost equal likelihood, find themselves in the offices of a pediatrician, a child psychologist, a neurologist, a speech pathologist, an otolaryngologist, a social worker, an educational tutor or a child psychiatrist. Indeed, depending on who first evaluates the child, he or she may receive diagnoses of mental retardation, developmental language disorder, disturbed family relations, learning disability, hyperkinesis, neurologic defects, or infantile autism. Clearly, a diagnostic framework in which all these areas of functioning could be addressed, would promote the best interdisciplinary professional communication.

Despite the apparent advantages of a multiaxial system of diagnosis and classification, the systems predominantly used in the past in the field of psychiatry have been uniaxial. This includes the ICDs, GAP, and DSM-I and DSM-II. DSM-III introduced a multiaxial classification system for the first time, although a multiaxial system had been discussed by the World Health Organization (Rutter, Shaffer & Shephard, 1975). The DSM-III multiaxial system is described below.

THE DSM-III MULTIAXIAL DIAGNOSTIC SYSTEM

Description of the System

The DSM-III scheme uses five axes. The first axis contains all the psychiatric clinical syndromes and those conditions that are not considered to be a mental disorder but could be the focus of evaluation and treatment (represented by V codes). These include such problems as borderline intellectual functioning and parent–child problems. Axis II in DSM-III contains the specific developmental disorders and the personality disorders. Thus, Axes I and II describe the clinical conditions.

The rationale for separating the specific developmental disorders and the personality disorders from the other clinical syndromes is a pragmatic one. Systematic studies of children suggest that if the child has a florid clinical syndrome such as conduct disorder and a developmental disorder such as reading disorder, the developmental disorder is more likely to be omitted from diagnoses in a unidimensional system. Likewise, an adult may have a florid clinical syndrome such as an acute episode of schizophrenic disorder along with a longstanding personality disorder. The longstanding personality disorder is more likely to be diagnosed if it is on a separate axis than if it is coded in a unidimensional diagnostic system.

Axis III of DSM-III is for physical disorders and conditions which are currently present and which exist outside of the mental disorders section of ICD-9. In DSM-III, only those physical disorders that are potentially relevant to either the understanding or the management of a particular disorder are considered for Axis III. Thus, a physical disorder such as epilepsy, diabetes, or asthma is only coded if it is necessary for the proper understanding and/or management of an Axis I or II condition.

In an autistic child who has a temporal lobe seizure disorder of longstanding duration, the coding of the temporal lobe seizure disorder is necessary for a complete understanding and management of the case. It should be pointed out that the Axis III conditions are not necessarily etiologic to the Axis I or Axis II disorders, although in some cases they may be. However, in most cases, Axis III disorders are associated problems that must be recognized for proper understanding and management of the Axis I and II conditions.

Axis IV may be viewed as the psychosocial complement of Axis III. Just as Axis III represents physical biologic conditions that should be coded for the proper understanding and/or management of Axis I or II conditions, so does Axis IV represent psychosocial factors that may also play the same role. In DSM-III, Axis IV codes the overall severity of psychosocial stressors on a 7-point dimensional rating scale. Any stress that is considered a significant contributor to the etiology or the exacerbation of an Axis I or II condition is coded. The severity coding is made on the basis of the reaction that an "average individual" would have to a particular stress, and the manual provides anchor points for each level of severity with examples for adults, children, and adolescents.

On Axis V of DSM-III, the highest level of adaptive functioning that the patient has experienced in the past year is coded. DSM-III conceptualizes adaptive functioning as consisting of a composite of three major areas: social relationships, use of leisure time, and functioning in the occupational setting. For children and adolescents, functioning in the school setting is substituted for functioning in the occupational setting. A 7-point rating scale is provided for a severity coding, and anchor points are given for examples with children, adolescents, and adults.

Case Illustrations

Two case illustrations are provided below, and it is shown how each of these cases would be diagnosed in the DSM-III multiaxial system and, conversely, in a uniaxial categorical diagnostic system (e.g., DSM-II). Case 1 is a 6-year-old boy who presents with a history of abnormal development since birth and current symptoms characteristic of infantile autism as described by Kanner. There is a clear history of seizures which are being treated. Testing has revealed a nonverbal IQ between 50 and 60. In addition, both of his older biological siblings have severe reading disorder, one of whom additionally has attention deficit disorder with hyperactivity.

It can be seen that this 6-year-old boy has three important clinical conditions, any one of which could have been diagnosed as a primary condition, depending on where the boy was brought for evaluation and who did the evaluation. At a mental retardation center for delayed development, the diagnosis in a uniaxial system might have been mental retardation with possibly some coding for autistic features. At a child neurology clinic for seizures, the primary and sole diagnosis might have been his seizure disorder with some possible coding of behavioral abnormalities. The IQ may have been overlooked. At a child psychiatric clinic, his sole diagnosis might have been infantile autism, with the seizure disorder and the IQ being de-emphasized.

Thus, in a uniaxial system, where only one parameter of functioning is addressed, the boy's diagnosis in a psychiatric setting would be somewhat limited. The diagnoses that this boy would have received in a uniaxial system and in the DSM-III multiaxial system are summarized in Table I. In the DSM-III multiaxial system in which the clinical psychiatric syndrome was coded on one axis, intellectual level was coded on another axis, and biologic factors were coded on another axis, all three of these clinical conditions would have been coded and noted. In addition, a multiaxial diagnostic system that allows one to code psychosocial and/or family factors would allow one to code the presence of developmental disorders in the two siblings.

Case 2 is a 12-year-old boy referred for difficulty in academic performance in school and avoidant behavior in interpersonal relationships. The history includes mild but nevertheless characteristic symptoms of infantile autism, special educational help, and speech and language therapy throughout most of the grade-school years. The year before evaluation, he was shifted into a regular class in junior high school, where his problems in academic performance became more manifest, and his difficulty in relating to his peers became more obvious. Language testing shows minor speech and vocabulary deviancies but good overall communicative language. The nonverbal IQ is 112, and there are no associated physical or neurologic disorders. Academic testing indicates reading skills several years below the level that would be predicted on the basis of chronologic age and IQ.

The boy is an only child of two very bright parents, both professionals and both of whom themselves had a good deal of avoidant behavior in interpersonal relationships. Neither

Table I. Uniaxial and Multiaxial Diagnoses of Autism

Case No.	Uniaxial psychiatric diagnosis	Multiaxial (DSM-III) psychiatric diagnosis
1	Autism	I. Autism II. Mental retardation III. Seizure disorder IV. Familial developmental disorders V. Major impairment in several areas
2	Autism (residual)	I. Autism II. Developmental reading disorder III. No physical disorder IV. Limited opportunities for social interactions V. Moderate impairment in social and school functioning

mother nor father had any particularly close friends. They spent most of the time together with their 12-year-old boy or were involved in their work.

Table I illustrates the way in which a uniaxial diagnostic system obscures the many clinical differences between these two boys. Both boys in a unidimensional diagnostic system might have been given a diagnosis of infantile autism. The second child might have been given a diagnosis of infantile autism residual state, although he was still demonstrating many of the characteristic problems that autistic children have. However, such a unidimensional diagnosis would have failed to capture the major differences between the two children. Recognition of these differences is critical for the appropriate treatment decisions to be made.

The younger boy is also significantly more mentally retarded and has a seizure disorder that needs to be treated. The prognosis based on his IQ is not nearly as hopeful as the prognosis for the older boy with an IQ in the normal range. In addition, the older boy has no physical or neurologic disorders that are handicapping in the way that the younger boy's seizure disorder is. The younger child has two siblings with developmental disorders suggesting there may be some type of family-genetic relationship between his autism and their developmental disorders. The older boy comes from quite a different family situation. Both parents have been described as avoidant or schizoid, and he has no siblings. He spends most of his time with his parents who, possibly because of their own nature, do not encourage peer relationships, although they do not discourage them either. Thus, family psychosocial factors may be hindering the older boy's potential in the development of significant peer relationships. This would be missed in any unidimensional diagnostic system that permitted only one diagnosis such as infantile autism. Also, the second child qualifies for a diagnosis of developmental reading disorder not present in the first boy. This too has important treatment implications, just as the seizure disorder has important treatment implications for the younger child.

Issues in the Establishment of a Multiaxial Diagnostic Scheme

The above case illustrations (summarized in Table I) show how a multiaxial system such as the one developed for DSM-III provides a richer description of patients. Because differences between patients in several domains can be captured, such a system may be more useful for clinical decision making. In particular, prognostic predictions and treatment plans can become clearer.

Furthermore, a system such as the DSM-III multiaxial scheme can lead to improved interdisciplinary communication. This is because, in a sense, each axis may be conceptualized as addressing a profession: Axis I addresses psychiatry; Axis II addresses developmental psychology, education and linguistics; Axis III addresses medicine and neurology; and Axis IV addresses social work and clinical psychology.

However, it must be mentioned that the DSM-III system is, in a large sense, an arbitrary one. There is no evidence that DSM-III has selected the optimal number of axes, the optimal content for each axis, or the optimal manner of coding the contents. Below, we discuss the issues that must be considered in formulating these decisions, and the significance of such decisions to the diagnosis of autism.

As stated at the beginning of this chapter, a goal of a diagnostic classification system is to be able to group patients with similar clinical pictures. Just how narrow these groupings are is a matter of achieving balance between being as comprehensive as possible and being practical. Theoretically, there are an endless number of axes that could be in a multiaxial diagnostic classification scheme. Although Kanner (1958) argued for the need to differentiate autistic children from both mentally retarded and other psychotic children, he also acknowledged that it would be a retrograde step to regard every patient as entirely individual (Kanner, 1959).

In deciding how narrow the classification system should be, a general rule is that an axis created in a system should represent a separate domain and should add something to the overall conceptualization of a disorder classified in a system. Thus, if one is considering multiaxial diagnostic schemes in which autism would be a primary diagnosis, the questions would be on which axis, axis 1 or axis 2, should autism be coded, and what other domains are important to be coded.

The two cases illustrated above indicate that coding of biologic factors such as a seizure disorder are of obvious importance. The coding of intellectual level is also of obvious importance because of its prognostic significance. Coding of psychosocial factors may be important. Overall ratings of adaptive functioning and severity of disorder might also be important. Other domains that have been proposed for inclusion in multiaxial systems include etiology, course of illness, psychodynamic factors, defense mechanisms, duration of symptoms, and overall severity for all Axis I and II conditions. Research is necessary to determine the value of adding such axes of classification. However, it is probable that the more axes that exist in the system, the less likely that some of them are to be used at all and used reliably.

In addition to the number and content of axes, there are a number of issues regarding the specific codings on various axes that are relevant to the diagnosis of autism. For example, Axes I and II of DSM-III are categorical codings of the presence or absence of specific disorders. In DSM-III, autism is coded on Axis I, although in the revision of DSM-III, autism will be coded on Axis II. In DSM-III-R, Axis II will be expanded to become a developmental disorders axis including learning disorders, speech and language disorders, coordination disorder, infantile autism, and mental retardation. It has been argued that mental retardation and autism should be on separate axes because they are more likely to be coded if they are on separate axes. Since mental retardation and autism overlap to a large degree, and since level of IQ does play an important prognostic role, this argument is quite reasonable. One solution would be to code autism on Axis I as it is in DSM-III and mental retardation on Axis II or to create a separate axis for intellectual level.

Another coding issue has to do with the representation of the severity of an illness. Overall severity of each disorder will be coded in DSM-III-R, although it is not coded in DSM-III. In DSM-III-R the separate axis for severity coding will be dropped; instead, the Axis I or II diagnoses will be specified by the addition of severity terms (such as mild, moderate, and severe in partial remission or in complete remission). The severity distinction will take into account the number, intensity, and duration of symptoms and signs of the illness. A term such as partial remission or complete remission will mean that the child may have the disorder in a modified form at the time of the current evaluation, but the full syndrome was present in the past. This is likely to be highly relevant for grownup autistic individuals who, when they reach late adolescence or young adult life, may not meet the specified criteria for autistic disorder that were present early in childhood.

The coding of physical disorders is also relevant for the diagnosis of autism since a significant number of autistic children suffer from physical complications. In DSM-III, Axis III is conceived as a categorical axis specifying the presence or absence of physical disorders using the International Classification of Diseases codings. One issue is whether a disorder should be coded if it is not necessary for the proper interpretation or management of an Axis I or II condition or whether all Axis III diagnoses present should be coded. Another issue is whether to use this axis to reflect only etiologic conditions. Another issue is what to do about a physical disorder or condition that was present in the past (but not currently present) and that may have played an important role in the development of an Axis I or II disorder.

Coding of Axis IV psychosocial stressors is among the most controversial aspects of DSM-III. Psychosocial stressors and the possible role that they play in the etiology of or the exacerbation of a psychiatric disorder could be coded in any one of several ways. The specific type of stress may be coded, the severity of an individual stress may be coded, or both the type and the severity of stress may be coded. The severity may be coded the way it is coded in DSM-III (i.e., the way an average individual reacts to a particular stressor), or it may be coded for amount of threat or life change that it causes for the particular patient. It is clear from the research literature that not all children or adolescents respond the same way to the same type of life stressor. Thus, coding overall severity of all stressors the way an "average individual" would respond is not only pragmatically difficult but probably scientifically incorrect. The type of stress, the severity of each of the stressors, and coding the severity for the particular patient (rather than for an average person's theoretical response) is probably the best way to use such a psychosocial axis.

Another coding issue has to do with the representation of global functioning. Specifying functioning within the past year will result in lower ratings for patients with predominantly enduring conditions such as autism than for patients with predominantly acute conditions, such as an episode of major depressive disorder. DSM-III-R proposes a global assessment of functioning scale to replace what is currently in DSM-III. The clinician will be able to indicate an overall judgment of the child's psychological, social, and occupational functioning on a continuum of mental health illness. A 9-point scale is proposed for functioning at the time of the evaluation and for the highest level of functioning for at least a few months during the past year. A global assessment of functioning scale taking into account previous scales such as the Global Assessment Scale and the Children's Global Assessment scale is being proposed. The recently revised Vineland may be a useful substitute for assessment of functioning in multiple domains for children and adolescents. These authors feel it is a mistake to lump such different areas globally as interpersonal relationships with peers, interpersonal relationships in the home, functioning in school, and others into one overall rating. It makes more sense to individually rate adaptive functioning in the most important areas of functioning.

SUMMARY

One of the fundamental usages of classification systems is that of communication. A phenomenologic system offers the best hope for a means of communication between individuals of different theoretical orientation. For example, people with different theoretical orientations may agree that a child has autism but may disagree on how the autism developed. The classification system should be based on as many facts as are generally agreed on, not on speculations made by different theoretical schools.

Symptomatology can be classified using either categorical or dimensional approaches. Categorical systems have been found useful in diagnosis of child and adolescent psychiatric disorders and in the diagnosis of autism and related disorders in particular. Dimensional systems do have certain advantages over categorical systems but also have certain disadvantages. They have not found much use in the classification of autism and related disorders primarily because of the rarity of these disorders and lack of the available scales to be used on a broad-based basis, such as are available for children with disruptive behavior disorders, such as attention-deficit disorder with hyperactivity.

Children may be classified using uniaxial or multiaxial schemes. Multiaxial classification schemes for child psychiatric disorders have been considered for many years, particularly since the early World Health Organization studies back during the late 1960s. However, DSM-III is the first official classification scheme to make use of a multiaxial scheme. It has many advantages, some possible disadvantages, and certain aspects that need to be worked out in greater detail. These have been discussed above with reference to autism. Future development of multiaxial diagnostic schemes should examine the utility of other types of axes as well as the reliability and validity of codings on specific axes.

REFERENCES

Achenbach, T. (1980). DSM-III in light of empirical research on the classification of child psychopathology. *Journal of the American Academy of Child Psychiatry, 19,* 395–412.

Cantwell, D. P. (1975). *The hyperactive child: Diagnosis, management, and current research.* New York: Spectrum.

Cantwell, D. P. (1980). The diagnostic process and diagnostic classification in child psychiatry—DSM-III. *Journal of the American Academy of Child Psychiatry, 19,* 345–55.

DeMyer, M. K., Hingtgen, J. N., & Jackson, R. K. (1981). Infantile autism reviewed: A decade of research. *Schizophrenia Bulletin, 7,* 388–451.

Feighner, J. P., Robins, E., Guze, S. B., Woodruff, R., Winokur, G., and Munoz, R. (1972). Diagnostic criteria for use in psychiatric research. *Archives of General Psychiatry, 26,* 57–63.

Goodwin, D. W., & Guze, S. B. (1979). *Psychiatric diagnosis.* New York: Oxford University Press.

Kanner, L. (1943). Autistic disturbances of affective contact. *Nervous Children, 2,* 217–250.

Kanner, L. (1958). The specificity of early infantile autism. *Keitscheift fur Zinderpsychiatrie, 25,* 108–13.

Kanner, L. (1959). The thirty-third Maudsley lecture: Trends in child psychiatry. *Journal of Mental Science, 105,* 581–93.

Klerman, G. L. (1983). Evaluation of diagnostic classification. Presented at the American Psychiatric Association Workshop, *DSM-III: An interim appraisal,* Washington, D.C., October 12–15.

Rutter, M., Shaffer, D., & Shepard, M. (1975). A multiaxial classification of child psychiatric disorders. Geneva: World Health Organization.

Spitzer, R. L., Endicott, J., & Robins, E. (1978). Research diagnostic criteria: Rationale and reliability. *Archives of General Psychiatry, 35,* 733.

Spitzer, R. L., & Williams, J. B. W. (1980). Classification of mental disorders and DSM-III. In H. I. Kaplan, A. M. Freedman, and B. J. Sadock (Eds.), *Comprehensive textbook of psychiatry* (Vol. III, pp. 1035–1072). Baltimore: Williams & Wilkins.

9

Psychometric Instruments Available for the Assessment of Autistic Children

SUSAN L. PARKS

INTRODUCTION

For many disorders of childhood, psychological assessment is viewed as a critical step in the formulation of an effective treatment plan. Descriptions of symptomatology are compiled, cognitive strengths and weaknesses evaluated, appropriate diagnoses made, and interventions begun. This logical progression has rarely been the experience of most families with an autistic child. Controversy over the diagnosis of autism has resulted in differing conceptions by various researchers and clinicians. Driven by these theoretical orientations, evaluations have tended to emphasize certain areas of deficit while ignoring other relevant features. Likewise, the special difficulties of autistic children have complicated the picture, making testing practices variable and undependable. The unfortunate labeling of autistic children as "untestable" has taken many years to overcome. But slowly and surely, the importance of thorough assessment has come to be recognized as invaluable. With that recognition has come the development of several instruments designed specifically for use with an autistic population. Most of these measures have been developed to aid the diagnostic process. Others have focused on targeting specific areas for intervention efforts. Both types of assessments are reviewed here. In addition, some modifications of more widely known standardized tests are also discussed.

DIAGNOSTIC INSTRUMENTS DESIGNED FOR AUTISM

Diagnostic Checklist for Behavior-Disturbed Children

One of the first attempts to quantify the syndrome of autism was a multiple choice questionnaire published by Rimland in 1964. Form E-1 consisted of 76 questions about the

This chapter is an expansion of an article that appeared in the *Journal of Autism and Development Disabilities*, *13*, 255–267, 1983.

SUSAN L. PARKS • Villa Maria Residential Treatment Center, Timonium, Maryland 21093.

child's birth history, speech patterns, and symptom development. Parents' responses to the questions indicated that their children's behavior patterns tended to become more idiosyncratic after the age of 5½ years (Rimland, 1968). Because Rimland was most interested in the core symptoms defined by Kanner (1943), he chose to focus on the first 5 years of life. Subsequent use of his Diagnostic Checklist for Behavior-Disturbed Children (Form E-2) contained 80 questions concerning social interactions, speech, reaction to stimuli, intelligence, family information, and psychological development. Each response is scored as plus one or minus one point, depending on whether the answer is characteristic of early infantile autism (+) or not (−). The child's score is the sum of all 80 questions. Reported data for 2218 questionnaires (Rimland, 1971) included scores ranging from −42 to +45. A cutoff point of +20 was set for diagnosing a child as autistic. Only 9.7% of the sample received scores of +20 or more, corresponding with Rimland's and Kanner's estimate that only 10% of those children labeled autistic are really exhibiting early infantile autism (Kanner, 1962, cited in Rimland, 1971; Rimland, 1964).

The Diagnostic Checklist suffers from several methodological problems. By relying on parental recall, it does not provide for any observation of the child. Objective definitions of terms are not provided, and the scoring key remains unpublished. These and other problems have been critiqued by Masters and Miller (1970). In addition, the reliability and validity of Form E-2 are subject to question. The reliability of parental reports has never been assessed. Test–retest reliability would establish the dependability of parents' memories if it could be demonstrated. Having parents complete separate forms and comparing responses would also be an appropriate test of awareness and recall. Prior and Bence (1975) have reported a comparison of parental and staff E-2 ratings of nine children attending school in Australia. Teachers and therapists were not blind to parents' responses, so this study cannot be considered a true test of reliability. However, it should be noted that staff members tended to report more abnormal behavior than did parents. The authors suggested that parents compared current behavior with previous lower functioning rather than using normal children's skill levels as a baseline.

Attempts to establish validity for the Diagnostic Checklist have focused on its discriminative ability. Forms E-1 and E-2 were able to distinguish between a group of early schizophrenic and autistic and nonpsychotic children (DeMyer, Churchill, Pontiers & Gilkey, 1971). Efforts by DeMyer et al. to differentiate between the autistic and schizophrenic children were successful only with Form E-1. Using Form E-2 yielded no significant differences among the subgroups of early schizophrenia, higher-functioning autism, and lower-functioning autism.

Another look at the discriminant validity of the Diagnostic Checklist has been reported by Davids (1975). Records of 66 former patients were read and scored using Form E-1. An autistic rating ranging from 1 to 4 was also determined for the psychotic children based on the history information. Form E-1 successfully distinguished the psychotic from the nonpsychotic children. Using the 4-point autistic rating, Form E-1 was also able to differentiate the autistic children from the other psychotic cases. Davids attempted to obtain retrospective E-1 responses from the parents of the children. Although the correlation of parental and record ratings was significant, more than 60% of the variance between scores remained unexplained. The parents' forms were not used to make the discriminations between diagnostic groups. Since the Diagnostic Checklist was designed to be completed by parents, it would have been interesting to see whether the results obtained were the same. Also, it should again be noted that Form E-1 was used by Davids, leaving the discriminative ability of E-2 still uncertain.

Rimland and others have used a biological approach to investigate the construct validity of his checklist. Initial reports of subgroups of autistic children indicated that those with high Form E-2 scores also exhibited high serotonin outflow (Boullin, Coleman, O'Brien & Rimland, 1971). Subsequent reports have contradicted this work (Yuwiler, Ritvo, Geller, Glousman, Schneiderman & Matsuno, 1975; Boullin, Freeman, Geller, Ritvo, Rutter & Yuwiler, 1982). The use of megavitamin therapy with autistic children has also been investigated by Rimland (1973). Hypothesizing a genetic error in metabolic functioning, children were supplied with large amounts of certain vitamins. Those children who improved on this regimen could be distinguished from those who did not by the magnitude of their E-2 scores.

The use of the Diagnostic Checklist as a variable in biological studies reflects the purpose of the instrument as originally developed by Rimland. He was primarily interested in studying those children exhibiting the core symptoms of autism as first described by Kanner (1943). The content validity of his instrument is therefore assumed by relying on Kanner's diagnostic criteria. Use of Form E-2 as a screening tool to obtain a research pool of "pure" autistic children may be viewed as an appropriate application of the instrument. Because of the changing nature of the diagnostic label autism, Rimland's checklist may not be of much help in describing the larger number of children being identified as autistic or in developing plans for the treatment of their symptoms.

Behavior Rating Instrument for Autistic and Atypical Children

The Behavior Rating Instrument for Autistic and Atypical Children (BRIAAC) is another instrument specifically developed for an autistic population (Ruttenberg, Dratman, Frankno & Wenar, 1966; Ruttenberg, Kalish, Wenar & Wolf, 1977). BRIAAC consists of eight scales that measure behavior in different areas: relationship to an adult, communication, drive for mastery, vocalization and expressive speech, sound and speech reception, social responsiveness, body movement, and psychobiological development. The scales were developed from observations of children enrolled in a psychoanalytically oriented therapy program. Scales are divided into 10 levels with descriptive behavior ranging from that of a "typical" autistic child to a normal 4-year-old. The rater observes the child's behavior and then distributes 10 points across the levels of each scale. All the scales are combined to give an overall rating and provide an interscale profile.

The most important feature of BRIAAC is the empirical derivation of its behavior descriptions from actual clinical notes. Similarly, scores on BRIAAC are based on observations of children and not reports of behavior. The scoring criteria, however, has not been well described and appears cumbersome. The discriminations needed for scoring are apparently trainable, for the properties of reliability and validity have both been studied. Interrater reliability for the initial four-scale BRIAAC was investigated using trained students as raters (Ruttenberg et al., 1966). Spearman rank correlation coefficients ranged from 0.85 to 0.88. Reliability coefficients for the revised eight-scale BRIAAC have also been reported (Wenar & Ruttenberg, 1976). Seven pairs of raters observed 113 autistic children. Although the methodology is vaguely described, the obtained correlation coefficients are high, ranging from 0.85 to 0.93.

The eight BRIAAC scales have been submitted to a test of internal consistency (Wenar & Ruttenberg, 1976). Correlations ranged from 0.54 to 0.86, indicating some common element among the scales, but also sufficient variation. Factor analysis yielded a single factor described as "resistance to realistic participation in various activities." Cohen and his colleagues (Cohen, Caparulo, Gold, Waldo, Shaywitz, Ruttenberg & Rimland, 1978) report a principal-component analysis that resulted in one factor accounting for 69% of the variance. Only the Psychosexual Development scale did not load significantly on this factor.

Validity studies of the BRIAAC scales have not yielded especially promising results. Ranked scores of 26 children have been correlated with another child study center's clinicians' ratings of disturbance (Wenar & Ruttenberg, 1976). Significant correlations were reported for BRIAAC total score and the subscales of Vocalization and Expressive Speech, Sound and Speech Reception and Relationship. These correlations are based on rankings, not actual scores, which makes the lack of significance of five of the eight scales comparisons look even more damaging.

Discriminant validity has also been investigated by Wolf, Wenar, and Ruttenberg (1972). BRIAAC scores were sufficient to distinguish between normal, mentally retarded, and autistic children. A control group of nonautistic but behavior-disturbed children was not included, which would have provided a more stringent test. Cohen et al. (1978) have reported the failure of BRIAAC scores alone to discriminate among diagnostic groups of primary and secondary autism, early childhood psychosis, developmental aphasia, and mental retardation. The number of subgroups and the possibility of diagnostic overlap in these particular categories may mitigate the negative findings. However, until a test of discriminant validity can demonstrate the capability of BRIAAC to distinguish between autistic and other disordered children, differential diagnosis should not be based solely on this measure.

The study by Cohen et al. (1978) contained an interesting comparison between BRIAAC scores and the Diagnostic Checklist. Only 2 of the 13 children diagnosed in the study as primary childhood autism had form E-2 scores of +20 or above. There was a nonsignificant relationship, therefore, between BRIAAC total scores and form E-2 scores. Again, the goals of these two measures must be addressed. The Diagnostic Checklist aims to identify a small group of children with a classic autism symptom history. BRIAAC focuses instead on current levels of behavioral functioning regardless of differences in history and etiology. Such an intent makes it an appropriate instrument for use in evaluating treatment effectiveness. Wenar and Ruttenberg (1976) reported such an investigation concluding that the scales of Sound and Speech Reception and Social Functioning seemed most sensitive to therapeutic change. Questions of maturation and developmental lag may obscure or perhaps explain many expected changes.

Behavior Observation System

The Behavior Observation Scale (BOS) has been under development since it was first reported in 1978 (Freeman, Ritvo, Guthrie, Schroth & Ball, 1978). Over the years, it has changed from a checklist of 67 objectively defined behaviors (1978 version) to its current status of 24 behaviors (Freeman, Ritvo & Schroth, 1984). The original goal of its developers was to develop a scale that would rely on objectively defined observable behaviors, adequately account for the influence of a child's age, and provide objective profiles of normal and abnormal children's scores (Freeman & Ritvo, 1981). Because autistic children are constantly changing and developing, their clinical state is also in continual flux. In order to assess children in a developmental context, adequate comparisons must be made with other children matched for mental and chronological age. The BOS was therefore designed for use with autistic, normal, and mentally retarded children.

The revised BOS consists of 24 behaviors divided into four groups: solitary, relationship to objects, relationship to people, and language. The child is videotaped through a one-way mirror in a room equipped with age-appropriate toys. The examiner brings the child into the room, gives directions to "do anything you want," and then remains seated in the room. Later the videotape is reviewed and behaviors are coded based on 10-sec intervals. Any of the 24 behaviors may occur during each interval and all that are observed are coded. Timing of the intervals is superimposed on the videotape, controlling for any stopwatch variation. The number of intervals during which a particular behavior was observed are counted and also the percentage of time the child spent facing the examiner. A weighting scheme allows for combining different behaviors to yield subscales.

Since one of the original purposes of Freeman et al. (1978) was to objectively define the behavior they were interested in observing, it is not surprising that they have consistently reported high interrater reliability. Correlation coefficients in the earliest work were listed as greater than 0.84 for 55 of the 67 behaviors (Freeman et al., 1978). Later reports increase the number of behaviors with correlation coefficients above 0.80 to 60 (Freeman & Ritvo, 1980; Freeman, Ritvo, Torich, Guthrie & Schroth, 1981). Most recently, Freeman et al. (1984) reported training undergraduate students to a criteria of 80% average agreement on each of the 24 behaviors. Actual interrater correlation coefficients are reported for each behavior during the data-collection process described. They range from 0.23 to 1.00, with a mean of 0.71.

Freeman and colleagues have been most interested in documenting the differences between the frequency of observed behaviors in normal, autistic, and mentally retarded children. They have repeatedly demonstrated the ability of the BOS to make this distinction (Freeman et al., 1978; Freeman, Guthrie, Ritvo, Schroth, Glass & Frankel, 1979; Freeman, Schroth, Ritvo, Guthrie & Wake, 1980; Freeman et al., 1981, 1984). However, they have also emphasized that there is a great deal of overlap among the behaviors exhibited by these three groups of children. Those behaviors which fail to distinguish among them are more dependent on age factors—both mental and/or chronological age (Freeman & Ritvo, 1980). Analyzing the frequency of occurrence of behaviors was found to be an inadequate measure for differentiating the groups of children when used by itself. Some behaviors with a low frequency were observed in many children; others were observed in all groups but with significantly different frequencies (Freeman et al., 1981). The fact that some low frequency behaviors occur at all may be important diagnostically (Freeman et al., 1984). Despite the ability of BOS to discriminate autistic from normal and mentally retarded children, no one behavior or subset of behaviors was able to differentiate with 100% accuracy. A discriminant analysis reported by Freeman et al. (1984) indicates high percentages of correct classification but not perfect assignment. The authors suggest that quantitative behavior alone may not be enough for diagnosis after all. Kanner (1943) included a disturbance in the quality of social interactions as one of the original criteria for the diagnosis of autism. Freeman et al. (1984) now acknowledge that qualitative, not just quantitative, data may be necessary for accurate diagnosis.

Childhood Autism Rating Scale

Like the BOS, construction of the Childhood Autism Rating Scale (CARS) was undertaken because of the limitations of the classification systems already in existence (Schopler, Reichler, DeVillis & Daly, 1980). Behavioral observations are used to score the 15 separate subscales included in the instrument: impairment in human relationships, imitation, inappropriate affect, bizarre use of body movement and persistence of stereotypes, peculiarities in relating to nonhuman objects, resistance to environmental change, peculiarities of visual responsiveness, peculiarities of auditory responsiveness, near-receptor responsiveness, anxiety reactions, verbal communication, nonverbal communication, activity level, intellectual functioning, and general impressions. The rationale for these scales is primarily based on consensual diagnostic criteria extracted from work by Kanner (1943), Creak (1964), Rutter (1978), and the National Society for Autistic Children (1978). As originally developed, raters complete the CARS after watching a structured interaction with the child through a one-way mirror. Examples and guidelines for scoring the separate scales are provided. Each scale ranges from normal to severely abnormal behavior on a continuum of seven points. Anchor points and definitions are objectively stated (Schopler *et al.*, 1980, Appendix). Ratings are influenced by the frequency and intensity of behavior as well as its peculiarity. Age appropriateness must also be considered while judging the "normality" of the exhibited behavior.

Completed ratings from a statewide sample of 537 children were used to empirically develop the scoring criteria (Schopler *et al.*, 1980). Possible scores can range from 15 to 60. Based on the distribution of scores from the standardization group, children with scores of <30 were described as "not autistic" ($N=266$). The diagnosis of severe autism was applied to children scoring 37 or higher who also had ratings of 3 or above on at least five of the scales ($N=125$). Children with scores between these extremes were classified as mild to moderately autistic.

Interrater reliability of the CARS has been well documented (Schopler *et al.*, 1980). Two independent raters observed and rated 280 cases resulting in correlation coefficients ranging from 0.55 on Intellectual Consistency to 0.93 on Human Relatedness. Overall reliability of the 15 scales averaged 0.71. A test of the internal consistency of the CARS yielded an extremely high coefficient alpha of 0.94. Validation of the CARS has been limited to comparisons with clinical ratings of psychosis. Judgments of clinicians obtained during the evaluation sessions correlated highly ($r=0.84$), as did independent assessments made by a child psychiatrist and psychologist ($r=0.80$) (Schopler *et al.*, 1980). How these evaluations were made is not described. So far no investigation of the discriminant validity of the CARS has been reported. Inclusion of control groups of mentally retarded and other developmentally disabled children would enable testing of the instrument's ability to provide a differential diagnosis.

A report by Schopler *et al.* (1980) includes another interesting comparison between diagnoses made with Rimland's Diagnostic Checklist and with CARS. Of the sample population, 450 had been evaluated with Form E-2. Only eight were diagnosed as autistic on the basis of Rimland's criteria, and three of those were described as nonautistic by CARS. Obviously, these differences reflect a large discrepancy between the definition of autism employed by the developers of these instruments.

Recently, Schopler, Reichler, and Rennar (1986) evaluated the validity of the CARS in conditions differing from those used to standardize the measure. Information obtained from interviews with the parents of 41 children were used to rate the CARS. These ratings were then compared with scores for the same children obtained during observations of structured sessions. Total scores and screening diagnoses were not significantly different. Similar results were obtained using classroom observations and chart reviews. Schopler *et al.* (1986) also reported a comparison of ratings made by expert and relatively untrained staff. After only a 1-hr training session, visiting professionals' ratings correlated significantly with those made by experienced observers. Although the number of children observed is not reported for each of the 18 "untrained" raters, the diagnostic screening classifications reached by the two groups agreed 92% of the time. These results suggest the CARS is appropriate for use as a widespread screening device. The measure can be employed in a variety of settings without the need for extensive staff training. Identification of children with autism can then be followed up with referrals for further assessment and treatment by professionals in the field.

Autism Behavior Checklist

Another instrument developed for the assessment of autistic children is the Autism Screening Instrument for Educational Planning (ASIEP) (Krug, Arick & Almond, 1979). Consisting of five separate components designed to measure different aspects of the disorder, only the Autism Behavior Checklist (ABC) has been evaluated psychometrically by the developers. The behaviors included in the checklist were selected from seven sources, including Rimland's Form E-2, Creak's (1964) criteria, BRIAAC items, and Kanner's (1943) criteria. Fifty-seven behavior descriptions are organized into five symptom groups: sensory, relating, body and object use, language, and social and self-help. Raters are asked to indicate the presence or absence of each behavior. Weighting factors for the various behaviors were assigned based on chi-square analyses of 1049 completed checklists (Krug, Arick & Almond, 1980). Sums of the weighted items can be transferred to profile charts and compared with standard profiles for children of the same chronological age. Little psychometric documentation of the ABC is available. Preliminary reports of interrater reliability and split half reliability are quite high: 95% agreement and a Spearman—Brown coefficient of 0.94 (Krug et al., 1980). The interrater reliability is based, however, on an excessively high number of raters observing only 14 children.

Developers of the ABC have described a successful attempt to differentiate between autistic and mentally retarded, emotionally disturbed, deaf–blind, or normal subjects (Krug et al., 1980). Details of the procedures used are not reported, and the number of children included in each comparison is also unknown. Since the number of autistic children's scores used is quite high (1049), the N for the control groups is certainly important when evaluating the comprehensiveness of the trial.

The ABC has also been used to evaluate a new sample of 62 persons already diagnosed as autistic (Krug et al., 1980). Although 86% of the group received scores within 1 SD of the mean for the standardization sample, it is not clear whether the raters were blind to the diagnoses. Since all individuals tested were autistic, that seems unlikely, and the study therefore cannot be construed as an independent evaluation of validity. Krug et al. (1980) promoted the ABC as a reliable instrument that can effectively screen for the presence of autism. Until further investigations using the ABC appear in the research literature, it would seem prudent to consider it a largely unknown entity.

DIAGNOSIS VERSUS INTERVENTION PLANNING

All the measures described in the preceding section were developed to assist in the identification and diagnosis of autistic children. Differential diagnosis in particular has been of special concern. Research designs and political decision-making processes may consider precise diagnostic labels vital for the accurate interpretation and funding of projects. The Diagnostic Checklist has been used repeatedly in research investigations aimed at distinguishing subgroups of autistic children. The Behavior Observation Scale, Childhood Autism Rating Scale, and Autism Behavior Checklist are similarly focused on separating autistic children from the larger pool of developmentally disabled children. Information collected through use of these instruments could perhaps be used to target areas of intervention. However, specific details needed for preparing treatment plans and evaluating their effectiveness are not readily available. In fact, the developers of two of these measures have already acknowledged the need for another sort of assessment tool.

Psychoeducational Profile

Before publication of the CARS, Schopler and colleagues had begun using a Psychoeducational Profile (PEP) (Schopler & Reichler, 1979) to plan educational and home teaching curricula for individual children. This inventory of behaviors can be used to identify children's abilities in a variety of areas including perception, motor performance, and cognitive skills. During the assessment, an examiner presents standard toys and activities to the child while also observing and recording responses. Test items include tasks appropriate for a 1-year-old to those a 7-year-old can accomplish. Because of the limitations of many autistic children, there is a greater emphasis on lower functioning skills. There is no preset order for administration of items, and the amount of language skill needed is minimal. These features circumvent a number of the problems frequently encountered when using standardized tests with autistic children. The child's performance of each task is rated as either passing, failing, or at an "emerging" level. In the latter case, the child shows some understanding of the task but does not have the skill necessary to complete it, or does so in an idiosyncratic way. At the conclusion of the test, scores are assigned in seven developmental scales. A profile of strengths and weaknesses can then be translated into an individualized program of intervention. By documenting the developing skills of a child, and not just his deficits, the educational objectives can be planned in a way that may more readily result in success for the child.

Schopler and Reichler (1979) report the use of the PEP with more than 565 children. However, they provide no information on the reliability of examiners. Since the Profile has been refined over the years and is used only for individual treatment planning, such a concern for standards of reliability may appear trivial. Without such reliability studies, however, the measure cannot be used to demonstrate therapeutic effectiveness unless the follow-up evaluations are completed by the same person who initially rated the child. Otherwise, any changes noted may be a result of interrater differences rather than actual improvements in behavior.

Another psychometric problem with the PEP is the lack of information provided about the control group of normals used to compile age-equivalent comparison profiles. The existence of such profiles is certainly commendable, since it allows for an evaluation of developmental factors. However, the instrument would benefit from greater detail in reports on the normative sample. Profiles of "typical" groups of autistic children might also be useful.

An attempt at validation of the measure has been undertaken by correlating scores on the PEP's overall level of performance with mental age scores from several standardized tests (Schopler & Reichler, 1979). Correlations were above 0.7 for the Merrill–Palmer Test of Mental Abilities, Vineland Social Maturity Scale, Bayley Scale, and Peabody Picture Vocabulary Test. Nonsignificant correlations were reported with the Wechsler scales and Leiter International Performance Scale. Details of procedures and number of subjects are not provided, but it appears that the PEP is measuring much of the same areas tapped by those tests with which it correlated well.

ASIEP: Components 2–5

Krug *et al.* (1979) also provided for a more detailed assessment of children labeled autistic by their Autistic Behavior Checklist. The ABC was the first component in a five-part approach to information gathering. The other components of the ASIEP include standardized instructions for direct sampling of behaviors. While not assessment instruments per se, these additional components provide specific guidelines for obtaining information useful for educational and treatment planning.

The Sample of Vocal Behavior consists of recording 50 spontaneous vocalizations in an unstructured setting. Analysis of the verbalizations considers the repetitiveness of sounds, communication value, and complexity of syntax. An age equivalency score of language can also be computed. Details of the scoring procedures have not been published apart from the test administration manual. A preliminary study using 61 students compared autistic and nonautistic groups on the various language scores (Krug *et al.*, 1981). Statistically significant differences were found at both preschool and school-age levels.

Component 3 is an assessment of social interaction between the child and an adult. Observable behaviors such as crying, tantrums, self-stimulation, and gestures are recorded using a time-sampling procedure. A total of 48 samples are observed and transferred to a profile of social interaction. Comparison profiles are available. Forty children were used as the standardization group for this component. Significantly different profiles were found for the categories of interaction, independent play, and no response. Aggressive negative responses did not differentiate the groups.

An Educational Assessment of Functional Skills is used to quantify the child's language, behavior, body concept, and imitative speech. This component requires communicative ability (either sign or speech), and no information about specific content is supplied. Initial comparisons were based on the scores of 41 autistic and 31 severely handicapped individuals. Mean total scores differed by 11 points but, since the range of the test is not specified, it is hard to evaluate the meaning of that difference.

The final component involves learning a black–white sequencing task. The child's learning acquisition rate is computed based on the responses to a specified set of procedures. Standardization data were collected by 41 professionals on 72 autistic or severely handicapped students. The large number of examiners used raises the possibility of varying application of the learning task despite the use of standard instructions. Significantly different profiles are again reported for the two groups.

The assessments described by Krug *et al.* (1979) have been deemed by the authors as reliable and capable of supporting differential diagnostic decisions. At this point, however, the components of ASIEP can best be considered in the developmental stage as far as psychometrics are concerned. No work on establishing interrater reliability has been reported, nor have there been any attempts to validate the components except by using another component of the ASIEP as the independent variable. Although the samples of behavior were to be used to track changes occurring as a result of educational interventions, no studies illustrating test–retest reliability or practice effects have been forthcoming. More detailed descriptions of the standardization samples and scoring procedures used would also be helpful. Clearly, more work needs to be done and reported in the research literature to establish the clinical value of this set of assessment tools.

Checklist for Autistic Children

The need for an instrument to assist in treatment planning and evaluation was a motivating force in the development of a unique system proposed by Mahita and Umezu (1973). The authors were involved with a behavior therapy program and needed an objective means of monitoring progress in treatment on a repeated basis. The Checklist for Autistic Children (CLAC) was designed to evaluate a child's behavior initially, to provide a resource in the design of a therapeutic program, to test for treatment effectiveness, and to differentiate subgroups of autistic children. The questionnaire covers 11 areas of behavior: eating, elimination, sleeping, activities of daily living, play, interpersonal relationships, speech and language, expressive behavior, manipulation of hands and fingers, autonomy, and emotional expression. Twenty-eight items are scored on a 5-point scale. Parents are asked to complete CLAC with the help of an evaluator. Ratings are then transferred to a diagram. On repeated administrations changes in the shape of the diagram are viewed as responses to treatment. Data on a group of 86 normal controls allows comparison to "normal" patterns.

CLAC suffers from several methodological problems. Although the list of items is provided, not all are well defined, and some require written descriptions rather than a multiple-choice response. The CLAC scheme offers no summary score and therefore would not be amenable to use as a general description. Reliance on the shape of the diagram results in good visual conceptions of a child's strengths and weaknesses but cannot be communicated easily. CLAC relies on parental report and does not employ objective observation. Given the behavioral nature of the intervention program, this seems most unusual. Furthermore, no information is provided on either reliability of raters or validity of the instrument. Control groups of normal and mentally retarded children matched for mental and chronological age would permit an evaluation of the influence of developmental changes (Freeman & Ritvo, 1981). The original intent of CLAC showed much promise and originality in addressing the need for an easily administered, repeatable measure of an autistic child's behavior. To date there has been no report in the U.S. literature to address these methodological shortcomings.

THE USE OF STANDARDIZED TESTS

The three assessment systems described above have each been focused more specifically on the issue of treatment planning and intervention evaluation. Obviously, many locally developed instruments are in use across the country as schools and treatment centers struggle with documenting individualized educational plans. The measures described here and the ones used in various school districts have enhanced clinicians' and educators' grasp of the strengths and weaknesses of the children they serve. However, the absence of widely recognized standardized test scores has limited the communication ability of many professionals and left unanswered core issues about intellectual IQ scores that may be vital for specific school placements. All communities do not have access to examiners trained in the administration of specialized assessments. Moreover, it may prove beneficial to have a child observed within the frame of reference of a familiar test with recognized age norms. While most assuredly not a panacea, the use of standardized tests is feasible with autistic children and can contribute to decision making and treatment planning processes.

Appropriate Selection of Instruments

The problems encountered in using standardized tests with autistic children have been repeatedly described. The special characteristics of autism may result in little motivation on the part of the child. He may be uninterested in interacting with an examiner, may demonstrate unusual reactions to test equipment, and may not be able to follow the shifts from one task to another. The lack of receptive and/or expressive language may prevent the child from completing items requiring verbal directions and responses. Another important consideration is the wide scatter of ability levels shown by most autistic children. Baker (1983) pointed out the difficulty of using a single instrument to assess the full range of skills and deficits. She has also issued an important warning regarding the interpretation of standardized IQ test scores. Since most tests are based on assumptions of normal developmental sequencing, baseline and ceiling items may be misleading and the usual methods of scoring useless.

Many of these handicaps can be minimized or avoided by selecting appropriate instruments and modifying procedures. Most autistic children can be adequately tested without great deviation of normal administration directions if the test items are consistent with their abilities (Alpern, 1967; Freeman & Ritvo, 1984). Test selection should be influenced by the child's developmental level, language skills, ability to relate, and length of attention span (Baker, 1983). Modification of procedures may include rearrangement of item sequences, increased use of gestures, inclusion of reinforcing activities interspersed with subtests, and the use of repetitive routines. Baker (1983) provided an excellent description of flexible test administration principles. By evaluating the child with both standard and modified procedures, much valuable information can be obtained.

Intelligence Tests

All the widely known tests of general intelligence can be used with an autistic population. Advantages and disadvantages of these instruments (Bayley Scale, Merrill–Palmer Test of Mental Abilities, McCarthy Scales, and Wechsler Scales) have been reviewed by Baker (1983). Successful use of tests for the deaf have also been reported (Maltz, 1981; Shah & Holmes, 1985). Two of these measures—Leiter International Performance Scale and Hiskey–Nebraska Test of Learning Aptitude—are included in Baker's review.

Tests of Social Skills

Freeman and Ritvo (1984) cautioned against assuming that intellectual and social functioning are highly correlated. Good performance on a structured cognitive assessment may not be accompanied by application of skills in a real-life situation. Nevertheless, the measurement of adaptive social behavior using standardized tests has not been well explored. The Vineland Social Maturity Scale has been utilized in several research investigations of autistic behavior (Alpern, 1967; Deckner, Soraci, Deckner & Blanton, 1981; Schopler & Reichler,

1979). It can be easily administered, since it relies on reporting from a caretaker. Scoring results in an overall social IQ that can be simply communicated. Because it is not based on direct observation of the child, however, the Vineland is subject to all the criticisms leveled at parental reports in earlier sections.

The Adaptive Behavior Scale (ABS) (Nihira, Foster, Shellhaas & Leland, 1975) has also been suggested for use with autistic children. It provides assessment of behavior in the classrooms. Percentile scores can be compared with norms from special education students. Sloan and Marcus (1981) investigated the reliability of parent and teacher ratings of the same child using the ABS. Significant correlations were found for many, but not all, of the various subscales. Behaviors in the first part of the test, which emphasize specific adaptive skills, tended to correlate much higher than those in the second part that require more value judgments by raters. Similar results were obtained when measuring behavior at the beginning and end of an academic year and also when comparing ABS scales with other standardized tests such as IQ and Vineland Social IQ. These findings argue against reliance on the ABS as a measure of social behavior. Sloan and Marcus (1981) suggest the need for investigation of other possible instruments and highlight the need for developing appropriate norms.

Concluding Remarks

It has been suggested that the use of a general category labeled severe developmental disability has mitigated the need for precise differential diagnosis (Power & Handleman, 1984). Since the difficulties of communication, retarded functioning, and problems with meaningful play are common to many children with mental retardation and autism, the insistence on differential labeling may seem arbitrary at best and destructive at worst. While acknowledging the overlap between autism and other developmental disorders (Bhatara, 1980), there are still sufficient reasons to argue for a complete, comprehensive assessment aimed at both a diagnostic decision and a thorough evaluation of behavioral strengths and weaknesses. Descriptions of inappropriate placement decisions like that detailed by Blau (1985) illustrate too well the continuing need for proper identification of autistic children in order to better serve their needs.

REFERENCES

Alpern, G. D. (1967). Measurement of "untestable" autistic children. *Journal of Abnormal Psychology, 72,* 478–486.
Baker, A. F. (1983). Psychological assessment of autistic children. *Clinical Psychology Review, 3,* 41–59.
Bhatara, V. (1980). Overlap of autism, mental retardation, and CNS dysfunction. *Psychiatric Annals, 10,* 298–304.
Blau, G. L. (1985). Autism—Assessment and placement under the education for all handicapped children act: A case history. *Journal of Clinical Psychology, 41,* 440–447.
Boullin, D. J., Coleman, M., O'Brien, R. A., & Rimland, B. (1971). Laboratory predictions of infantile autism, based on 5-hydroxytryptamine efflux from blood platelets and their correlation with the Rimland E-2 score. *Journal of Autism and Childhood Schizophrenia, 1,* 63–71.
Boullin, D. J., Freeman, B. J., Geller, E., Ritvo, E., Rutter, M., & Yuwiler, A. (1982). Toward the resolution of conflicting findings. (Letter to the Editor.) *Journal of Autism and Developmental Disorders, 12,* 97–98.

Cohen, D. J., Caparulo, B. K., Gold, J. R., Waldo, M. C., Shaywitz, B. A., Ruttenberg, B. A., & Rimland, B. (1978). Agreement in diagnosis: Clinical assessment and behavior rating scales for pervasively disturbed children. *Journal of the American Academy of Child Psychiatry, 17,* 589–603.

Creak, M. (1964). Schizophrenic syndrome in childhood: Further progress report of a working party (April, 1964). *Developmental Medicine and Child Neurology, 6,* 530–535.

Davids, A. (1975). Childhood psychosis: The problem of differential diagnosis. *Journal of Autism and Childhood Schizophrenia, 5,* 129–138.

Deckner, C. W., Soraci, S. A., Deckner, P. O., & Blanton, R. L. (1981). Consistency among commonly used procedures for assessment of abnormal children. *Journal of Clinical Psychology, 37,* 856–62.

DeMyer, M. K., Churchill, D. W., Pontius, W., & Gilkey, K. M. (1971). A comparison of five diagnostic systems for childhood schizophrenia and infantile autism. *Journal of Autism and Childhood Schizophrenia, 1,* 175–89.

Freeman, B. J., Guthrie, D., Ritvo, E., Schroth, P., Glass, R., & Frankel, F. (1979). Behavior Observation Scale: Preliminary analysis of the similarities and differences between autistic and mentally retarded children. *Psychological Reports, 44,* 519–24.

Freeman, B. J., & Ritvo, E. R. (1981). The syndrome of autism: A critical review of diagnostic systems, follow-up studies, and the theoretical background of the Behavior Observation Scale. In J. E. Gilliam (Ed.), *Autism, diagnosis, instruction, management, and research.* Springfield, IL: Charles C.Thomas.

Freeman, B. J., & Ritvo, E. R. (1984). The syndrome of autism: Establishing the diagnosis and principles of management. *Pediatric Annals, 13,* 284–88, 290, 294–296.

Freeman, B. J., Ritvo, E. R., Guthrie, D., Schroth, P., & Ball, J. (1978). The Behavior Observation Scale for Autism: Initial methodology, data analysis, and preliminary findings on 89 children. *Journal of the American Academy of Child Psychiatry, 17,* 576–588.

Freeman, B. J., Ritvo, E. R., & Schroth, P. C. (1984). Behavior assessment of the syndrome of autism: Behavior Observation System. *Journal of the American Academy of Child Psychiatry, 23,* 588–94.

Freeman, B. J., Ritvo, E. R., Tonich, I., Guthrie, D., & Schroth, P. (1981). Behavior Observation System for Autism: Analysis of behaviors among autistic, mentally retarded, and normal children. *Psychological Reports, 49,* 199–208.

Freeman, B. J., Schroth, P., Ritvo, E., Guthrie, D., & Wake, L. (1980). The Behavior Observation Scale for Autism (BOS): Initial results of factor analyses. *Journal of Autism and Developmental Disorders, 10,* 343–6.

Kanner, L. (1943). Autistic disturbances of affective contact. *Nervous Child, 2,* 217–50.

Krug, D. A., Arick, J. R., & Almond, P. J. (1979). Autism Screening Instrument for Educational Planning: Background and development. In J. Gilliam (Ed.), *Autism: Diagnosis, instruction, management, and research.* Austin: University of Texas at Austin Press.

Krug, D. A., Arick, J., & Almond, P. (1980). Behavior checklist for identifying severely handicapped individuals with high levels of autistic behavior. *Journal of Child Psychology and Psychiatry, 21,* 221–9.

Maltz, A. (1981). Comparison of cognitive deficits among autistic and retarded children in the Arthur adaptation of the Leiter International Performance Scales. *Journal of Autism and Developmental Disorders, 11,* 413–26.

Makita, K., & Umezu, K. (1973). An objective evaluation technique for autistic children: An introduction of CLAC scheme. *Acta Paedopsychiatrica, 39,* 237–53.

Masters, J. C., & Miller, D. E. (1970). Early infantile autism: A methodological critique. *Journal of Abnormal Psychology, 75,* 342–3.

National Society for Autistic Children. (1978). National Society for Autistic Children definition of autism. *Journal of Autism and Childhood Schizophrenia, 8,* 162–7.

Nihira, K., Foster, R., Shellhaas, M., & Leland, H. (1975). *AAMD Adaptive Behavior Scale, 1975 Revisions: Manual.* Washington, D. C.: American Association on Mental Deficiency.

Powers, M. D., & Handleman, J. S. (1984). *Behavioral assessment of severe developmental disabilities.* Rockville, MD: Aspen Systems Corp.

Prior, M., & Bence, R. (1975). A note on the validity of the Rimland Diagnostic Checklist. *Journal of Clinical Psychology, 31,* 510–13.

Rimland, B. (1964). *Infantile autism: The syndrome and its implications for a neural theory of behavior.* New York: Appleton-Century-Crofts.

Rimland, B. (1968). On the objective diagnosis of infantile autism. *Acta Paedopsychiatarica, 35,* 146–61.

Rimland, B. (1971). The differentiation of childhood psychoses: An analysis of checklists for 2,218 psychotic children. *Journal of Autism and Childhood Schizophrenia, 1,* 161–74.

Rimland, B. (1973). The effect of high dosage levels of certain vitamins on the behavior of children with severe mental disorders. In D. R. Hawkins and L. Pauling (Eds.), *Orthomolecular psychiatry.* San Francisco: W. H. Freeman.

Ruttenberg, B. A., Dratman, M. L., Frankno, J., & Wenar, C. (1966). An instrument for evaluating autistic children. *Journal of the American Academy of Child Psychiatry, 5,* 453–78.

Ruttenberg, B. A., Kalish, B. I., Wenar, C., & Wolf, E. G. (1977). *Behavior rating instrument for autistic and other atypical children.* (rev. ed.). Philadelphia: Developmental Center for Autistic Children.

Rutter, M. (1978). Diagnosis and definition in childhood autism. *Journal of Autism and Childhood Schizophrenia, 8,* 139–61.

Schopler, E., & Reichler, R. J. (1979). *Individualized assessment and treatment for autistic and developmentally disabled children. Vol. I: Psychoeducational profile.* Baltimore: University Park Press.

Schopler, E., Reichler, R. J., DeVellis, R. F., & Daly, K. (1980). Toward objective classification of childhood autism: Childhood Autism Rating Scale (CARS). *Journal of Autism and Developmental Disorders, 10,* 91–103.

Schopler, E., Reichler, R. J., & Renner, B. R. (1986). *The Childhood Autism Rating Scale (CARS): For diagnostic screening and classification of autism.* New York: Irvington.

Shah, A., & Holmes, N. (1985). Brief report: The use of the Leiter International Performance Scale with autistic children. *Journal of Autism and Developmental Disorders, 15,* 195–203.

Sloan, J. L., & Marcus, L. (1981). Some findings on the use of the Adaptive Behavior Scale with autistic children. *Journal of Autism and Developmental Disorders, 11,* 191–9.

Wenar, C., & Ruttenberg, B. A. (1976). The use of BRIAAC for evaluating therapeutic effectiveness. *Journal of Autism and Childhood Schizophrenia, 6,* 175–91.

Wolf, E. G., Wenar, C., & Ruttenberg, B. A. (1972). A comparison of personality variables in autistic and mentally retarded children. *Journal of Autism and Childhood Schizophrenia, 2,* 92–108.

Yuwiler, A., Ritvo, E., Geller, E., Glousman, R., Schneiderman, G., & Matsuno, D. (1975). Uptake and efflux of serotonin from platelets of autistic and nonautistic children. *Journal of Autism and Childhood Schizophrenia, 5,* 83–98.

III

General Assessment Issues

10

Behavioral Assessment of Autism

MICHAEL D. POWERS

INTRODUCTION

Behavioral assessment is a multimethod approach for gathering information about behavior using procedures that are both empirically validated and developmentally sensitive (Ollendick & Hersen, 1984). In contrast to traditional assessment methods, behavioral assessment emphasizes environmental and organismic control over behavior, reliance on the direct observation of behavior and subsequent deemphasis on inference, consideration of temporal and contextual bases within which the target behavior is embedded (Mash & Terdal, 1981), and the use of multiple assessment methods. The purposes of behavioral assessment are twofold: (1) to aid treatment plnning by providing predictive information with respect to the potential efficacy of one intervention over another, and (2) to monitor and evaluate the effects of the intervention, once implemented.

Contemporary conceptualizations of behavior therapy identify behavioral assessment as critical to the process of change. As a treatment planning process, behavioral assessment precedes behavioral intervention. However, as a tool for treatment evaluation, behavioral assessment proceeds throughout treatment. Thus, a unique feature of the behavioral assessment enterprise is its ability to serve predictive, formative, and summative evaluation functions. While considerable progress has been made in the identification of formative and summative evaluation strategies in behavioral assessment in recent years, the ability of behavioral assessment to predict appropriate interventions and fulfill its role in treatment planning lags behind (Durand & Carr, in press) and remains an area for future work.

This chapter describes the process of behavioral assessment with persons with autism. After noting characteristics of the behavioral assessment of autism and a framework for practice, assessment methods are detailed. The chapter concludes with a discussion of special issues in the behavioral assessment of children and adults with autism.

MICHAEL D. POWERS • Preschool Autism Project, Department of Special Education, University of Maryland, College Park, Maryland 20742.

CHARACTERISTICS OF BEHAVIORAL ASSESSMENT OF CHILDREN AND ADULTS WITH AUTISM

The goals of the behavioral assessment of children and adults with autism are identical to those for persons with other disabling conditions: (1) identification of target behaviors; (2) determination of controlling variables, both environmental and organismic; (3) development and implementation of a treatment plan; and (4) evaluation of the effects of treatment (Nelson & Hayes, 1981; Powers, 1985; Powers & Handleman, 1984). Because of the special educational needs and learning and behavioral characteristics of individuals with autism, eight characteristics of the behavioral assessment of autism emerge when translating these goals into practice.

Developmentally Based

Autism is characterized as a disorder of development. Historically, however, developmental considerations have been underrepresented in behavioral assessment (Edelbrock, 1984; Harris & Ferrari, 1983). Because children with developmental disabilities such as autism exhibit disturbances in developmental rate or sequence of language, social, cognitive, perceptual, and adaptive functions, attention to both normal and atypical developmental sequelae across the life span is critical. Finally, the idiosyncratic developmental characteristics of the person with autism being evaluated must be considered.

Multidimensional

The complexity of the clinical manifestation of autism demands consideration of multiple aspects of the target behavior beyond the operational definition of a discrete event. In addition to providing an operational definition that is clear, objective, and complete (Hawkins & Dobes, 1975) the clinician must consider various contextual aspects of the target behavior. These include client affect before, during, and after performance of the behavior; sensory or perceptual factors that occasion or inhibit the target behavior; interpersonal and social components and consequences; communicative intent; learning history; and functional consequence of the behavior for the client and for significant others.

Multiple Sources of Data

To account for the complexity of behavior observed and to provide opportunities for convergence or discrepancies of observation, multiple data sources should be considered. These include not only behavioral observations by various relevant others in the client's environment, but also information from psychological evaluations, family interviews, and DSM-III-R diagnosis. When intervention is based on an understanding of the complex factors motivating or contributing to the behavior rather than simply on response topography (i.e., "how it looks"), treatment will be more highly individualized.

Interdisciplinary Collaboration

The behavioral assessment of persons with autism ultimately should provide guidelines for treatments to accelerate or decelerate behavior as well as insight into the client's learning contingencies. Recent work on the biobehavioral aspects of autism (e.g., DeMyer, Hingtgen & Jackson, 1981), communication (e.g., Schopler & Mesibov, 1985), and instructional methods (e.g., Koegel, Rincover & Egel, 1982) highlights the need for integrating evaluation data from a variety of disciplines when assessing a person with autism.

Molecular and Molar Levels of Analysis

Behavioral assessment should focus on two levels of analysis. At the molecular level, the clinician considers the specific target behavior and its controlling variables and provides information useful to program planning (e.g., IEP or IHP development). At the molar, level the target behavior is considered within relevant developmental and ecological contexts. Attempts to assess a target behavior without considering both specific aspects of that behavior and relevant contextual information will likely lead to well-defined target behaviors responsive to modification only in highly controlled analogue settings, or to poorly understood target behaviors that will resist modification in natural environments because the contingencies motivating them are unknown.

Emphasis on Strengths and Needs

While there are many good arguments for the use of syndromal diagnosis (see Powers, 1984), the ultimate goal of assessment is to guide instruction. Thus, the behavioral assessment of autism emphasizes the careful and complete description of behavioral excesses, deficits, and strengths as they relate to educational planning. It is insufficient merely to describe those behaviors which should be reduced in order to facilitate learning; one must also determine functional strengths, skills, and preferences that can be incorporated into the educational plan so that a prosocial functional behavior replaces a behavioral excess or deficit.

Functional Approach

Behavioral assessors participate in the process of selection and prioritizing of treatment goals. In addition to selecting goals that are socially valid (Kazdin, 1977; Wolf, 1978), clinicians should emphasize the selection, assessment, and treatment of target behaviors that promote participation in integrated community settings. By selecting the "criterion of ultimate functioning" (Brown, Nietupski & Hamre-Nietupski, 1976) as the conceptual framework for the behavioral assessment of autism, clinicians will guarantee the ultimate utility of their efforts and promote client transition to less restrictive educational and living environments.

Systems Emphasis

Various investigators have argued for the expansion of behavioral assessment and treatment domains when providing services to persons with developmental disabilities such as autism (Christian, Hannah & Glahn, 1984; Emery, Binkoff, Houts & Carr, 1983; Harris, 1983; Powers, 1988; Powers & Handleman, 1984; Schopler, Lansing & Waters, 1983; Schopler & Reichler, 1979, Schopler, Reichler & Lansing, 1980). This expanded approach beyond a single context (e.g., home, school) emphasizes assessment, treatment, and evaluation across various systems of interaction within which the person with autism operates. Explicit consideration of client, family, environmental, and interactional variables thus becomes essential to a comprehensive behavioral assessment and treatment plan. While several characteristics of a systems approach can be identified (see Powers, 1988), one critical feature relevant to the present discussion is the reciprocity between various aspects of the autistic person's environment, and the impact of these components on behavior. For example, the systems emphasis of behavioral assessment facilitates recognition, assessment, and treatment of the reciprocal social influences of autism. As a disorder of social interactive functioning, autism engenders severe deficits of social perception and functioning in an individual (Kozloff, 1973). However, such deficits have an impact on nonautistic significant others (e.g., teachers, siblings, bus drivers) as well. Assessment of the reciprocally determined behavior of those people and environmental conditions that interact with the person with autism permits both a broader base for treatment (Emery et al., 1983), and access to a wider variety of change agents, thereby promoting generalization and maintenance.

Numerous variables in any given client converge to produce the highly individualized behavioral, cognitive, and environmental profile to which we respond. These include health factors; biological variables; prior learning histories (Powers & Handleman, 1984); peer reactions (McHale & Simeonsson, 1980); classroom curriculum (Donnellan, 1980); the present position of the child within the family's lifecycle (Harris & Powers, 1984); the presence and capabilities of siblings (Lobato, 1983; McHale, Simeonsson & Sloan, 1984); the family's response to raising a developmentally disabled child (Harris, 1982); expectations of reward and punishment (Franzini, 1979); expectations of personal efficacy (Bandura, 1977); the family's readiness for change (Powers & Handleman, 1984); and the family's technical skill in managing their child's behavior (Harris, 1984). Consideration of each client, family, community, and school-related variable with each individual disabled by autism is rarely possible, nor is the above list exhaustive; additional factors such as community reactions, physical characteristics of living and educational environments, and maternal insularity have not been included. All, however, have been found to determine the behavior of some developmentally disabled persons. To the extent that each of these components might provide information relevant to problem maintenance or problem resolution, they deserve attention in the behavioral assessment process.

ADVANTAGES OF BEHAVIORAL ASSESSMENT

Behavioral assessment is idiographic in application. Response covariations and controlling variables are understood to be specific to the individual. In contrast, nomethetic assessment methods (e.g., standardized psychological tests when such tests are used to compare persons with autism to a norm population; DSM-III-R diagnosis) lead to generalizations about an individual's performance. While nomothetic data are useful because they summarize clinically relevant information, help narrow intervention options, and facilitate communication among professionals (Nelson & Barlow, 1981), sole reliance on nomothetic data would lead to ill-defined treatment plans. By combining idiographic and nomothetic descriptions of behavior, behavioral assessment facilitates the development of individualized treatments.

Through the use of the SORKC analysis (stimulus–organismic-response–contingencies of reinforcement-consequence) (Kanfer & Saslow, 1969), the behavioral assessment of autism takes on a comprehensive focus. This model is an improvement over the earlier ABC (antecedent–behavior–consequence) framework because of the inclusion of two assessment domains important to autism: contingencies and schedules of reinforcement (K) and organismic variables (O). This latter variable has particular relevance to assessment of the person with autism because it permits consideration of individual physiological conditions and prior learning histories in the assessment and treatment planning process.

FRAMEWORK FOR THE BEHAVIORAL ASSESSMENT OF AUTISM

The framework for the behavioral assessment of persons with autism consists of four steps: (1) identification of the target behavior; (2) determination of controlling variables, both environmental and organismic; (3) development of the treatment plan; and (4) evaluation of the effects of treatment. The first two steps focus on the specific target behavior under consideration. The third step considers the target behavior within its developmental and ecological molar contexts, while the fourth step emphasizes the evaluation of the interventions based on both molecular and molar analysis. Specifically, this last step includes outcome evaluation, social validation (e.g., Schreibman, Koegel, Mills & Burke, 1981), and program evaluation (Maher & Bennett, 1984; Powers & Handleman, 1984).

Identification of the Target Behavior

Before intervention, a target behavior must be identified, clarified, and defined operationally. Teachers and parents must be provided assistance in prioritizing target behaviors for intervention where several exist in the service of reducing potential treatment failures or negative effects due to overextended resources, burnout, or confusion. A second task is to assess parent or teacher requests for their reasonableness and social validity. Some behaviors may be believed by caregivers to warrant attention when such treatment would actually be inappropriate. Education about developmental expectations of autistic and nonhandicapped children may help them determine the social validity of potential target behaviors identified for possible treatment.

Determination of Controlling Variables

Determination of variables that control a target behavior is accomplished through the SORKC analysis described earlier. Three major classes of controlling variables have been described: current environmental variables (stimuli and consequences), organismic variables, and contingencies of reinforcement (Nelson & Hayes, 1979). Additional variables important to the behavioral assessment of autism include schedules of reinforcement and response dimensions.

Stimuli (S)

Environmental conditions that precede performance of the target behavior and that are presumed to exert control over the target behavior are termed stimulus antecedents. Antecedents can be further categorized as either discriminative stimuli or as elicitors. A discriminative stimulus "sets the stage" for a specific response, because the individual has learned that this response will occasion a particular consequence. By contrast, elicitors represent the class of stimulus antecedents that evoke physiological or automatic emotional responses (e.g., tachychardia, tantrums). Elicitors are of special interest to the behavioral assessment of autism because of the autistic person's characteristic deviance in response to sensory stimuli. Where sensory hyperreactivity is observed to preceed a targeted behavioral excess (e.g., self-injury), a clinically meaningful stimulus antecedent may have been identified. Other antecedent stimuli to be considered when assessing an individual with autism include interactions with other children and adults, social situations, and environmental conditions such as physical space, time of day, place, and temperature.

Recent research suggests the importance of considering the instructional or interactive situation as a complex array of stimuli when assessing the individual with autism (Koegel, Rincover & Egel, 1982). Specifically, the clinician must determine the motivation for the performance of a particular target behavior by the individual when he or she is confronted with the instructional or interactive task. Four potential motivating conditions have been described: escape and avoidance, access to social attention, sensory reinforcing consequences, and access to preferred activities and tangible rewards (cf. Carr, 1977; Carr & Durand, 1985a,b; Iwata, Dorsey, Slifer, Bauman & Richman, 1982). Determining motivators for a particular target behavior has important implications for treatment selection and the prediction of intervention outcomes. For example, treatments that reduce behavioral excesses and deficits without considering what motivated the client to emit the behavior in the first place (e.g., escape from a difficult task demand, or a desire for adult attention) may lead to client performance of a new maladaptive to fulfill the same motivational function.

Organismic Variables (O)

These frequently neglected variables have special relevance to the behavioral assessment of persons with autism. Included here are biological states such as sensory impairments, fatigue, and health (Nelson & Hayes, 1979), genetic, biochemical, or neurologic variables (Mash & Terdal, 1981), and prior learning histories (Powers & Handleman, 1984). Organic conditions that have a specified effect on the form and function of behavior and that are known to co-occur with autism, such as Tourette's syndrome (Realmuto & Main, 1982) and seizures (Deykin & MacMahon, 1979), should be included in the behavioral assessment process, so that the intervention that follows reflects the specific behavioral excesses or deficits under the control of biologic or genetic factors.

Responses (R)

Comprehensive behavioral assessment of a client%s response to antecedent or conse-quent stimuli should include specification of at least five dimensions: duration, frequency, topography, magnitude, and pervasiveness. Duration refers to the elapsed time between the onset and the offset of each behavior. Frequency refers to how often a behavior occurs, while topography refers to the physical characteristics of the behavior (e.g., "how it looks"). Magnitude represents the degree of social validity attached to the target behavior by signifi-cant others, while pervasiveness provides an index of the form and type of multiple environ-ments within which the behavior occurs.

Contingencies of Reinforcement (K)

These variables refer both to the schedules of reinforcement (Ferster & Skinner, 1957) and to the contingencies of reinforcement that influence the topography, rate, correctness, durability, or potency of a client's response. Schedule of reinforcement refers to the timing, density, and delivery of reinforcers as well as to the ratio of reinforcers to correct responses. Koegel and Rincover (1974) and Koegel, Schreibman, Britten, and Laitinen (1979) demon-strated the importance of reinforcement schedules in teaching individuals with autism. Con-tingencies of reinforcement are those particular conditions under which reinforcement occurs that influence the probability of a correct response. Numerous contingencies of reinforcement relevant to the behavioral assessment of autism have been identified. These include stimulus variation during the task (Dunlap & Koegel, 1980), variation of intertrial interval (Koegel, Dunlap & Dyer, 1980), variation of reinforcement (Egel, 1980, 1981), stimulus-specific reinforcement (Litt & Schreibman, 1981), level and predictability of supervision (Dunlap & Johnson, 1985), and the use of sensory reinforcers (Durand & Carr, 1985; Iwata et al., 1982; Rincover & Newsom, 1985).

Consequences (C)

The behavior of persons with autism is often under the control of reinforcing and aversive consequences. Consequences that are reinforcing to one person may be aversive to another, however. For this reason, consequences must be defined functionally in behavioral assessment: Reinforcing consequences increase the likelihood that the behavior preceeding it will increase or maintain over time, and aversive consequences increase the likelihood that behavior will decrease over time.

A note of caution on terminology and philosophical values is warranted. The importance of emphasizing individual reinforcing and aversive consequences with an autistic person cannot be overstated. Research has demonstrated that some interventions traditionally viewed as aversive (e.g., restraint) are in fact reinforcing for some persons with severe developmen-tal disabilities (Favell, 1983; and Favell, McGimsey & Jones, 1978). Similarly, reinforcer preferences may be highly idiosyncratic (Favell & Cannon, 1977). It therefore represents a leap-of-faith to assume, a priori, the reinforcing or aversive nature of any consequence. Recent years have witnessed an increased use of the qualifier "nonaversive" with a variety of behavior reduction procedures with persons with autism and other severe developmental disorders. Given the idiosyncratic preferences of many autistic individuals, the question of "nonaversiveness" can be restated as "nonaversive to whom?" Here issues of philosophy and science collide. One current philosophical position shared by many clinicians is that aversive procedures violate client rights to humane and normalizing interventions and should therefore be prohibited. In some jurisdictions (e.g., the District of Columbia) such beliefs have been translated into law. Other jurisdictions adopt a more cautious approach, evaluating the aversiveness of a proposed intervention on a more individualized basis. One problem with the latter approach is that the actual aversiveness of a treatment to the client with whom it is applied is an empirical issue: if the rate, intensity, duration, magnitude, or pervasiveness of the target behavior decreases contingent upon the intervention, then the intervention was aversive. Many clinicians could predict aversiveness from prior knowledge of, or experience with, the treatment procedure, particularly interventions at the most restrictive end of the aversiveness continuum (e.g., contingent electric shock). But decisions come harder as clinicians move toward the midpoint of the continuum. As a result, reliance on empirical validation is not sufficient. One must also be prepared to assess and demonstrate the social validity (Wolf, 1978) of the target behavior and the proposed intervention from the perspective of significant others and community members who are reflective of local norms. The aversive or nonaversive nature of a proposed intervention can then be specified individually (to whom: staff? the client? parents? other professionals? and under what circumstances?). Failure to evaluate the social validity of proposed target behaviors and interventions is contrary to "best practice" in behavioral assessment. However, the assumption of the social validity (or invalidity) of targets or treatments has more far-reaching implications because of the potential violation of an autistic persons's right to effective treatment (see Martin, 1975; and McClannahan & Krantz, 1985).

Development of the Treatment Plan

The goal of this third step is to obtain information on the multiple situational contexts within which the target behavior occurs. Several assessment domains and related tasks have been identified for this molar analysis (Kanfer & Saslow, 1969; Powers & Handleman, 1984). These include (1) clarification of the problem situation to determine who supports or objects to the target behavior; (2) assessment of reinforcers and punishers that are salient for the client; (3) motivational assessment (i.e., access to attention, escape, sensory consequences, access to material rewards); (4) determination of those who have been successful in delivering positive and negative consequences in the past; (5) assessment of social status for affiliations and community resources that might contribute to acquisition and maintenance of adaptive behavior to replace the maladaptive target behavior; (6) assessment of the extent of self-control, conditions motivating effective self-control, and conditions that cause a breakdown in the client's ability to exert self-control; (7) assessment of social relationships for significant others who elicit appropriate prosocial behavior, as well as inappropriate behavior; (8) determination of reinforcers that are operative in social situations; (9) assessment of prevailing sociocultural norms related to the target behavior in the various environments within which the client operates; and (10) assessment of the client's physical environments for reduced or enhanced opportunities for reinforcement.

While some assessment tasks may not be relevant to particular clients with autism, failure to account for ecologic constraints and resources may increase the likelihood that

environmental resources will go unused, or that interventions will proceed without consideration of ecologic constraints, inhibiting generalization and maintenance.

Evaluation of the Effects of Treatment

Evaluation of an intervention for a client with autism is both formative and summative in
nature and takes place within a variety of contexts. Throughout treatment, dependent measures are obtained to provide guidance on treatment plan modification. Dependent measures
selected for this formative evaluation must be practical, yet objective, valid, and reliable.
Behavioral assessment methods include direct observation of the target behavior in the
natural environment (e.g., using interval, event, duration recording); the use of enactment
analogues (i.e., artificial situations representing typical environmental conditions); perma-
nent products (e.g., nursing notes, incident reports, the number of soiled diapers in a
receptacle at day's end); and behavioral checklists of client excesses, deficits and strengths.
Measurement of dependent variables must then be incorporated into an appropriate experimental or quasi-experimental evaluation design to demonstrate a functional relationship
between treatment and rate of behavior before and after intervention (Kazdin, 1982b; Kratochwill, 1985; Powers & Handleman, 1984; Voeltz & Evans, 1983).

The multidimensional, multisituational nature of behavioral assessment in autism demands evaluation of treatment effects beyond the single case. The social validity of treatment
gains for significant others must be determined (e.g., Kazdin, 1977; Wolf, 1978). Negative
effects (e.g., Mays & Franks, 1985) and unanticipated positive effects may be evident and
should be evaluated. Finally, procedural reliability (Billingsley, White & Munson, 1980)—
the extent to which program implementors followed the intervention protocol correctly—
may have bearing on the results of treatment and should be addressed.

BEHAVIORAL ASSESSMENT METHODS

In order to meet adequately the goals of facilitating treatment planning as well as the
evaluation of intervention plans, clinicians conducting a behavioral assessment of an individual with autism must access data from a variety of sources including direct observation of
the target behavior, syndromal diagnosis, psychological test data, parent and teacher interviews, and objective behavioral rating scales. Consideration of data from multiple sources
facilitates an understanding of the target behavior within relevant contexts, may confirm or
disconfirm hypotheses, and may identify additional areas within the client's social ecology
requiring treatment.

Idiographic Methods

Idiographic methods of assessment emphasize the specification of response rate, setting,
person, event, and organismic controlling variables so that resultant interventions will be
highly individualized. Within the behavioral assessment enterprise the direct observation of
behavior is the principle method for gathering idiographic data. Direct observation techniques
include time sampling, interval, duration, and frequency recording; all emphasize the impor-

tance of highly valid and reliable measures, and deemphasize inferences in the data evaluation process. A comprehensive description of the advantages and disadvantages of direct
observation deserves book-length exposition; for that the reader is referred elsewhere (Kazdin, 1980; and Barton & Ascione, 1984). Suffice to say that the direct observation of client
behavior remains one of the mainstays of behavioral assessment. Recent criticisms of the
tendency for simplified direct observation methods to obscure meaningful behavioral interrelationships and response chains (e.g., Kazdin, 1982a; Voeltz & Evans, 1982) has resulted in
increased emphasis on the definition and measurement of collateral behavior (Voeltz &
Evans, 1982), the use of sequential recording and analysis (Barton & Ascione, 1984),
archival analysis (Bornstein, Bridgwater, Hickey & Sweeney, 1980) and real-time computer
analysis (Romanczyk, 1983).

Direct observation as a behavioral assessment method requires a subsequent decision as
to observation setting. Observations can be carried out in either naturalistic or analogue
settings depending on the treatment design and available resources. Each has advantages and
disadvantages. Assessment in the natural environment provides data more likely to reflect
performance under "typical" conditions than data obtained in analogue or experimental
settings. However, naturalistic assessment increases the potential for client reactivity to
assessment devices or strategies. Kazdin (1979) describes several methods for decreasing the
obtrusiveness of behavioral assessment in natural environments including use of one-way
mirrors, videotaping observations for later analysis, use of archival data, and assessment of
physical traces including job tasks completed, objects stolen, and litter.

Regardless of observation setting, the use of direct observation techniques raises the
possibility of numerous sources of measurement error including expectation biases, reactivity, consensual drift among observers, and biasing factors influencing the reliability of the
observations. Kazdin (1980) describes these issues and methods for their remediation in
detail.

Nomothetic Methods

Nomothetic assessment emphasizes the comparison of an individual client to a global
descriptive assessment system that summarizes the performance or characteristics of many
persons. Conclusions about the individual's performance based on nomothetic methods are
useful because they guide the clinician's behavior, summarize research and clinical information, facilitate communication among professionals, suggest response covariations and controlling variables for further assessment, and promote comparison of clinical samples by
providing additional descriptive information about subjects (Hartmann, Roper & Bradford,
1979; Nelson & Barlow, 1981; Nelson & Hayes, 1981).

Two nomothetic assessment methods have particular relevance to the behavioral assessment of children and adults with autism: psychological assessment and syndromal diagnosis.
As most individuals with autism have had or will have a psychological evaluation conducted
for purposes of determining eligibility for special educational or vocational services and
related program planning, these data provide potentially useful information to be incorporated into the behavioral assessment enterprise.

The psychological assessment of persons with autism and other severe developmental
disabilities has three goals: (1) the observation and evaluation of behavioral repertoires using
traditional instruments (Weschler Intelligence Scale for Children—Revised; Weschler, 1974)

and those designed specifically for individuals with autism (e.g., Psychoeducational Profile; Schopler & Reichler, 1979); (2) data analysis to yield a profile of functional strengths and weaknesses across the domains of cognitive, perceptual, motor, language, and social functioning; and (3) synthesis of data from these domains with diagnostic and behavioral assessment data to provide specific intervention strategies across school, family, and community systems. These goals emphasize the unique status of the person with autism and focus on the collection of data that will be helpful in remediating the presenting problem. The extreme heterogeneity of persons with autism make the development of norms difficult. As a result of the uneven patterns of individual development and idiosyncratic responding of many persons with autism, an ipsative approach to evaluation is necessary. In contrast to normative use of assessment instruments, an ipsative approach emphasizes comparison of a client's particular response to his or her total set of responses during the assessment. While a normative comparision may be made for regulatory or insurance purposes with an educational or diagnostic classification as the outcome, such a label is of secondary importance in behavioral assessment.

During a psychological evaluation, the tests employed can be conceptualized as standardized stimulus formats against which an individual's performance is assessed, and also as a means of determining response style, selective attention to multiple stimulus cues, response to rapid versus slow pacing, prompting, prompt fading, and explicit reinforcement, and the client's ability to profit from instrumental enrichment over the course of the testing session. In addition to gathering clinical data on learning characteristics the examiner may have the opportunity to observe, assess, and modify various behavioral excesses and deficits that interfere with learning (e.g., stereotypy, self-injury). To the extent that hypotheses can be tested during the evaluation session, the results obtained will be useful for program planning purposes.

Syndromal diagnosis provides information useful to the behavioral assessment of persons with autism. In particular, the Diagnostic and Statistical Manual of Mental Disorders (3rd edition, revised) (DSM-III-R, American Psychiatric Association, 1987) provides a useful adjunct to the behavioral assessment process, promoting a synthesis between the two systems. In providing nomothetic descriptions of client behavior, DSM-III-R diagnosis performs an initial, broad-band assessment function. A determination of controlling variables for each specific DSM-III-R criterion met by the client is then made using a SORKC analysis. Relevant assessment methodologies for each criterion are subsequently identified and implemented, leading to a functional analysis of each criterion identified. This in turn leads to treatment hypotheses, intervention plans, evaluations, and follow-up.

Several advantages to the use of this synergistic model have been noted (Powers, 1984). The use of feedback loops inherent in the behavioral assessment process is facilitated, enabling information obtained at any phase of the diagnosis and assessment to influence decision-making at other points. Cues to additional areas warranting assessment may become evident. Diagnosis, along with behavioral assessment methods, becomes one part of an information system producing data on the autistic person's behavior, which then guides the appropriate and comprehensive treatment of that behavior. These data can then be summarized and communicated efficiently to other professionals. Thus, important characteristics of this information system include its functional-analytic capacities, its use of feedback loops for decision-making, and its ability to generate, synthesize, use, and disseminate nomothetic data for clinical and research purposes. This last point renders the integration of findings in child psychiatry more feasible due to a common classification system (Kazdin, 1983), facilitating interdisciplinary collaboration in the diagnosis, assessment, and treatment of autism.

Behavioral Interviewing

In order for the behavioral assessment to begin, the presenting problem must be clarified in an interview, the end result of which is an operationally defined target behavior understood within its ecologic context. During the initial interview(s), the clinician addresses herself to two goals: (1) gathering detailed information about the unity, duration, latency, topography, and interresponse time of the target behavior, and (2) assessing relevant home, school, and community contexts within which the behavior is performed in order to evaluate environmental controlling variables.

Six objectives have been identified for the behavioral interview of the family or teacher of a child with autism: (1) to establish rapport; (2) to clarify the reason for referral; (3) to assess the family's (or teachers') interactional style; (4) to obtain a social history; (5) to obtain a developmental history; and (6) to determine the family's (or teachers'') resources and readiness for change. While the low validity and reliability of parent and teacher reports compromise the utility of some of these data, the data obtained during the behavioral interview represent a clinically useful sample of behavior (Ollendick & Cerny, 1981).

Establishing Rapport

Clinicians must be sensitive to, and prepared to validate, feelings of frustration of teachers and parents with regard to the presenting problem. Issues of loss, denial, extended grieving, and other concerns related to parental perceptions of their child's handicap often must be acknowledged. Finally, early implications by the clinician that the parents or teacher were somehow responsible for the problem should be avoided. While behavioral assessment may in fact identify a functional relationship between the behavior of the autistic child and the parents' behavior, premature description of this relationship may weaken already frail feelings of personal efficacy. As caregiver perceptions of self-efficacy are integral to the process of change, they should be protected initially, fostered, and developed.

Clarifying the Reason for Referral

Clarification of the referral question represents an attempt to define further the precise nature of the problem and to identify environmental factors that may contribute to or inhibit the performance of the target behavior. Several dimensions are relevant, including family perceptions, natural history of the problem, situational specificity, and drug–behavior interactions. Table I elaborates eight areas for assessment.

Assessing Interactional Style

Harris (1982) identifies several interactional patterns of families with autistic members, including enmeshment, underinvolvement, leniency, and outright rejection. Importantly, these patterns represent the coping responses of family members to the family member with autism. To the extent that interaction patterns are sometimes maladaptive or destructive

Table I. Assessment Domains for Problem Clarification

Assess parental concerns and perceptions of the problem(s) experienced.

Assess the natural history of the problem including when it began, relevant environmental antecedents, and consequences.

Assess for situational specificity or generalized nature of the problem (e.g., school, home, community)

Assess sibling and extended family perceptions of the problem.

Conduct a brief ABC (antecedent–behavior–consequence) analysis of the last few times the behavior was observed.

Assess for previous attempts at problem resolution.

Assess for medication use, duration and dose, recent changes in dosage, and parental perceptions of interaction of behavior and medication.

Assess family members for the degree of symptom reduction necessary for them to consider the problem "manageable."

---

further assessment and intervention may be warranted. Where such patterns are within the boundaries of normal family process, family strengths and resources that may facilitate problem resolution can be identified and incorporated into the treatment plan.

While less well described, the social ecology of service delivery organizations that the person with autism operates within present similar concerns and represent opportunities for behavioral assessment. At the most basic level, classrooms may have little structure imposed by the teacher, too much structure, or an inconsistent combination of both. In the less desirable of these situations, even the most carefully conceived behavioral intervention may fail due to a low level of congruence with the organizational structure.

Obtaining a Social and Developmental History

These data provide relevant background information across a variety of areas, including family demographics; birth history; early history; recent development; developmental milestones; educational and vocational history; current status in social, communication, self-help, and other areas; a symptom checklist for screening purposes; and relevant release of records forms. As completion of this task can be time-consuming, some clinicians have found it more expedient to have parents fill out a social and developmental history form at home and mail it to the clinician prior to the initial interview.

Determining Resources and Readiness for Change

In some families, a change in the presenting problem may be desired, but few individuals may be available to carry out the treatment program. In others, cultural or religious values may counsel tolerance of problematic behavior even when such behavior is not in the best interest of the person with autism. In either case, failure to determine ahead of time these impediments to planned change can result in treatment failures. Powers and Handleman (1984) describe several areas for consideration when evaluating the resources and readiness for change of families and teachers. The availability of resources and the willingness to

Table II. Behavioral Rating Scales and Checklists

| Name | Domains assessed | Total No. of items | Ratings based on: | | Special competencies needed for administration or scoring | Measures of severity for each item included? | Validity | Reliability |
			Direct observations	Third-party report				
Behavior Observation System (Freeman et al., 1984)	Solitary behavior Relation to objects/toys Relation to examiner Language	24	X		Trained raters; computer analysis of raw data	No	Satisfactory	Satisfactory
Autism Descriptors Checklist (Fisch et al., 1985)	Interpersonal relationships Communication and affect Sound and speech reception Vocalization and expressive speech Visual behavior Learning and memory Maintenance of sameness Self-care Stereotypy Body movement	70 (Interview edition) 58 (Direct observation edition)	X	X	Trained raters for the direct observation edition	Yes 6-point scale	Satisfactory	Satisfactory
Real Life Rating Scale (Freeman et al., 1986)	Sensorimotor Social relationship to people Affectual responses Sensory response Language	47	X		Trained raters	Yes 4-point scale	Satisfactory	Satisfactory
Childhood Autism Rating Scale (Schopler et al., 1980)	Relationship with people Imitation Affect Body awareness	15	X		Trained raters	Yes 7-point scale	Satisfactory	Satisfactory

Instrument	Content assessed	Number of items		Raters	Scoring	Reliability	Validity
Diagnostic Checklist for Behavior-Disturbed Children (Form E-2) (Rimland, 1971)	Relation to nonhuman objects; Adaptive to change; Visual responsiveness; Auditory responsiveness; Near-receptor responsiveness; Anxiety reaction; Verbal communication; Activity level; Intellectual functioning; General impressions; Items assess language and social functioning; family history; affective, motor, cognitive, and perceptual development; various other behaviors believed characteristic of autism	80	X	None	No	Satisfactory	Not reported
Behavior Rating Instrument for Autistic and Atypical Children (Ruttenburg et al., 1977)	Relationship; Communication; drive for mastery; vocalization; sound and speech; social responsiveness; Body movement; Psychobiologic development	Each scale has 10 progressive levels, one of which is selected	X	Trained raters	Yes; Scale of 1–10	Satisfactory	Satisfactory
Autism Behavior Checklist (Krug, Arick & Almond, 1979)	Sensory; Relating; Body and object use; Language; Social and self-help skills	57	X	Trained raters	No	Unsatisfactory	Unsatisfactory

commit those resources to bring about planned change in the individual with autism must be assessed. Behavioral expectations and philosophical, religious, and culturally based positions can also have an impact on success. Congruence with family or classroom values is often an unspoken precondition of treatment; lack of congruence may undermine the intervention process. Family characteristics that may promote or impede change include the stability of the marital and sibling relationships, maternal insularity (e.g., Wahler, 1980), a disabling disorder in the parental subsystem (e.g., alcoholism, depression), the "tradition of flexibility" within the family, divorce, death, and family relocations. Perceived need or "system pain" (Powers & Franks, 1988) motivating the request for change must be evident. Presenting problems with insufficient system pain will often be accompanied by low levels of parental or teacher perceptions of obligation to actually do something about the problem. Finally, the expected benefits of planned change which families or teachers believe will accrue if they participate in intervention must be considered. Not surprisingly, a perceived sense of control over their lives is a yield valued by many parents and teachers seeking treatment for a person with autism.

Rating Scales and Checklists

Behavioral assessment of persons with autism can be augmented by use of behavioral rating scales and checklists designed specifically for this population. Rating scales are typically descriptive in nature, but may also serve diagnostic functions (e.g., *The E-2 Scale;* Rimland, 1971; *The Childhood Autism Rating Scale;* Schopler, Reichler, DeVellis & Daly, 1980). All identify behavioral correlates of autism for consideration by the rater, often with options for noting severity of the symptom. Ultimately, beyond any possible diagnostic functions behavioral rating scales provide listings of potential target excesses and deficits for program planning purposes, and identify behavioral strengths and weaknesses. Several rating scales and objective behavioral assessment systems are discussed below and are summarized in Table II.

Behavioral Observation System

The BOS is designed to differentiate autistic from nonautistic children, identify subgroups, and provide a coherent and consistent basis for describing autistic children for research purposes (Freeman *et al.*, 1984, p. 588). The BOS contains 24 items that provide a valid, reliable, and objective means for describing the behavior of children suspected of autism. The 24 behaviors are divided into four general categories: Solitary behaviors; Relation to Objects/Toys; Relation to Examiner; and Language. Precise behavioral definitions are provided for each item. Advantages of the revised BOS include its objectively defined categories, validity, and reliability. Additionally, because of its use of sequential coding of observed behavior and subsequent computer analysis, the BOS holds promise for identifying response patterns and behavioral interrelationships for subtypes of autism. Disadvantages include the lack of reported diagnostic cutoff scores and questionalbe ability to differentially diagnose autism from other childhood psychopathologic states (excluding mental retardation).

Autism Descriptors Checklist

The ADC is both a parent report retrospective checklist and a behavioral coding system designed to discriminate subgroups of autism based on developmental symptomatology (Fisch, Cohen, Wolf & Friedman, 1985). It consists of 70 items in the parent interview edition and 58 in the direct observation edition. The behavioral items on the ADC are divided into 10 categories: Interpersonal Relationships; Communication and Affect; Sound and Speech Reception; Vocalization and Expressive Speech; Visual Behavior; Learning and lemory; Maintenance of Sameness; Self-Care; Stereotyped Behavior; and Body Movement. Operational definitions for each behavioral item are not provided. Advantages of the ADC are that items are scored against the client's relevant developmental time period, the inclusion of severity ratings, and the availability of two assessment formats (parent report and direct observation). Disadvantages include the lack of reported cutoff scores for various subtypes of autism and questionable ability to differentiate autism from conditions other than mental retardation.

Ritvo–Freeman Real-Life Rating Scale

The RLRS is an adaptation of the BOS (Freeman *et al.*, 1984) intended for use in nonclinical settings by professionals. The RLRS contains 47 well-defined target behaviors for videotape observation and coding by trained raters. These items are scattered among five scales: Sensory Motor; Social Relationship to People; Affectual Response; Sensory Response; and Language. Scoring is accomplished by rating the child at the end of a 30-min standard observation session.

Advantages of the RLRS include its emphasis on nonclinical settings for observation, well defined target behaviors, and good validity and reliability. Disadvantages are limited to the scaling method used. Given the potential for enormous differences in client behavior rating a score of 3 (i.e., from behavior observed 7 times to behavior observed "constantly"), it is possible that by averaging item scores highly deviant performance in one or two areas will be obfuscated. To a certain extent, this problem can be solved by individual item analysis.

Childhood Autism Rating Scale

The CARS is a diagnostic instrument designed to discriminate subgroups of autistic children from children with other developmental disabilities (Schopler, Reichler, DeVellis & Daly, 1980). The CARS is rated by an experienced examiner after observation of a structured psychoeducational diagnostic evaluation. Each of the following 15 items is evaluated on a 7-point scale: Relationship with People; Imitation; Affect; Body Awareness: Relation to Non-human Objects; Adaptation to Change; Visual Responsiveness; Auditory Responsiveness; New Receptor Responsiveness; Anxiety Reaction; Verbal Communication; Nonverbal Communication; Activity Level; Intellectual Functioning; and General Impressions. Advantages of the CARS include its attention to developmental level, the provision of diagnostic cutoff scores, reliability, and validity, and its applicability to persons with autism across the lifespan (see Mesibov, *this volume*, for a discussion of the use of the CARS with adolescents and adults). Disadvantages include the reliance on post hoc, rather than real-time, analysis of behavior.

Diagnostic Checklist for Behavior-Disturbed Children, Form E-2

The E-2 scale is a retrospective, multiple-choice parent report designed to diagnose early infantile autism (Rimland, 1971). The 80 items included assess language and social functioning, family history, affective, motor, cognitive, and perceptual development, and various behaviors characteristic of autism such as responsiveness to various stimuli and obsessive and perseverative behavior. The E-2 scale generates three scores: speech, behavior, and total. Possible total scores range from -42 to $+45$, with $+20$ set as the cutoff score for the diagnosis of early infantile autism (Rimland, 1971). Disadvantages of the E-2 scale surround the lack of any reliability or validity studies (Parks, 1983), low intecorrelation (.35) between the Speech and Behavior scores (Deckner, Soraci, Deckner & Blanton, 1982) and the tendency of parent ratings to underrepresent pathology when compared to those of teachers (Prior & Bence, 1975). At this time, the recommendation that Form E-2 of the Diagnostic Checklist for Behavior-Disturbed Children be used only for screening purposes appears most prudent (DeMyer, Churchill, Pontius & Gilkey, 1971; Parks, 1983).

Behavior Rating Instrument for Autistic and Atypical Children

The BRIAAC is a direct observation instrument for use with autistic and other low-functioning developmentally disabled children (Ruttenberg, Kalish, Wenar & Wolf, 1977). There are eight scales, each with operationally defined behavioral descriptions at ten possible levels. These include: Relationship; Communication; Drive for Mastery; Vocalization; Sound and Speech; Social Responsiveness; Body Movement; and Psychobiological Development. Advantages of the BRIAAC include excellent validity and reliability, its use of objectively defined behaviors, and the developmental progression from normal-to-extremely deviant behavior across each of the domains assessed. The major disadvantages to the BRIAAC include its post hoc (as opposed to real time) coding system, and its difficulty in differentiating among subtypes of autism, mental retardation, and related pervasive developmental language disorders (Cohen, Caparulo, Gold, Waldo, Shaywitz, Ruttenberg & Rimland, 1978).

Autism Screening Instrument for Educational Planning

The ASIEP (Krug, Arick & Almond, 1979) was designed to measure different aspects of autistic symptomatology:

Component 1. Overt behavioral symptoms
Component 2. Vocalizations
Component 3. Interactions
Component 4. Educational assessment
Component 5. Prognosis of learning rate

Overt behavioral symptoms are measured using the Autism Behavior Checklist (ABC), while performance in components 2–5 is evaluated by sampling behavior in quasistandardized formats described by the authors. Only the ABC has been evaluated for reliability and validity (Krug et al., 1980).

The ABC consists of 57 items sampling behavior across five domains: sensory, relating, body and object use, language, and social and self-help skills. While interrator reliability is high, it is based on a very small sample ($N=14$). The ABC would benefit from an analysis of discriminant validity based on the direct observation of groups of children and adults with and without, rather than the demographic analysis of checklists method used by the authors (Krug et al., 1980). For the present, the ABC is insufficient as a diagnostic tool, and best regarded as a screening device for behavior often associated with autism (Table II).

Integration of Behavioral Assessment Data

For behavioral assessment to be a worthwhile process, decision-makers must use the information obtained to promote and expand the habilitative options of persons with autism. When translating this policy into practice, however, certain assumptions are warranted. First, the use of disparate behavioral assessment methods precludes the opportunity for data "averaging." The final plan resulting from consideration of multiple sources of data will necessarily be a product of clinical judgment. For some clients, interviews with parents and nomothetic data from psychological testing may influence a decision to intensify home-based parent training efforts. For others, the severity of self-injurious behavior may argue for a comprehensive approach to treating the problem whereby the family and school both shift gears and commit resources to ameliorate the problem. Behavioral assessors must resist the urge to determine final single common pathways to the measurement of change, and accept the responsibility to evaluate change by the most empirical standard available for each method used.

Second, multiple methods of data collection require multiple methods, and levels, of data analysis. Few would argue that retrospective data from parent interviews are less reliable than direct observation of client behavior repeated over time. However, careful clinical interviewing can provide otherwise inaccessible information about family resources, preferences for treatment, and cultural and religious values. Each data source has merit. The inclusion of clinical assessment into the process of behavioral assessment in no way weakens the process; rather, it provides context. To reconcile differences in assessment method, the clinician must evaluate change at many levels. Individual treatment outcomes can be evaluated with single-case designs. At the small system level, teacher attitudes or burnout may need to be followed before and after intervention, or parent stress may need to be monitored. At the larger system level community norms may be evaluated through social validation, and educational norms and expectations by program evaluation methods. The evaluation of data from these varied sources requires flexibility of the clinician and the willingness to seek points of behavioral convergence across data rather than applying a personal theoretical agenda to data analysis. To the extent that different behavioral assessment methods identify target behaviors and supporting hypotheses for treatment and then establish a method for ongoing data analysis, the assessment–intervention–evaluation cycle will be well served.

SPECIAL ISSUES IN THE BEHAVIORAL ASSESSMENT OF AUTISM

Conducting a behavioral assessment on a person with autism demands consideration of several factors beyond selection of an assessment framework and appropriate behavioral assessment methods. Additional assessment dimensions are related to idiosyncratic aspects of the disability of autism per se and to the need to allow assessment questions to be sufficiently broad so that data obtained are not provided out of context to educational and vocational program planners.

Assessment of Communicative Function

Recent work by Carr (1985) and Carr and Durand (1985a, 1986b) described the communicative nature of disruptive behavior in some children and adults with autism. They propose that disruptive behavior (including tantrums, aggression, and self injury), when motivated by attention from others or escape, may be a primitive means of communicating the desire for adult attention or to exit a demanding situation. Teaching a more functional, socially valid communication form to replace the disruptive behavior thus becomes a focus of treatment.

When conducting a behavioral assessment the form and social function of the target behavior must be evaluated for communicative intent. Where disruptive behavior is hypothesized to serve on communicative function, the teaching of more appropriate responses should be incorporated into the treatment plan. Durand and Carr (1982, 1983) offer additional assessment and treatment guidelines.

Social Validity

In recent years behavior therapists have been turning their attention increasingly toward the assessment of the social and clinical importance of target behavior selection, intervention options, and treatment results. Social validation techniques (Kazdin, 1977; Wolf, 1978) for the formal evaluation of these areas have been developed and used to document the social or applied significance of empirical findings with persons with autism (Runco & Schreibman, 1983; Schreibman, Koegel, Mills & Burke, 1981). Such techniques represent an important part of the behavioral assessment process.

Throughout and after treatment the effects of intervention can be evaluated through social validation. Kazdin (1977) describes two procedures: social comparison, whereby the client's performance is compared to that of a nonhandicapped peer, and subjective evaluation, whereby global judgments are obtained from persons with whom the client interacts regularly regarding the social importance of the effects of treatment.

The use of social validation techniques with persons with autism has certain limitations. For example, identification of a normative group of autistic children for social comparison purposes might be difficult due to the extreme heterogeneity within the disorder. In such cases subjective evaluation of targets selected, interventions chosen, and results obtained may be more appropriate. Documentation that the target behavior is clinically important and that other less invasive interventions have proved unsuccessful may be the best one can do. Sole reliance on the opinions of others for target behavior selection and acceptable levels of post-treatment behavior may be influenced by parental, teacher, or school agenda or biases, and should thus be approached cautiously. Finally, the clinician should remain vigilant of community norms. The acceptability of different treatment alternatives can vary widely across jurisdictions.

While social validation data are often obtained for target behavior selection and treatment outcome (cf. Schreibman et al., 1981; Runco & Schreibman, 1983), few studies have evaluated the social validity of the treatment procedures selected (see Schutz, Rusch & Lamson, 1979, for an exception). An investigation of the social validity of various behavioral interventions, and a determination of the perceived appropriateness of specific procedures for particular target behaviors remains an important area for future research.

Response Interrelationships

Unplanned positive and negative effects of treatment are sometimes observed with individuals with autism (Koegel & Covert, 1972; Lichstein & Schreibman, 1976). These response covariations or interrelationships occur because several behaviors may exist as part of a single response class, whereby changes in the antecedent or consequent stimuli for one behavior will occasion a change in other behaviors. Within a response class, one behavior may serve an "executive" function over others. Wahler's (1975) investigations led to the description of these executive behaviors as keystones. A response may function as a keystone because it exposes the client to the natural community of reinforcers, effectively signaling a potential increase in the density of reinforcement, or because the response is an essential preparatory response upon which other behaviors are based (Voeltz & Evans, 1982).

Voeltz and Evans (1982) argue that the equivocal results of many behavioral treatments with persons who are autistic or otherwise severely disabled may be the result of failure to assess for response interrelationships prior to beginning treatment. They offer several suggestions: (1) assess for naturally occurring behavioral chains that terminate in the target behavior. Intervention may be possible at an earlier, less obtrusive point in the chain; (2) assess preparatory responses necessary for behavioral performance of the target response; (3) determine whether behaviors hypothesized to be interrelated have similar social functions; (4) determine, through a functional analysis, whether a more appropriate behavior can be taught or substituted to fulfill the same function as the target response; (5) the use of multiple baseline designs across behaviors and alternating treatments for outcome evaluation may obscure the interpretation of response interrelationships. Alternatively, consider the monitoring of multiple responses over time for treatment evaluation.

Educational Validity

Educational validity (Voeltz & Evans, 1983) refers to the internal, empirical, and social validity and procedural reliability of a given educational intervention for a person with a severe disability. Each area has special relevance to the education of individuals with autism and should be included in the initial and ongoing phases of behavioral assessment.

Internal validation refers to the process of demonstrating whether a functional relationship exists between the behavioral intervention and obtained levels of the target behavior. Empirical validation represents the determination whether the treatment will be beneficial to the student's eventual outcome. Thus, interventions offered must be developmentally appropriate but must also address the criterion of ultimate functioning (Brown et al., 1976) and account for generalization and maintenance across environments as well as environmental agents including teachers, peers, parents (Christian & Luce, 1985). Social validation represents an assessment of the social and clinical significance of target behaviors, interventions, and outcomes. Moreover, skills taught must be valued in the environment in which the client is expected to perform (Libert, Haring & Martin, 1981). Procedural reliability (cf. Billingsley, White & Munson, 1980) refers to the extent to which the intervention program was implemented as intended.

In emphasizing the importance of educational validity, Voeltz and Evans (1983) offer suggestions for behavioral assessment. Teachers must conduct ecologic functional analyses to identify conditions in effect during treatment. Once treatment has begun, ongoing monitoring of these characteristics and teacher behavior will help determine the relative effectiveness of the intervention on the client's behavior. The amount of teacher time actually spent implementing the treatment should be assessed and monitored; treatment failures where there was insufficient teaching time provided are uninterpretable.

Educational validation emphasizes the pragmatic differences between clinical or research settings and schools. As such, attention to internal, experimental, and social validity and procedural reliability assure the practical relevance of behavioral interventions to children with autism in educational settings.

CONCLUSIONS

Like the developmental disorder itself, the behavioral assessment of autism is multidimensional. Specific clinical manifestations of autism make necessary consideration of multiple sources of data and verification of progress in social, communication, perceptual, and motor domains. No one method of data collection is adequate; rather, behavioral assessment utilizing many methods with subsequent determination of areas of congruence, strengths, and needs is most beneficial to treatment planning. The special advantage of behavioral assessment make its use with autistic children and adults comprehensive, evaluable, and systematic, and well suited to the development of individualized treatment programs. Where the selection of target behaviors, acceptable methods of treatment, and response rates are determined empirically with emphasis on the social, interpersonal, and ecologic dimensions of client behavior, behavioral assessment represents an important skill in the armamentarium of clinicians serving both children and adults with autism as well as their families.

ACKNOWLEDGMENTS. Preparation of this chapter was supported in part by HCEEP grant G008630278 from the U. S. Office of Education.

REFERENCES

American Psychiatric Association (1987). *Diagnostic and statistical manual of mental disorders* (3rd ed.-revised) Washington, D. C.: American Psychiatric Association.
Bandura, A. (1977). Self-efficacy: Toward a unifying theory of behavioral change. *Psychological Review, 84,* 191–215.
Barton, E. J., & Ascione, F. R. (1984). Direct observation. In T. H. Ollendick & M. Hersen (Eds.), *Child behavioral assessment: Principles and procedures* (pp. 166–94). New York: Pergamon.
Billingsley, F., White, O. R., & Munson, R. (1980). Procedural reliability: A rationale and an example. *Behavioral Assessment, 2,* 229–41.
Bornstein, P. H., Bridgwater, C. A., Hickey, J. S., & Sweeney, T. M. (1980). Characteristics and trends in behavioral assessment: An archival analysis. *Behavioral Assessment, 2,* 125–33.

Brown, L., Nietupski, J., & Hamre-Nietupski (1976). The criterion of ultimate functioning and public school services for severely handicapped students. In M. A. Thomas (Ed.), *Hey, don't forget about me: Education's investment in the severely, profoundly, and multiply handicapped* (pp. 2–15). Reston, VA: Council for Exceptional Children.

Carr, E. G. (1977). The motivation of self-injurious behavior: A review of some hypotheses. *Psychological Bulletin, 84,* 800–16.

Carr, E. G. (1985). Behavioral approaches to language and communication. In E. Schopler & G. B. Mesibov (Eds.), *Communication problems in autism* (pp. 37–57). New York: Plenum.

Carr, E. G., & Durand, V. M. (1985a). The social-communicative basis of severe behavior problems in children. In S. Reiss & R. Bootzin (Eds.), *Theoretical issues in behavior therapy* (pp. 219–54). New York: Academic Press.

Carr, E. G., & Durand, V. M. (1985b). Reducing behavior problems through functional communication training. *Journal of Applied Behavior Analysis, 18,* 111–26.

Christian, W. P., Hannah, G. T., & Glahn, T. J. (Eds.) (1984). *Programming effective human services.* New York: Plenum.

Christian, W. P., & Luce, S. C. (1985). Behavioral self-help training for developmentally disabled individuals. *School Psychology Review, 14,* 177–81.

Cohen, D. J., Caparulo, B. K., Gold, J. R., Waldo, M. C., Shaywitz, B. A., Ruttenberg, B. A., & Rimland, B. (1978). Agreement in diagnosis. *Journal of the American Academy of Child Psychiatry, 17,* 589–603.

Deckner, C. W., Soraci, S. A., Deckner, P. O., & Blanton, R. L. (1982). The Rimland E-2 assessment of autism: Its relationship with other measures. *Exceptional Children, 49,* 180–2.

DeMyer, M. K., Churchill, D. W., Pontius, W., & Gilkey, K. M. (1971). A comparison of five diagnostic systems for childhood schizophrenia and infantile autism. *Journal of Autism and Developmental Disorders, 1,* 175–89.

DeMyer, M. K., Hingtgen, J. N., & Jackson, R. K. (1981). Infantile autism reviewed: A decade of research. *Schizophrenia Bulletin, 7,* 388–451.

Deykin, E. Y., & MacMahon, B. (1979). The incidence of seizures among children with autistic symptoms. *American Journal of Psychiatry, 13,* 1310–12.

Donnellan, A. M. (1980). An educational perspective of autism: Implications for curriculum development and personnel development. In B. Wilcox & A. Thompson (Eds.), *Critical issues in educating autistic children and youth* (pp. 53–88). Washington, D. C.: U. S. Dept. of Education, Office of Special Education.

Dunlap, G., & Johnson, J. (1985). Increasing the independent responding of autistic children with unpredictable supervision. *Journal of Applied Behavior Analysis, 18,* 227–36.

Dunlap, G., & Koegel, R. L. (1980). Motivating autistic children through stimulus variation. *Journal of Applied Behavior Analysis, 13,* 619–27.

Durand, V. M., & Carr, E. G. (1982, August). *Differential reinforcement of communicative behavior: An intervention for the disruptive behaviors of developmentally disabled children.* Paper presented at the meeting of the American Psychological Association, Washington, D. C.

Durand, V. M., & Carr, E. G. (1983, October). *Differential reinforcement of communicative behavior: Classroom intervention and maintenance.* Paper presented at the meeting of the Berkshire Association for Behavior Analysis and Therapy, Amherst, MA.

Durand, V. M., & Carr, E. G. (1985) Self-injurious behavior: Motivating conditions and guidelines for treatment. *School Psychology Review, 14,* 171–6.

Durand, V. M., & Carr, E. G. (in press). Autism. In V. B. VanHasselt, P. S. Strain, & M. Hersen (Eds.), *Handbook of developmental and physical disabilities.* New York: Pergamon.

Edelbrock, C. (1984). Developmental considerations. In T. H. Ollendick & M. Hersen (Eds.), *Child behavioral assessment: Principles and procedures* (pp. 20–37). Elmsford, NY: Pergamon.

Egel, A. L. (1980). The effects of constant vs. varied reinforcer presentation on responding by autistic children. *Journal of Experimental Child Psychology, 30,* 455–63.

Egel, A. L. (1981) Reinforcer variation: Implications for motivating developmentally disabled children. *Journal of Applied Behavior Analysis, 14,* 345–50.

Emery, R. E., Binkoff, J. A., Houts, A. C., & Carr, E. G. (1983). Children as independent variables: Some clinical implications of child-effects. *Behavior Therapy, 14,* 398–412.

Favell, J. E. (1983, May). *Self-injurious behavior: An overview.* Invited address presented at the National Conference on self-injurious behavior, Valley Forge, PA.

Favell, J. E., & Cannon, P. (1977) Evaluation of entertainment materials for severely retarded persons. *American Journal of Mental Deficiency, 81,* 357–61.

Favell, J., McGimsey, J., & Jones, M. (1978). The use of physical restraint in the treatment of self-injury and as positive reinforcement. *Journal of Applied Behavior Analysis, 11,* 225–41.

Ferster, C. B., & Skinner, B. F. (1957). *Schedules of reinforcement.* New York: Appleton-Century-Crofts.

Fisch, G. S., Cohen, I. L., Wolf, E. G., & Friedman, E. (1985). The autistic descriptors checklist (ADC): A preliminary report. *Journal of Autism and Developmental Disorders, 15,* 233–4.

Franzini, L. R. (1970). Neglected variables in behavioral case assessment. *Behavior Therapy, 1,* 354–8.

Freeman, B. J., Ritvo, E. R., & Schroth, P. C. (1984). Behavior assessment of the syndrome of autism: Behavior Observation System. *Journal of the American Academy of Child Psychiatry, 23,* 588–94.

Freeman, B. J., Ritvo, E. R., Yokota, A., & Ritro, A. (1986). A scale for rating symptoms of patients with the syndrome of autism in real life settings. *Journal of the American Academy of Child Psychiatry, 25,* 130–6.

Harris, S. L. (1982) A family systems approach to behavioral training with parents of autistic children. *Child and Family Behavior Therapy, 4,* 21–35.

Harris, S. L. (1983). *Families of the developmentally disabled: A guide to behavioral intervention.* Elmsford, NY: Pergamon.

Harris, S. L. (1984). Intervention planning for the family of the autistic child: A multilevel assessment of the family system. *Journal of Marital & Family Therapy, 10,* 157–66.

Harris, S. L., & Ferrari, M. (1983). Developmental factors in child behavior therapy. *Behavior Therapy, 14,* 54–72.

Harris, S. L., & Powers, M. D. (1984). Behavior therapists look at the impact of an autistic child on the family system. In E. Schopler & G. Mesibov (Eds.), *The effects of autism on the family* (pp. 207–20). New York: Plenum.

Hartmann, D. P., Roper, B. L., & Bradford, D. C. (1979). Some relationships between behavioral and traditional assessment. *Journal of Behavioral Assessment, 1,* 3–21.

Hawkins, R. P., & Dobes, R. W. (1975). Behavioral definitions in applied behavior analysis: Explicit or implicit. In B. C. Etzel, J. M. LeBlanc, & D. M. Baer (Eds.), *New developments in behavioral research: Theory, methods, and applications.* Hillsdale, NJ: Lawrence Erlbaum.

Iwata, B. A., Dorsey, M. F., Slifer, K. J., Bauman, K. E., & Richman, G. S. (1982). Toward a functional analysis of self-injury. *Analysis and Intervention in Developmental Disabilities, 2,* 3–20.

Kanfer, F. H., & Saslow, G. (1969). Behavioral Diagnosis. In C. M. Franks (Ed.), *Behavior therapy: Appraisal and status.* New York: McGraw-Hill.

Kazdin, A. E. (1977). Assessing the clinical or applied importance of behavior change through social validation. *Behavior Modification, 1,* 427–51.

Kazdin, A. E. (1979). Unobtrusive measures in behavioral assessment. *Journal of Applied Behavioral Analysis, 12,* 713–24.

Kazdin, A. E. (1980). *Behavior modification in applied settings.* Homewood, IL: Dorsey Press.

Kazdin, A. E. (1982a). Symptom substitution, generalization, and response covariation: Implications for psychotherapy outcome. *Psychological Bulletin, 91,* 349–65.

Kazdin, A. E. (1982b). *Single-case research designs: Methods for clinical and applied practice.* New York: Oxford.

Kazdin, A. E. (1983). Psychiatric diagnosis, dimensions of dysfunction, and child behavior therapy. *Behavior Therapy, 14,* 73–99.

Koegel, R. L., & Covert, A. (1972). Relationship of self-stimulation to learning in autistic children. *Journal of Applied Behavior Analysis, 5,* 381–7.

Koegel, R. L., Dunlap, G., & Dyer, K. (1980). Intertrial interval duration and learning in autistic children. *Journal of Applied Behavior Analysis, 13,* 91–9.

Koegel, R. L., & Rincover, A. (1974). Treatment of psychotic children in a classroom environment: I. Learning in a large group. *Journal of Applied Behavior Analysis, 7*, 45–59.

Koegel, R. L., Rincover, A., & Egel, A. L. (1982) (Eds.), *Educating and understanding autistic children*. San Diego: College Hill Press.

Koegel, R. L., Schreibman, L., Britten, K., & Laitinen, R. (1979). The effects of schedule of reinforcement on stimulus overselectivity in autistic children. *Journal of Autism and Developmental Disorders, 9*, 383–97.

Kozloff, M. (1973). *Reaching the autistic child: A parent training program*. Champaign, IL: Research Press.

Kratochwill, T. R. (1985). Case study research in school psychology. *School Psychology Review, 14*, 204–15.

Krug, D. A., Arick, J., & Almond, P. (1979). *Autism screening instrument for educational planning*. Portland, OR: ASIEP Educational Co.

Krug, D. A., Arick, J., & Almond, P. (1980). Behavior checklist for identifying severely handicapped individuals with high levels of autistic behavior. *Journal of Child Psychology and Psychiatry, 21*, 221–9.

Libert, K. A., Haring, N. G., & Martin, M. M. (1981). Teaching new skills to the severely handicapped. *Journal of the Association for the Severely Handicapped, 6*, 5–13.

Lichstein, K., & Schreibman, L. (1976). Employing electric shock with autistic children: A review of the side effects. *Journal of Autism and Childhood Schizophrenia, 6*, 163–73.

Litt, M. D., & Schreibman, L. (1981). Stimulus-specific reinforcement in the acquisition of receptive labels by autistic children. *Analysis and Intervention in Developmental Disabilities, 1*, 171–86.

Lobato, D. (1983). Siblings of handicapped children: A review. *Journal of Autism and Developmental Disorders, 13*, 347–64.

Maher, C. A., & Bennett, R. E. (1984). *Planning and evaluating special education services*. Englewood Cliffs, NJ: Prentice-Hall.

Martin, R. (1975). *Legal Challenges to behavior modification*. Champaign, IL: Research Press.

Mash, E. J., & Terdal, L. G. (1981). Behavioral assessment of childhood disturbance. In E. J. Mash and L. G. Terdal (Eds.), *Behavioral assessment of childhood disorders*. New York: Guilford.

Mays, D. T., & Franks, C. M. (Eds.) (1985). *Negative outcome in psychotherapy and what to do about it*. New York: Springer.

McClannahan, L. E., & Krantz, P. J. (1985). Some next steps in rights protection for the developmentally disabled. *School Psychology Review, 14*, 143–9.

McHale, S. M., & Simeonsson, R. J. (1980). Effects of interaction on nonhandicapped children's attitudes toward autistic children. *American Journal of Mental Deficiency, 85*, 18–24.

McHale, S. M., Simeonsson, R. J., & Sloan, J. L. (1984). Children with handicapped brothers and sisters. In E. Schopler & G. B. Mesibov (Eds.), *The effects of autism on the family* (pp. 327–42). New York: Plenum.

National Society for Autistic Children and Adults (1978). Definition of the syndrome of autism. *Journal of Autism and Childhood Schizophrenia, 8*, 162–6.

Nelson, R. O., & Barlow, D. H. (1981). Behavioral assessment: Basic strategies and initial procedures. In D. H. Barlow (Ed.), *Behavioral assessment of adult disorders*, New York: Guilford.

Nelson, R. O., & Hayes, S. C. (1979). Some current dimensions of behavioral assessment. *Behavioral Assessment, 1*, 1–16.

Nelson, R. O., & Hayes, S. C. (1981). An overview of behavioral assessment. In M. Hersen & A. Bellack (Eds.), *Behavioral assessment: A practical handbook* (2nd ed.). New York: Pergamon.

Ollendick, T. H., & Cerney, J. A. (1981). *Clinical behavior therapy with children*. New York: Plenum.

Ollendick, T. H., & Hersen, M. (1984). An overview of child behavioral assessment. In T. H. Ollendick & M. Hersen (Eds.), *Child behavioral assessment: Principles and procedures*. Elmsford, NJ: Pergamon.

Olley, J. G. (1980). Organization of educational services for autistic children and youth. In B. Wilcox & A. Thompson (Eds.), *Critical issues in educating autistic children and youth* (pp. 13–23). Washington, D. C.: U. S. Dept. of Education, Office of Special Education.

Parks, S. L. (1983). The assessment of autistic children: A selective review of available instruments. *Journal of Autism and Developmental Disorders, 13,* 255–67.

Powers, M. D. (1984). Syndromal diagnosis and the behavioral assessment of childhood disorders. *Child and Family Behavior Therapy, 6,* 1–15.

Powers, M. D. (1985). Behavioral assessment and the planning and evaluation of interventions for developmentally disabled children. *School Psychology Review, 14,* 155–61.

Powers, M. D., (Ed.) (1988). Expanding systems of service delivery for persons with developmental disabilities. Baltimore: Paul H. Brookes.

Powers, M. D., & Franks, C. M. (1988). Behavior therapy and the educative process. In J. C. Witt, S. N. Elliott & F. M. Gresham (Eds.), *Handbook of behavior therapy in education* (pp. 3–36). New York: Plenum.

Powers, M. D., & Handleman, J. S. (1984). *Behavioral assessment of severe developmental disabilities.* Rockville, MD: Aspen.

Prior, M., & Bence, R. (1975). A note on the validity of the Rimland Diagnostic Checklist. *Journal of Clinical Psychology, 31,* 510–13.

Realmuto, G. M., & Main, B. (1982). Coincidence of Tourette's disorder and infantile autism. *Journal of Autism and Developmental Disorders, 12,* 367–72.

Rimland, B. (1971). The differentiation of childhood psychoses: An analysis of checklists for 2,218 psychotic children. *Journal of Autism and Developmental Disorders, 1,* 161–74.

Rincover, A., & Newsom, C. D. (1985). The relative motivational properties of sensory and edible reinforcers in teaching autistic children. *Journal of Applied Behavior Analysis, 18,* 237–48.

Romanczyk, R. G. (1983, May). Self-injurious behavior: Models and the myth of a response class. Invited address presented at the National conference on self-injurious behavior, Valley Forge, PA.

Runco, M. A., & Schreibman, L. (1983). Parental judgments of behavior therapy efficacy with autistic children: A social validation. *Journal of Autism and Developmental Disorders, 13,* 237–48.

Ruttenberg, B. A., Kalish, B. I., Wenar, C., & Wolf, E. (1977). *The Behavior Rating Instrument for Autistic and Other Atypical Children.* Chicago, IL: Stoelting.

Schopler, E., Lansing, M., & Waters, L. (1983). *Individualized assessment and treatment for autistic and developmentally disabled children. Vol. III: Teaching activities for autistic children.* Baltimore: University Park Press.

Schopler, E., & Mesibov, G. B. (1985) (Eds.). *Communication problems in autism.* New York: Plenum.

Schopler, E., & Reichler, R. J. (1979). *Individualized assessment and treatment for autistic and developmentally disabled children. Volume I: Psychoeducational Profile.* Austin: Pro-Ed.

Schopler, E., Reichler, R. J., DeVellis, R. E., & Daly, K. (1980). Toward objective classification of childhood autism: Childhood Autism Rating Scale (CARS). *Journal of Autism and Developmental Disorders, 10,* 91–103.

Schopler, E., Reichler, R. J., & Lansing, M. (1980). *Individualized assessment and treatment for autistic and developmentally disabled children: Volume II: Teaching strategies for parents and professionals.* Baltimore: University Park Press.

Schreibman, L., Koegel, R. L., Mills, J. I., & Burke, J. C. (1981). Social validation of behavior therapy with autistic children. *Behavior Therapy, 12,* 610–24.

Schutz, R. P., Rusch, F. R., & Lamson, D. C. (1979). Evaluation of an employers procedure to eliminate unacceptable behavior on the job. *Community Services Forum, 1,* 4–5.

Van Houten (1979). Social validation: The evolution of standards of competency for target behaviors. *Journal of Applied Behavior Analysis, 12,* 581–91.

Voeltz, L. M., & Evans, I. M. (1982). The assessment of behavioral interrelationships in child behavior therapy. *Behavioral Assessment, 4,* 131–65.

Voeltz, L. M., & Evans, I. M. (1983). Educational validity: Procedures to evaluate outcomes in programs for severely handicapped learners. *Journal of the Association for the Severely Handicapped, 8,* 3–15.

Wahler, R. G. (1975). Some structural aspects of deviant child behavior. *Journal of Applied Behavior Analysis, 8,* 27–42.

Wahler, R. G. (1980). The insular mother: Her problems in parent–child treatment. *Journal of Applied Behavior Analysis, 13,* 207–19.

Wechsler, D. (1974). *Wechsler Intelligence Scale for Children—Revised.* New York: Psychological Corp.

Wolf, M. M. (1978). Social validity: The case for subjective measurement or how applied behavior analysis is finding its heart. *Journal of Applied Behavior Analysis, 11,* 203–14.

11

Intellectual and Developmental Assessment of Autistic Children from Preschool to Schoolage
Clinical Implications of Two Follow-up Studies

CATHERINE LORD and ERIC SCHOPLER

INTRODUCTION

The recognition that intellectual functioning and developmental level are valid measures in autism was one of the major steps in the field during the late 1960s (Schopler, 1976, 1982). Intellectual level can be assessed in autistic children; to a great extent, it has an equivalent meaning for children with autism as it has for other handicapped people (Rutter & Schopler, 1987). IQ has been shown to be related to outcome in autistic persons; it is associated with the acquisition of a variety of different kinds of skills (Lotter, 1974; Rutter, 1985). A nonverbal intelligence test is now an essential part of any assessment of an autistic child or adolescent (Parks, 1983).

On the other hand, there are many difficulties with using developmental and intelligence tests as if they were straightforward measures of a single variable. These difficulties pertain to all populations, not just autistic children and adolescents. However, there are specific aspects of autism that can make the use of intelligence tests particularly problematic. The purpose of this chapter is to discuss what we have learned from two follow-up studies about the stability and predictability of the IQs of young children with autism. The empirical basis for this chapter was provided by research carried out at Division TEACCH (Lord & Schopler, 1988a, b). In these studies, we observed the changes in scores of autistic children tested at relatively young ages, that is under 6 years, over a follow-up period of approximately 5 years. In this chapter, we use these data to provoke a discussion of some of the uses and the limitations of early intelligence testing of autistic children.

The focus of this chapter is on IQs and developmental quotients generated in early childhood, i.e., prior to age 6. Earlier studies by Rutter and Lockyer (1967; Lockyer &

CATHERINE LORD • Department of Pediatrics, University of Alberta, and Department of Psychology, Glenrose Rehabilitation Hospital, Edmonton, Alberta T5G 0B7, Canada.   ERIC SCHOPLER • Division TEACCH, The University of North Carolina at Chapel Hill, Chapel Hill, North Carolina 27599-7180.

Rutter, 1969, 1970; DeMyer *et al.*, 1973, 1974; Freeman, Ritvo, Needleman & Yakota, 1985) have shown that testing autistic children over about age 4 is reliable and yields relatively stable scores. However, relatively little is known about how stable scores are for preschool children, particularly those age 4 years and younger. Early intervention projects and greater recognition of the syndrome of autism have contributed to more and more children being referred and assessed at earlier ages. In a clinic in Edmonton modeled after the TEACCH program, the average age for first assessment of an autistic child is about 3½ years. Often these children have received some kind of assessment at other clinics before they are referred to us.

Testing younger children is different in many ways from testing children who are above age 6. Not only are the younger children more limited in absolute skills, they are much less likely to be familiar with a school or testing kind of environment, they are less likely to understand specific aspects of the situation such as the examiner's language and they are less likely to share the examiner's general expectations of how they should behave while being tested. Many 2 and 3 year olds have little experience of being asked to play or carry out activities with a strange adult. Although tests for preschool children or infants are designed to take these factors into account, the entire experience of coming to a clinic or to a hospital to be "evaluated" on the basis of interactions with a stranger is a novel one for almost all young children.

In addition, normal variability in language skills affects the ability of very young children to communicate with unfamiliar people far more than the equivalent variability when children are older. Extremes of language delay, such as those experienced by most children with autism, can make communicating even the most basic ideas (e.g., that this assessment will end very soon) difficult.

Furthermore, tests used with very young children are different from tests which most school-oriented psychologists have been trained to administer. Scores on these tests, such as the Bayley Scale of Mental Development (Bayley, 1969), are notoriously less stable for all populations than are scores of tests typically used with school-age children (Ebert & Simmons, 1943; Hindley & Owen, 1978; Sattler, 1982). Thus, in assessing younger children, one has to take into account not only differences in the general developmental level of the children, but also differences in language level and in specific tests employed.

Altogether, we addressed two main questions in this chapter. First, is the stability and usefulness of intelligence tests similar for children with autism as for language-delayed and mentally handicapped children who are not autistic? Second, what are some of the specific concerns in testing children under the age of 6 and in interpreting their results? How does a child's age and developmental level at initial assessment, and his/her level of language interact with characteristics of specific tests to affect the stability and predictability of scores?

DESCRIPTION OF SAMPLES

Two studies are reported. The first is a comparison of 71 autistic children (60 males, 11 females) to 71 nonautistic communication disordered and mentally handicapped children who were individually matched to the autistic children on both assessments for chronological age, race, sex, and for performance IQ/developmental quotient (range: 30–105), language status and test at the initial assessment, and time between the first assessment and a later assessment (Lord & Schopler, 1987a). All children were first assessed between ages 2 years and 5 years, and reassessed a minimum of 24 months later between ages 6 and 12 years. Table I provides a summary of scores for these children.

Table I. Raw Scores and Difference Scores for IQs and SQs
of Autistic and Nonautistic Children at Two Ages

Group	IQ				SQ			
	4 yrs.	10 yrs.	r	M Absolute difference	4 yrs.	10 yrs.	r	M Absolute difference
Autistic	60.74	64.98	.79	12.01	55.91	50.83	.70	12.30
	(11.46)	(19.95)		(8.07)	(19.22)	(24.05)		(8.08)
Nonautistic	62.26	63.99	.79	10.86	67.20	66.36	.64	11.36
	(15.70)	(18.42)		(8.21)	(22.47)	(24.78)		(9.93)

The second study was a follow-up study of 213 autistic children first tested under age 6 and again a minimum of 2 years later, at a maximum of 12 years of age (Lord & Schopler, 1987*b*). This group included the 71 autistic children in the other study, plus 142 autistic children whom we had not been able to match to nonautistic children. Longitudinal comparisons were made for the 213 children grouped according to the age of first assessment, with the interval between first and second assessments held constant (between 2–0 and 6–11 years, with means between 4–6 and 4–7 years) for each of the three longitudinal comparisons.

Thus, children who were first assessed at ages 2 or 3 and later assessed between ages 6 and 8 are henceforth referred to here as the 3- to 7-year-old group and compared with children who were first assessed at age 4 or 5 and later seen between ages 8 and 10 (referred to as the 4- to 9-year-old group) and to children who were first assessed at age 6 or 7 and seen again at ages 10 to 12 (referred to as the 6- to 10-year-old group). Summary data from these children are provided in Table II.

In order to eliminate the subjects so severely retarded that diagnosis of autism was tenuous, and in order to control for differences in range at high and low ends, only those children who received performance IQ/developmental quotients between 30 and 105 during the initial assessment were included. All children were living at home with at least one biologic or adoptive parent, and all subjects (autistic and nonautistic) had at least 6 weeks of regular outpatient treatment, which consisted primarily of training parents as educational therapists (Schopler, 1987).

Table II. Relationship between IQ/DQ Scores at Ages 2–7
to Scores 4–5 Years Later for Autistic Children

Age (years/months)			IQ or DQ			M Absolute difference	Median IQ difference	SQ	
Time 1	Time 2	N	Time 1	Time 2	r			Time 1	Time 2
3–2	7–8	72	56.64	63.52	.68	15.33	12	60.47	59.31
(5.9)	(5.8)		(19.96)	(22.04)		(16.77)		(15.88)	(14.76)
4–7	9–1	70	58.18	60.90	.81	12.18	11	56.48	52.79
(3.3)	(6.4)		(22.62)	(20.40)		(8.71)		(14.67)	(13.29)
6–6	11–1	71	58.39	57.65	.83	11.10	9	50.76	47.40
(3.7)	(6.1)		(22.19)	(21.71)		(8.72)		(17.01)	(19.90)

Children were classified as autistic on the bases of concordant clinical impressions of two psychologists using Rutter (1978) criteria and a CARS (Schopler, Reichler & Renner, 1986) score of more than 30 on both assessments. The nonautistic sample consisted of a heterogeneous group of language-delayed children with behavioral problems. Only children with CARS scores less than 20 who received clinical judgments of "not autistic" were included in this sample in order to exclude "autistic-like" children. Many children in this group were generally mentally handicapped, as well as language-delayed.

The measure of receptive language used in these analyses was whether a child received a basal score on the Peabody Picture Vocabulary Test, form A or B, which preceded the revised version (Dunn, 1959). There were obvious limitations to this measure (Tsai & Beisler, 1984), but it was one of the few measures of early language which could be reliably determined from retrospective data. A child who passed at least eight consecutive items on the PPVT received an age equivalent of 23 months or higher. Thus, when we refer to a child below as having "no language," we are referring to a child for whom an attempt was made to administer a PPVT who did not receive a basal. Children referred to below as "having language" scored at this level, i.e., just under 2 years, or higher on the PPVT.

Both follow-up studies used clinical samples. While the use of clinical samples provided us with access to a relatively large number of subjects, results must be interpreted recognizing that the data were acquired from ongoing clinical assessments. Thus, most obviously, the assignment of tests to children was not random. Rather, a child was given the test intended to be for children closest to the chronologic age on which they could receive a basal. Since the use of more than one test is unavoidable if children across any significant age or IQ span are to be evaluated, we believed that this difficulty was one to be acknowledged, but worth working around. It was possible to limit the contribution of this problem in group comparisons by matching according to test at initial assessment. In addition, data were available for all children on the Vineland Social Maturity Scales (Doll, 1965) at both times of testing, so that comparisons could be made between same-test SQ changes and IQ changes occurring with different instruments.

Similarly, the timing of the first and second assessments was not random in this sample, but was determined by individual children's clinical needs. However, we had no reason to believe that the reasons for timing were any different across samples of children that were compared (see Lord & Schopler, 1988a, for further details).

All testing was carried out by experienced examiners trained in the TEACCH program (Schopler, 1987). The intelligence and developmental tests most frequently administered at each age were identified. Only children assessed with these particular tests, listed below, were included in the sample. For the first assessment, these tests consisted of the Bayley Infant Scales of Mental Development (Bayley, 1969) and the Merrill–Palmer Scale of Mental Tests (Stutsman, 1943). For the second assessment, scores were included from the Merrill–Palmer, the Leiter International Performance Scale (Arthur, 1952) and the performance scale of the Wechsler Intelligence Scale for Children, revised version (Wechsler, 1974).

DIFFERENCES BETWEEN AUTISTIC AND NONAUTISTIC CHILDREN

Shown in Table I are data collected to address the first question, that is, are there differences in the correlations over time and the absolute stability of IQs from preschool to early school age in autistic and nonautistic communication and/or mentally handicapped children? Obviously the answer is no. The children were matched in IQ for time 1; scores for both groups then remained quite stable over an average of 6 years. Correlations for both groups were high and virtually identical. There was relatively little difference in either the average absolute change in IQ for the autistic and nonautistic children, or in the median difference in IQ for the two groups. Nor was there a difference across diagnostic groups in the relationship between IQ and language status, as measured by a basal score or higher on the PPVT.

While differences in IQ between the autistic and nonautistic children were minimal at both ages, there were marked differences in scores on the early version of the Vineland Social Maturity Scale (Doll, 1965). The same autistic children whose IQ scores reported in Table I were 60–65 over the course of this study received a mean social quotient at time 1 of 56 and time 2 of 51. By contrast, nonautistic children with similar IQ scores received a mean Vineland score at time 1 of 67 and at time 2 of 66. These are statistically and clinically significant differences between groups for SQ for both times, even though the autistic and nonautistic children were matched very closely on performance IQ. For both groups, the correlations between social quotients at time 1 and 2 were quite high, ranging between 0.64 to 0.70.

By contrast, when autistic and nonautistic children were considered in separate groups, there were no significant group differences in the extent (i.e., the correlations) of the relationship between scores on the various developmental and intellectual assessments and the Vineland. Thus, correlations between the Vineland and the Merrill–Palmer were 0.79 (autistic) and 0.69 (nonautistic), with correlations between the Leiter and the Vineland ranging from 0.67 (autistic) to 0.54 (nonautistic).

The similarity in the predictability of IQ from a concurrent measure was particularly interesting because the direction of the relationship between IQ and SQ for the two diagnostic groups differed for all tests but the Bayley. Thus, nonautistic children were more likely to score slightly higher on the Vineland than on the IQ test, while autistic children were likely to score significantly higher on the performance test. This is similar to the result obtained by Lockyer and Rutter (1970). The exception in our study was the Bayley, for which all but six out of 94 autistic and nonautistic children received higher quotients on the Vineland.

To summarize these comparisons, there were no significant differences in the amount of change or the direction of change in IQ when a group of autistic children were compared to a group of nonautistic children matched on various measures including initial IQ at age 4. Correlations between IQ scores at the two assessments were high and equivalent across the two groups. In addition, correlations between IQ and social quotients when both measures were administered at the same time and correlations for individual IQ measures across time were relatively high and not significantly different for the two groups. However, although the children had been well matched on performance IQ, the groups did differ in Vineland scores both during preschool years, and again at the later school-age assessment.

EFFECT OF AGE OF ASSESSMENT ON PREDICTABILITY AND STABILITY OF IQ IN AUTISTIC CHILDREN

The next question was the relationship between age at initial assessment and the predictive value of IQ over a 4- to 5-year period for autistic children. Data addressing these questions were presented in Table II for the three different longitudinal samples of between 70 and 72 autistic children. Age changes in the stability and predictability of IQ scores from preschool to school age were generally quite straightforward. Scores became more stable and predictability over time increased as the autistic children grew older. This was the case both for mean scores by age group and for the absolute amount of change experienced by individual children.

Yet, even for the youngest group, that is, the 3-to 7-year-old comparison, the correlation between IQ scores from the two assessments was significant and similar to correlations of other samples of children in this age range (Sattler, 1982). While mean scores were significantly different over time for this age group, in fact, the change was only an average of 7 points for the group and 15 points for individuals. Thus, even for the 2- and 3-year-old autistic children, developmental and intellectual assessments could yield information that was reliable into the school years.

On the other hand, the magnitude of change and, more important, the direction of change differed across age groups of autistic children. The IQs of the youngest children (3- to 7-year-old comparisons) were more likely to increase compared to the IQs of the oldest children (6- to 11-year-old comparisons), which were more likely to decrease in all parametric analyses. These differences related not just to chronologic age, however, but also to developmental level and the test employed. For example, low functioning (IQ = 30–49) children's scores tended to increase in the early years only, and high functioning (IQ = 70–105) childrens scores tended to decrease, particularly in the later school years. Below, we consider first the contribution of developmental level and language status to these age effects. A discussion of specific test effects follows.

RELATIONSHIP OF AGE AND DEVELOPMENTAL LEVEL TO PREDICTABILITY AND STABILITY OF IQ

Beginning with questions concerning the magnitude and direction of change in IQ of individual children, it was clear that patterns of change were quite different for each of the three longitudinal comparisons. From 3 to 7 years, all changes of 20 points or greater were increases and occurred within the group initially categorized as severely retarded (IQ: 30–49). From 4 to 9 years, changes of 20 points occurred for all 3 groups in both directions. From 6 to 11 years, all changes of 20 or more points were decreases. This pattern held true across all three IQ groups. For the later two comparisons, the pattern of IQ changes across IQ groups was similar, with about 20% of severely retarded children, 15% of mildly retarded children and 10% of nonretarded children showing changes of more than 20 points. Differences could not be accounted for simply by regression to the mean (see Lord & Schopler, 1988*b*, for further details).

The same pattern emerged both for parametric analyses and when dichotomous distributions were used to group children according to whether their IQs increased or decreased over time. For example, for the 3- to 7-year-old comparison, 21 out of 22 severely retarded children and 26 out of 32 mildly retarded children showed increases in IQ, in contrast to 8 out of 18 nonretarded children. For the 4- to 9-year-old comparison, 19 out of 25 low-functioning children showed increases, while decreases occurred for 16 out of 28 mildly retarded children and 14 out of 17 nonretarded children. For the 6- to 11-year-old comparison, low-functioning and mildly retarded groups both were almost equally split in increases and decreases, whereas 12 out of 13 of the nonretarded children showed decreases.

Table III shows the distribution of the entire sample of 213 subjects at different IQ ranges for the initial and later assessments. The point of this analysis is to give clinicians, who often report and interpret scores in terms of level or range rather than in absolute points,

Table III. Distribution of Full Sample of Autistic Children
According to IQ Scores at Time 1 and Time 2

	IQ range at time 2			
IQ range at time 1	Severe (<50)	Mild (50–69)	Nonretarded (>70)	Total
Severe (30–49)[a]	31	24	7	62
Moderate (50–69)	27	40	36	103
Nonretarded (70–105)[a]	2	10	36	48
Totals:	60	74	79	213

[a]These scores reflect the IQ ranges for the initial assessment used to select subjects. If scores fell beyond these ranges (i.e., <30 or >105) in the later assessment, children were still included.

an indication of how reliable these levels were. It is important to remember that the size of these changes varied from 1 to 20 points, depending on where a particular score fell within the range.

This distribution was clearly not random. Within each IQ range, the greatest proportion of children always remained in the same range in which they had scored during their initial assessment. However, many children changed IQ levels as well. At each level, one third to one half (39–52%) of the children remained in the same IQ range for the second assessment as they had scored in the first. Changes of more than one category were much less common than changes of one category: 7 out of 62 children who initially scored in the severely retarded range scored in the nonretarded range at the later assessment. Only 2 out of 48 children who initially scored above 70 later scored below 50. From the opposite perspective, of 79 children who scored as nonretarded during the second assessment, 36 (46%) of them had scored in the same range previously, but 43 had not, including 7 (9%) who had initially scored as severely retarded. Overall, nonretarded children had the least amount of change in mean IQ points and were most likely to remain in the same range (i.e., 75% did so). Severely retarded children showed the greatest amount of change in IQ points. Mildly retarded children were least likely to remain in the same range (i.e., 39% did so). However, this last finding was clearly a function of the way in which we defined mild retardation in this study (with both upper and lower limits).

ROLE OF CHANGE IN LANGUAGE STATUS IN CHANGES IN IQ

Given the findings of differential effects of both age and initial IQ level, it was important to evaluate the relationship between change in language status and change in IQ within the context of these two other factors. Planned comparisons were performed in order to evaluate change in IQ over time for groups of children defined by age at each assessment, initial adaptive level and change in language status. As shown in Table IV, the pattern of significant planned comparisons across time reflected the same general trends of greatest change in younger and severely retarded youngsters that had emerged in earlier analyses.

Thus, children who did not achieve a PPTV basal score at either assessment who scored as severely retarded showed significant increases in IQ at the earlier ages (i.e., 3–7 and 4–9 comparisons) and no change on the last comparison. For all other ages and IQ groups,

Table IV. Mean IQs According to Age of Assessments, SQ Level, and
Changes in Language Status[a,b]

Comparisons[c,d]	SQ 31–49		SQ 50–69		SQ >70	
	1	2	1	2	1	2
3- to 7-year-old ($N = 72$)						
$N \times N^2$	37.78	54.25[e]	59.25	55.82	75.58	53.55[e]
	(10.39)	(11.59)	(9.87)	(8.15)	(5.94)	(6.34)
$N \times L$	37.80	60.21[e]	57.40	70.26[e]	84.25	79.00
	(6.05)	(5.64)	(12.97)	(10.61)	(4.87)	(6.16)
$L \times L$	. . . . . .	. . . . . .	69.00	78.00	93.50	90.00
			(19.06)	(19.25)	(6.50)	(6.00)
4- to 9-year-old ($N = 70$)						
$N \times N$	33.37	47.94[e]	59.46	52.31	. . . . . .	. . . . . .
	(6.23)	(7.01)	(16.05)	(14.09)		
$N \times L$	34.41	46.67[e]	65.43	66.86	77.17	77.86
	(11.40)	(16.58)	(14.17)	(11.60)	(23.80)	(22.87)
$L \times L$	48.59	47.21	66.80	60.40	82.14	80.21
	(7.03)	(6.85)	(8.97)	(8.33)	(10.97)	(13.17)
6- to 11-year-old ($N = 71$)						
$N \times N$	34.41	32.08	58.56	57.54	. . . . . .	. . . . . .
	(7.05)	(8.74)	(16.50)	(14.52)		
$N \times L$	34.06	47.52[e]	56.75	57.75	. . . . . .	. . . . . .
	(1.08)	(2.53)	(14.17)	(13.92)		
$L \times L$	44.00	47.67	60.08	59.17	81.20	74.05[e]
	(7.83)	(6.55)	(8.35)	(10.40)	(10.81)	(10.81)

[a]For overlapping longitudinal samples.
[b]$t > 2.58$, $p < .01$ tailed.
[c]N, no basal; L, basal or higher on PPVT.
[d]First letter indicates language status at time 1; second letter indicates language status at time 2.
[e]Score at time 2 significantly different from score at time 1 according to planned comparisons.

children without language at either time showed no change or showed decreases in IQ, none of which were significant except nonretarded children in the 3- to 7-year-old comparison, who showed a significant decrease in IQ from a mean of over 75 to 53.

Changes in IQ associated with the acquisition of some receptive language (i.e., the group $N \times L$ in Table IV) were significant only for severely retarded children across age groups and for the youngest group of mildly retarded children. In most cases, language status at time 1 did not affect IQ at time 2 for either the lowest- or the highest-functioning children, although the direction of patterns was generally reversed for the two groups. Thus, IQs of severely retarded children in the early years almost always went up, whether they made language gains. The IQs of higher functioning children almost always went down slightly.

Two caveats are important, however. First, though some of these changes were quite large, the mean IQ at time 2 for all but the youngest group of children remained within the range of severe mental retardation. Second, this upward trend was beginning to reverse itself in the last longitudinal comparison. Most of the severely retarded subjects still remained without language at this point. Thus, most changes were not in and out of mental retardation or even over a range of mental retardation, but within 10 or 15 points. Many of the upward trends did not extend beyond the early schoolage years.

For nonretarded children, IQ changes were generally slight and downward, except for those children who did not acquire language between 3- and 7-year-old, and for older children (i.e., 6- to 11-year-old comparisons), where the decreases were more marked and statistically significant. A similar pattern of no change or slight decreases was found for mildly retarded children regardless of language status, except for children who acquired some language between 3 and 7 years of age. These children showed concommitant significant gains in IQ over that interval. The youngest group of children who had language at time 1 also showed increases in IQ, although these were not significant. Analyses of IQ changes, as a function of changes in language status for individual children, revealed similar results (Lord & Schopler, 1988*b*).

PREDICTION OF CHANGE IN LANGUAGE STATUS BY IQ RANGE

The relationship between IQ and language can also be considered from the opposite perspective, i.e., to what extent can it be predicted whether a child will acquire a minimal level of receptive language, on the basis of IQ score at an early assessment? This relationship was assessed in two stages. First, the number of children in each IQ range falling into each category of language status was determined. These distributions were significantly different

Table V. Proportion of Children Grouped by Initial IQ
and Age with Various Language Statuses

	IQ		
Language status	31–50	51–69	≥70
With language at time 1			
3- to 7-year-old	0	.03	.22
4- to 9-year-old	.12	.21	.65
6- to 11-year-old	.40	.46	1.00
With language at time 2			
3- to 7-year-old	.41	.53	.61
4- to 9-year-old	.48	.46	1.00
6- to 11-year-old	.60	.86	1.00
Gained language between time 1 and time 2			
3- to 7-year-old	.41	.52	.50
4- to 9-year-old	.41	.70	1.00
6- to 11-year-old	.33	.74	—

Table VI. Relationship between IQ Scores on the Same or Different Tests
for Autistic Children[a,b]

Tests	N	M age		IQ		r
		Time 1	Time 2	Time 1	Time 2	
Different tests						
Bayley–MP	126	3–2	6–4	38.98	56.11	.53[a]
MP–Leiter	168	5–0	8–7	60.36	63.68	.59
MP–WISC-R	31	5–3	9–3	69.61	66.25	.55
Leiter–WISC-R	25	9–0	11–11	66.33	64.92	.51
Same tests						
Bayley–Bayley	42	3–8	5–9	35.69	24.74	.75
MP–MP	137	4–11	8–2	42.61	39.55	.78
Leiter–Leiter	60	6–5	11–10	59.51	56.34	.86
Vineland–Vineland	213	6–0	11–9	56.71	52.76	.73

[a]All correlations are significant at $p < .01$. Correlations between the same test are all significantly higher than correlations between different tests.
[b]MP, Merrill–Palmer.

for all three longitudinal comparisons. As shown in Table V, the proportion of children who acquired a minimal level of language by the second assessment (i.e., $N \times L$ and $L \times L$) increased as IQs went up.

Secondly, the proportion of children in each IQ grouping who, not having some language at time 1, acquired some language by time 2, was also computed for each longitudinal comparison. Chi squares were significant only for the 4- to 9-year-old comparisons. *All* the children who scored above 70 at age 4 who did not achieve a PPVT basal at that age eventually scored as having some receptive language by age 9, compared with fewer than one half of children with IQs between 51 and 69. As shown by the proportions reported in Table V, similar patterns occurred at earlier and later ages, but statistics assessing these distributions did not yield significant differences.

RELATIONSHIP BETWEEN IQ SCORES ON THE SAME AND DIFFERENT TESTS FOR AUTISTIC CHILDREN

The last question concerns the role of specific tests in the stability and the predictive value of intelligence testing of young autistic children. Data addressing this question are presented in Table VI. Because these studies contained a relatively large sample of children 4 years and younger, of particular interest was the use of the Bayley Scales of Mental Development and the Merrill–Palmer Scales of Mental Development. These tests are important because they are quite different from each other in content and construction. However, it is possible to administer each of them to young children unfamiliar with school-like procedures and with the constraints built into the standardization of most tests intended for older and more advanced (socially, linguistically, and cognitively) children. The tests share the advantages of having visually interesting materials, allowing the modification of the order of items and including demonstration for many tasks. However, they differ in several ways.

The Bayley Scale of Mental Development is a test designed primarily for children with mental ages under 2½ years. Although most of the items on the Bayley do not require language, about one third of the items after the age of 1 year measure behavioral responses to language or involve expressive language. Language items become more frequent as age increases. The Bayley also differs from the other tests in that it includes direct assessment of social behaviors, such as whether a child smiles at himself in a mirror or repeats an action that the examiner laughs at. These items constitute about one fifth of the entire test, with most of them rated as under one year of age in occurrence. The Bayley also primarily involves items that can be carried out in 10–30 sec. Relatively few items are timed.

In contrast, the Merrill–Palmer is primarily a performance test, involving puzzles and peg boards. Many of the items are timed. It can be scored as a nonverbal test by excluding language items in computations. In fact, for these studies, results were analyzed both ways, including language items and treating them as refusals. There was no difference in results, probably because the language items are relatively few in number and most prevalent at early ages.

Given that our samples were clinical, tests were not assigned to children on a random basis. There were definite selection effects as to which children were given which test. For example, if a child was still being given a Bayley at age 6, it was generally because that child could not receive a basal on the Merrill–Palmer. The highest functioning children were given the most chronologically age-appropriate tests and generally showed the most frequent changes in tests over time. Thus, children who continued to be given the same preschool test generally showed decreases in IQ as well as lower IQs at both testings than children able to move on to a test for an older age group. In a way, the stability of the scores found for children with IQs above 70 was particularly impressive, since these children were most likely to have been assessed on different tests on the two different occasions.

Conclusions from Table VI are relatively straightforward. All the correlations between tests were significant; correlations for the same test given twice were statistically higher than correlations between two different tests. Thus, some of the slippage in stability of IQ over time lay in the fact that children were given different tests as they got older. However, correlations across tests were quite high, especially given the relatively small number of children in these samples. These correlations were similar to correlations for the same tests given to nonautistic children (Lord & Schopler, 1988a).

All the children included in these analyses were given the Bayley first and the Merrill–Palmer at a later date, so some of the instability of the Bayley could have been attributable to age at initial assessment. However, we were able to find a small number of children who received both Bayleys and Merrill–Palmers within a 6-month period. All these children scored from 5 to 40 points higher on the Merrill–Palmer than they did on the Bayley. Thus, at least some of this relationship seemed to be due to the fact that autistic children, especially when tested at very young ages, tended to do particularly poorly on the Bayley in ways that did not necessarily reflect their later IQ on performance tasks. This finding seems especially important because, in a few cases, the changes were so marked that children went from being classified as severely mentally retarded to having scores within the normal range of nonverbal intelligence when they were reassessed with Merrill–Palmers. We were also able to find a small number of children who were given Merrill–Palmers at ages 2 and 3 and again within 12 months. Almost all these children also showed increases in IQ with repeated assessments. However, these differences were much smaller (i.e., under 10 points) than the comparisons with the Bayley.

CONCLUSIONS AND SUMMARY

What could be concluded from these results in terms of the predictive usefulness of developmental or IQ assessments of very young autistic children? First, IQ scores of very young autistic children and nonautistic children were relatively stable over 5- to 6-year periods of time spanning preschool to early schoolage, given a number of caveats. The most clear cut of these limitations was that while the Bayley may be useful for determining current developmental level, developmental quotients computed as ratio IQs under 50 were not necessarily stable over long periods of time. Correlations between the Bayley and other tests were significant, but most children with very low scores showed some improvement. Given how many children improved and the extent of some of the changes, these scores should certainly not be used alone to determine prognosis or placements for autistic children under the age of 5.

Improvements were probably related in part to the very young age of the children at initial assessment. Thus, Freeman and colleagues (Freeman *et al.*, 1985) also reported that autistic children tested for the first time under 3 years of age accounted for all the shifts in level of functioning observed in their study. However, also significant was the social and communication-oriented nature of the Bayley and its interaction with initial developmental level. In fact, the only other study where lower-functioning children showed increases in IQ was one study by Mittler, Gillies and Jukes (1966) who compared initial scores (at a mean age of 7 years) on early versions of the Stanford–Binet (Terman & Merrill, 1973), another verbally oriented test, to later scores (at a mean age of 15 years) on the Wechsler Intelligence Scale for Children, which has a performance scale as well as verbal subtests.

It also bears repeating that several other studies in which follow-up has continued into early adolescence have shown decreases in cognitive and adaptive functioning (Waterhouse & Fein, 1984), particularly for lower-functioning children (DeMyer *et al.*, 1974; Gillberg & Steffenburg, 1987; Lockyer & Rutter, 1969). This trend may have been beginning to emerge in the 6- to 11-year comparisons in this study, but since the maximum age included here was 12 years, the evidence is limited. Two other differences between the present samples and previous research may also account for the different pattern of results. First, the Lockyer and Rutter (1969, 1970) papers used Vineland SQs as the outcome measure, compared with a variety of tests (including a substantial number of Merrill–Palmers) as the initial score. Thus, in moving from performance scores to an adaptive measure, their results were biased in the opposite direction to the changes we observed in children initially tested on the Bayley and later given a performance test. Second, we deliberately excluded subjects whose initial IQs or developmental quotients fell at 30 or below. Had these children been included in our "severely retarded" group, the pattern might have been quite different.

Next, as found by other researchers, language status at the time of assessment was clearly related to how well a child performed on a nonverbal test at that same time (Freeman *et al.*, 1985). That is, children who understood at least a few words tended to do better at that time on IQ tests than children who did not understand any language. Language status (at least as measured on the PPVT) did not predict any changes in IQ except at very early ages, i.e., when the first assessment was under age 4 and when the child was not scoring in the severely retarded range on the developmental scale or performance test. However, it is important to remember that in these studies we had only a single and limited measure of language (Tsai & Beisler, 1984).

Changes in language status were particularly linked to increases in IQ for children who scored in the mildly retarded range at age 3 and who acquired language between that time and age 7. These children showed marked IQ increases. By contrast, children who did well on the

Bayley or Merrill–Palmer at ages 2 or 3 but failed to acquire language by age 7 showed significant decreases in IQ over this period. For children who scored below 50 IQ or DQ at age 2 or 3, it was difficult to predict who would acquire language or to predict which children would do better in further intellectual assessments.

Altogether, care must be taken not to conclude that two to three year old autistic children with poor scores on the Bayley will remain nonverbal and function as severely mentally retarded, because of results of these very early assessments (under age 3). Although it is unlikely that an autistic child who scores below 50 and does not understand enough words to score on the PPVT at age 3 will later score as nonretarded; from our data, this child does have a 40% chance of having a receptive vocabulary of at least a 2-year-old level by age 7 and a 50% chance of scoring above the severe level of retardation at a later age.

Finally, one can ask which of our findings seem to be specific to autism and which have to do with general characteristics of using developmental and intellectual tests with very young children. On the whole, most of the results seemed to be related to the young age of the children, their low developmental levels and their language status rather than specifically to autism. However, the finding that autistic children had consistently lower social quotients and that the social quotients were associated with language status suggested that adaptive skills and/or social quotients are important measures in realistically assessing the strengths and deficits of young children with autism.

In conclusion, we would like to contend that early assessments of intelligence can be useful and can provide reliable information about young children with autism. However, great care needs to be taken in making long-term predictions for individuals on the basis of such scores. Caution must be used in interpreting results of any single test. It is also important to remember that a priori, only children who were consistently assessed as autistic were included in the autistic samples, so that although many children made marked improvements in intellectual test scores between ages 3–5 and 6–12 years, these children were still significantly handicapped by their autism. Studies by others (Lockyer & Rutter, 1969; 1970; Waterhouse & Fein, 1984) indicating that intellectual skills of some autistic individuals decreased at or during adolescence suggest a curvilinear trend, with the highest scores achieved during early school years as in this sample (i.e., at 6–9 years of age). A positive note, however, is that it may be the case that the intellectual handicaps of some very young nonverbal autistic children are sometimes overestimated if early test results are taken too literally. When coupled with the diagnosis of autism, the presence and/or severity of mental retardation may be difficult to assess with precision if the child's developmental level and experience requires administration of the Bayley Mental Scales.

Although we did not directly assess this possibility in these studies, the earlier finding by Lockyer and Rutter (1969) of the good predictability yielded by incomplete assessments (many of which were Merrill–Palmers and which, in contrast to the Bayley, tended to yield overestimates for their sample) suggests that a combination of tests, such as the Bayley, the Merrill–Palmer, a language screening test (even if incomplete), and an adaptive scale may yield the most stable and useful results.

ACKNOWLEDGMENT. This research was funded in part by grants from the Natural Sciences and Engineering Research Council of Canada and the Alberta Heritage Foundation for Medical Research to the first author. Preliminary results from this project were presented at the annual TEACCH Conference on Autism in Durham, North Carolina, in May 1986. Requests for reprints may be addressed to Catherine Lord, Department of Psychology, Glenrose Rehabilitation Hospital, Edmonton, Alberta T5G 0B7.

REFERENCES

Arthur, G. (1952). *The Arthur Adaptation of the Leiter International Performance Scale*. Chicago: The Psychological Service Center Press.

Bayley, N. (1969) *Manual for the Bayley Scales of Infant Development*. New York: Psychological Corporation.

DeMyer, M. K., Barton, S., Alpern, G. D., Kimberlin, C., Allen, J., Yang, E., & Steele, R. (1974). The measured intelligence of autistic children. *Journal of Autism and Childhood Schizophrenia, 4*, 42–60.

DeMyer, M. K., Barton, S., DeMyer, W. E., Norton, J. A., Allen, J., & Steele, R. (1973). Prognosis in autism: A follow-up study. *Journal of Autism and Childhood Schizophrenia, 3*, 199–245.

Doll, E. A. (1965). *Vineland Social Maturity Scale*. Circle Pines, MN: American Guidance Service.

Dunn, L. M. (1959). *Manual for the Peabody Picture Vocabulary Test*. Minneapolis: American Guidance Service.

Ebert, E., & Simmons, K. (1943). The British foundation study of child growth and development. *Monograph of the Society for Research in Child Development, 8*, 35.

Freeman, B. J., Ritvo, E. R., Needleman, R., & Yokota, A. (1985). The stability of cognitive and linguistic parameters in autism: A five-year prospective study. *Journal of the American Academy of Child Psychiatry, 24*, 459–64.

Gillberg, C., & Steffenburg, S. (1987). Outcome and prognostic factors in infantile autism and similar conditions: A population-based study of 46 cases followed through puberty. *Journal of Autism and Developmental Disorders, 17*, 273–88.

Hindley, C. B., & Owen, C. F. (1978). The extent of individual changes in IQ for ages between 6 months and 17 years, in a British longitudinal sample. *Journal of Child Psychology and Psychiatry, 19*, 329–30.

Lockyer, L., & Rutter, M. (1969). A five to fifteen-year follow-up study of infantile psychosis. III. Psychological aspects. *British Journal of Psychiatry, 115*, 865–82.

Lockyer, L., & Rutter, M. (1970). A five to fifteen-year follow-up study of infantile psychosis. IV. Patterns of cognitive ability. *British Journal of Social and Clinical Psychology, 9*, 152–63.

Lord, C., & Schopler, E. (1988a). Stability of assessment results of autistic and nonautistic language-impaired children from preschool years to early school age. Manuscript in review.

Lord, C., & Schopler, E. (1988b). The role of age of assessment, developmental level, and test in the stability of intelligence scores in autistic children from preschool years through early school age. Manuscript in review.

Lotter, V. (1974). Factors related to outcome in autistic children. *Journal of Autism and Childhood Schizophrenia, 4*, 263–77.

Mittler, P., Gillies, S., & Jukes, E. (1966). Prognosis in psychotic children: Report of a follow-up study. *Journal of Mental Deficiency Research, 10*, 73–83.

Parks, S. L. (1983). The assessment of autistic children: A selective review of available instruments. *Journal of Autism and Developmental Disorders, 13*, 255–68.

Rutter, M. (1978). Diagnosis and definition of childhood autism. *Journal of Autism and Developmental Disorders, 8*, 139–61.

Rutter, M. (1985). Infantile autism and other pervasive disorders. In M. Rutter & L. Hersov (Eds.), *Child and adolescent psychiatry: Modern approaches* (pp. 545–66). London: Blackwell Scientific Publications.

Rutter, M., & Lockyer, L. (1967). A five to fifteen year follow-up study of infantile psychosis. I. Description of sample. *British Journal of Psychiatry, 113*, 1169–82.

Rutter, M., & Schopler, E. (1987). Autism and pervasive developmental disorders: Concepts and diagnostic issues. *Journal of Autism and Developmental Disorders, 17*, 159–86.

Sattler, J. M. (1982). *Assessment of children's intelligence and special abilities*. Boston: Allyn & Bacon.

Schopler, E. (1976). Towards reducing behavior problems in autistic children. In L. Wing (Ed.), *Early childhood autism* (pp. 221–46). London: Pergamon.

Schopler, E. (1982). Evolution in understanding and treatment of autism. *Triangle, 21*, 51–7.

Schopler, E. (1987). Specific and nonspecific factors in the effectiveness of a treatment system. *American Psychologist, 42*, 376–83.

Schopler, E., Reichler, R. J., & Renner, B. R. (1986). *The Childhood Autism Rating Scale (CARS) for Diagnostic Screening and Classification of Autism.* New York: Irvington.

Stutsman, R. (1931). Guide for administering the Merrill–Palmer Scale of Mental Tests. In L. M. Terman (Ed.), *Mental measurement of preschool children* (pp. 139–262). New York: Harcourt, Brace & World.

Terman, L. M., & Merrill, M. A. (1973). *Stanford-Binet Intelligence Scale Form L-M.* Boston: Houghton-Mifflin.

Tsai, L., & Beisler, J. M. (1984). Research in infantile autism: A methodological problem in using language comprehension as the basis for selecting matched controls. *Journal of the American Academy of Child Psychiatry, 23*, 700–3.

Waterhouse, L., & Fein, D. (1984). Developmental trends in cognitive skills for children diagnosed as autistic and schizophrenic. *Child Development, 55*, 236–48.

Wechsler, D. (1974). *Wechsler Intelligence Scale for Children—Revised.* New York: The Psychological Corporation.

12

Assessing the Quality of Living Environments

MICHAEL L. JONES

INTRODUCTION

Traditional theories of autism treat behavior disorders and delayed development as symptoms of internal deficits. These deficits have been expressed in terms of physiological factors (e.g., brain pathology) or hypothetical concepts of information processing (e.g., sensory overload). Most theories further stipulate, however, that the correlation between symptoms and internal deficits is not perfect because of the mediating role of the environment. Environmental factors must be acknowledged to account for the fact that an individual with a mild deficiency, reared in a depriving environment, might show severe developmental delay (Bijou & Dunitz-Johnson, 1981).

There is another more compelling reason to acknowledge environmental factors. There is currently little we can do to correct internal deficits but we can correct environmental deficits that contribute to developmental problems associated with autism. Most successful treatment efforts for people with autism involve control and manipulation of environmental factors. Thus, even people with severe manifestations of internal deficits, reared in an optimal environment, may be expected to demonstrate substantial development gains.

The focus of this chapter is on identifying and correcting environmental deficits that may contribute to problems in development. In examining environmental deficits, a basic question must be asked: What behaviors does the environment foster and maintain? In many cases, the environment encourages those behaviors we consider to be problematic. We should also ask: What behaviors should the environment foster and maintain? In general, these behaviors can be described under the general heading of behavioral engagement. This chapter describes behavioral engagement, its importance to progressive development, its environmental determinants—variables that can be manipulated to promote engagement and thus development—as well as methods for evaluating the quality of the environment by examining opportunities provided for behavioral engagement.

MICHAEL L. JONES • Bureau of Child Research, University of Kansas, Lawrence, Kansas 66045.

THE IMPORTANCE OF BEHAVIORAL ENGAGEMENT

Behavioral engagement refers to the amount of time an individual spends interacting with the environment in a developmentally appropriate manner (McWilliams, Trivette & Dunst, 1985). Engagement may consist of simply attending to events in the environment, actively manipulating and exploring the environment, or interacting with others in the environment. Ideally, engagement is initiated independently and results in feedback from the environment (i.e., indication that response has affected the environment).

In whatever form, appropriate behavioral engagement is important for a number of reasons. First, it is the basis for learning adaptive behavior. Adaptation occurs in response to interaction with the environment. More frequent interaction with the environment has a practice effect and leads to fluency in responding.

Second, appropriate engagement provides a context for teaching. The best time to teach is when an individual is engaged with the subject matter. High engagement results in more opportunities for this "incidental" teaching to occur (Hart & Risley, 1976).

Third, appropriate engagement is important because it is inversely related to undesirable engagement. When individuals are not engaged in appropriate behaviors, they are either doing nothing or engaging in undesirable behavior. Conversely, engagement is preventative in the sense that high levels of appropriate engagement preclude inappropriate or nonengagement.

Fourth, behavioral engagement is important to the effectiveness of many behavior management techniques. For example, time-out procedures are only effective if "time in" consists of an engaging environment. Further, only minimal time out procedures will be necessary if time in is highly engaging. In an environment rich with engagement opportunities (e.g., the typical home), removal to an environment that is only slightly less engaging (e.g., "Go to your room!") may be effective. Whereas, in a depriving environment (e.g., the typical institutional dayroom), "time out" must be truly barren (e.g., the institutional time out room).

Finally, engagement is important for humanitarian reasons. People have a right to live in an environment that is appropriately engaging. We have an obligation to the people in our charge to provide them with an environment that maximizes their development.

BEHAVIORAL ENGAGEMENT AND ENVIRONMENTAL QUALITY

Various criteria have been proposed for evaluating the quality of treatment environments (Jones, Risley & Favell, 1984). Ultimately, assessment of environmental quality should be based on a functional analysis of behavior within the environment and the degree to which preferred behavioral outcomes are achieved. Thus, environmental assessment should focus on evaluating the relationship between behavioral engagement and the immediate, manipulable factors that determine its occurrence.

A useful criterion for evaluation is the extent to which the environment offers opportunities for engagement; if necessary, prompts engagement; and provides appropriate consequences for engagement. An engaging environment is one in which there are ample antecedents for engagement, rules of the setting permit and encourage engagement, and engagement responses are consistently reinforced.

The first step in programming an engaging environment should be evaluating the existing environment to determine its impact on engagement. Evaluation is important in at least four respects. First, it is necessary to identify inadequacies in the environment (e.g., times and locations where engagement opportunities are low). Evaluation of the existing environment may be used to justify intervention efforts and identify the focus of such efforts. Evaluation also permits systematic, proactive planning for change rather than reactive change to address a crisis situation (Jones, Lattimore, Ulicny & Risley, 1986).

Second, evaluation of the treatment environment provides a measure of success or failure for interventions attempted to improve engagement. Measures of engagement and related environmental determinants (i.e., engagement opportunities) are useful indicators of treatment effectiveness (McWilliams et al., 1985). Third, repeated evaluation and subsequent feedback to setting managers are vital to maintain quality. Without ongoing assessment and feedback, slippage in environmental quality is inevitable.

Fourth, information about behavioral engagement and its environmental determinants may be important in assessing autism and other developmental disabilities. In line with traditional theories of autism, the focus in assessment has been on identifying internal deficits (Jones, Risley & Favell, 1984). For example, neurologic assessment attempts to identify brain pathology and associated behavioral disorders. Intelligence testing measures cognitive processes presumed to be linked to performance.

Limited attention to environmental factors is highlighted by the intelligence quotient formula (mental age/chronologic age=IQ) which asserts that chronologic age is equivalent to normal experience with the environment. This is often not the case with severely disabled individuals who reside in group living environments. A more realistic assessment of performance deficits should consider opportunities for normal interaction with the environment as the denominator.

It is important to emphasize that evaluation of the treatment environment must include an assessment of behavioral engagement with the environment. The quality of engagement opportunities can only be determined by the levels of engagement they produce. For example, a common assumption about environmental quality is that high levels of material and activity availability are indicative of quality. But this is true only to the extent that the available materials and activities result in higher levels of engagement. Several studies have shown that simply improving material and activity availability may not be sufficient. Improved engagement depends on the engagement potential of the materials and activities provided (Favell & Cannon, 1977; Jones, Favell, Lattimore & Risley, 1984). The only way to tell if engagement opportunities are engaging is to assess behavior.

Valid measures of environmental quality may best be derived from direct observations of behavior in its environmental context. An *ecobehavioral* strategy should be used to obtain these measures—one that documents ongoing behavior and immediate environmental factors that may influence it. There are a number of methodologic considerations in employing an ecobehavioral assessment strategy. These considerations are detailed in an earlier publication (Jones, Risley & Favell, 1984) and are summarized below.

First among these is the *locus* or reference point of measurement. This locus may be either environment-centered or person-centered. Environment-centered measures ignore the behavior of individuals and focus on the surrounding environment and more global pattern of behavior. Person-centered measures focus on behavior and the individual's interactions with the immediate environment. A person-centered locus may be the most effective measure for describing the immediate opportunities available for engagement.

A second consideration is for *sampling frequency* of measuring environment and behavior events. For example, behavior may be measured as an ongoing, continuous stream of events or as discrete samples of events over time. Continuous ongoing measurement is ideal but unrealistic. Ongoing behavior and environmental events can be accurately assessed by taking periodic time samples. Three methodologic conditions must be met, however, in order to obtain valid estimates from time samples: samples must be random, instantaneous, and of sufficient frequency (Klesges, Woolfrey & Vollmer, 1985).

Randomness can be achieved by taking samples based on some arbitrary time criterion rather than predetermined factors in the setting. Time sampling must be instantaneous so that discrete samples, rather than multiple episodes of behavior, are observed at each sampling interval. Time samples must be made often enough to minimize sampling error. As with any sampling procedure, the number of samples required to obtain a representative picture will be determined by the heterogeneity of the population sampled.

If these conditions are met, observed events may be quantified by duration rather than rate because the proportion of time a behavior is observed during time-sample observations corresponds to the absolute proportion of time occupied by the behavior. For example, if clients are observed engaging appropriately in activities during 50% of the observations taken throughout an 8-hr day, it may be assumed that clients spend 50% of an 8-hr day engaged in appropriate activity (Jones, Lattimore, Ulicny & Risley, 1986).

A third consideration is selecting behavioral and environmental variables to assess. In terms of client behavior, the primary focus is appropriate and inappropriate engagement. Behavior may be classified in one of three ways: appropriate, inappropriate, or nonengagment. Alternatively, behavior may be classified in an open data system, whereby a brief, narrative description of behavior is recorded. This recording system offers maximum flexibility and allows observers to assess any situation without resorting to an extensive system of predetermined behavior scoring codes. This flexibility may be important when it is difficult, at best, to determine in advance all the events (and corresponding codes) that might be encountered. Furthermore, this procedure results in descriptive data that may be coded and analyzed in a number of ways after the fact. The resulting archival data may be reanalyzed without the limitations imposed by an idiosynchratic coding system.

There are two environmental variables of primary interest as opportunities for engagement. First, availability of engaging materials and activities should be measured. This involves assessing their immediate availability to clients during each instantaneous time sample. It is important to document the type of material or activity available as thoroughly as possible, as well as the manner in which it is provided. Based on the record of client behavior during the observation, it is possible to determine exactly which materials and activities are associated with appropriate engagement.

The second environmental variable of primary interest is clients' interactions with staff. Ideally, interactions should be conducted so they are learning activities for clients and provide maximum opportunities for independent responding. Thus, in addition to noting the frequency of contacts between staff and clients, the specific nature of interactions should be documented. Staff should have pleasant verbal interactions with clients whenever possible (including basic care activities) to promote language development. They should also provide the least possible assistance necessary to engage clients in an ongoing activity. This will encourage independent responding rather than passive participation by the client. Thus, social interactions may be classified along two dimensions: (1) presence or absence of a positive or corrective verbal interaction (i.e., social versus nonsocial), and (2) presence or absence of an opportunity to respond independently (i.e., assistive versus custodial interaction).

In addition to time-sampling data, it is useful to gather information on a number of variables that may control the environmental conditions observed. This information will be useful in determining the cause of environmental deficiencies. Additional information about the setting should include: personnel policies, staff scheduling, supervisory structure, degree and type of staff training, nature of interactions between departments, flow of responsibility for client treatment, and existing guidelines and procedures for handling disruptive behavior.

An Example of an Ecobehavioral Assessment

To illustrate an ecobehavioral assessment strategy, an example is drawn from ongoing research on treatment environments for profoundly multiply handicapped individuals. This research involves comparing engagement opportunities available in different environments for disabled and nondisabled individuals in an attempt to establish normative standards for environmental quality.

Study of behavioral engagement across populations of disabled and nondisabled individuals may provide additional insight into the relationship between environmental and organismic factors in developmental disabilities. For example, information about differences in engagement of disabled and nondisabled persons under similar environmental conditions would help determine the extent to which internal deficits account for limited engagement. With normative data available for comparison, measures of behavioral engagement under optimal environmental conditions would identify persons at risk of delayed or abnormal development.

Similarly, engagement data collected across environments may provide normative standards for engagement in various settings. Such standards would provide a useful index of environmental quality. Assessment of engagement opportunities—and inhabitants' actual engagement—in a given setting would identify functionally depriving environmental conditions.

Three samples of nine subjects participated in the study. Two samples included profoundly mentally retarded, nonambulatory, multiply handicapped individuals living in institutional settings. The two samples did not differ in level of functioning (average develop-

Table I. Manifest Observation Categories

Position: specific body position of client (e.g., sitting)

Attention: object, environmental feature, or person client is attending to (i.e., looking at) most prominently

Hands: object, environmental feature, or person client is contacting with his/her hands (may be two objects)

Behavior: brief description of client's behavior at instant of observation

Client problem: any problems with client's behavior (e.g., self injury, aggression) noted

Staff problem: whether staff's behavior or lack of behavior poses a problem for client (e.g., abusive or neglectful situation) noted

Staff proximity: location of nearest staff/person to client

Social interaction: client's involvement in a social interaction, person involved, and type of interaction

Situation code: context of observed activity, if any (e.g., basic care, training, leisure activity)

Material availability: presence of a manipulable stimulus material (e.g., toy, training materials, grooming or other self-care materials) within arm's reach of client

mental age of 6 months) or type and severity of handicapping onditions. However, they resided in settings that were judged to be significantly different in quality of treatment (qualitative judgments are corroborated by recent reviews for AC/MRDD accreditation).

The third sample consisted of developmentally normal infants (average age: 6 months), attending a private daycare center for children aged 1–18 months. Nondisabled infants were selected as a normative sample because of similar developmental functioning and similar care requirements.

Direct observations were made in each setting using an adaptation of the Resident Activity MANIFEST (Jones & Risley, 1984). The MANIFEST uses a time-sampling procedure whereby individuals are observed instantaneously at designated intervals (i.e., every 30 min). Specific data are recorded concerning clients' behavior and a number of environmental conditions. Observational categories scored with the MANIFEST are described in Table I.

For the present example, MANIFEST data are aggregated across all subjects for each time period. Two analyses are of primary interest: (1) opportunities for behavioral engagement, and (2) active behavioral engagement. Opportunities for engagement consisted of Material Availability, Social Interaction with Staff, and Structured Activity Availability. Active behavioral engagement consisted of scorings in the Behavior category of 2.0: manipulation by hand of objects or specific environmental features, 3.0: manipulation by mouth of food, or eating utensils, 9.0: self-care activities, and 10.0: ambulation activities.

Figures 1, 2, and 3 show the distribution of both opportunities for engagement (shaded background) and actual engagement (plotted points) across time of day in the Day Care Center, MR Setting One, and MR Setting Two, respectively. Data represent the percent of subjects having opportunities and/or engaged during each observation.

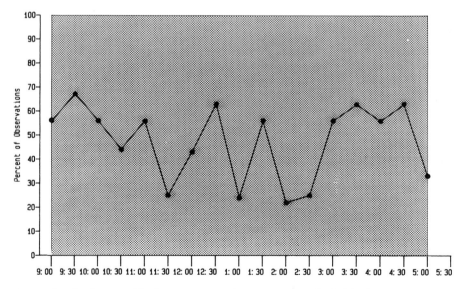

Fig. 1. The distribution of both opportunities for engagement (shaded background) and actual engagement (plotted points) across time of day in the day-care center.

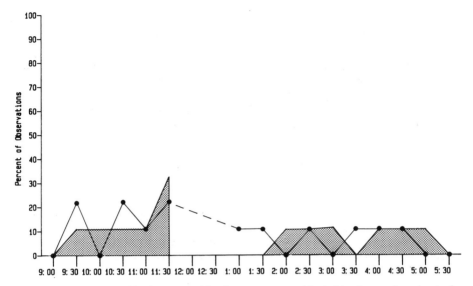

Fig. 2. The distribution of both opportunities for engagement (shaded background) and actual engagement (plotted points) across time of day in the MR Setting One.

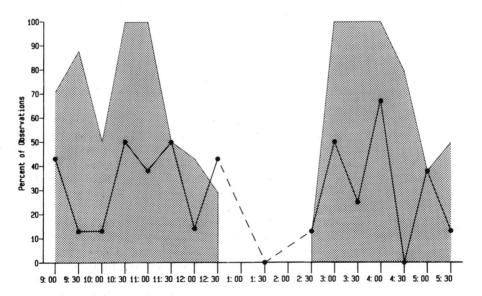

Fig. 3. The distribution of both opportunities for engagement (shaded background) and actual engagement (plotted points) across time of day in the MR Setting Two.

This example highlights global differences in engagement between retarded and non-retarded populations and between retarded populations in different settings. The study also emphasizes rather dramatic differences between settings in opportunities for engagement. The two MR settings differed from the day-care setting not only in quantity but in type of engagement opportunities as well. The Day Care setting was characterized by high levels of both material availability and structured activities. MR Setting Two differed from Setting One primarily in material availability. Although engagement in Setting Two was twice that in Setting One, it did not approximate "normal" levels of engagement.

PROGRAMMING AN ENGAGING ENVIRONMENT

Evaluation of the existing treatment environment should identify a number of areas for improvement. Changes to improve the setting should be addressed systematically. Our research in various settings with different populations has led us to adopt several guiding "principles" for programming an engaging treatment environment. They apply to design of both the physical environment and the activities, or program, of the setting.

Principles of Living Environment Design

The concept of open environment design is foremost among these principles. An open environment has a minimum of visual and physical barriers among activities. Most or all activities are conducted within a single, large area but with clear delineations between activity areas. Ideally, activity areas are designated by changes in floor surface, arrangement of furnishings, and so on, to provide clear but unobtrusive boundaries.

The open environmental design has several advantages. Clients can more freely explore and choose from among several available activities. The design also facilitates supervision of both clients and staff and permits easier transition between sequential activities. Finally, the open design provides greater flexibility in use of space. Activity areas may be rearranged as needs change over time. In short, activities shape the space, rather than space shaping activities.

Several potential problems with the open design should be noted. There must be an adequate match between the setting's physical and program design. An open physical plan requires an open program design. The difference between a workable open environment and a barren dayroom is determined largely by program design. This is an advantage in one respect, since many settings (e.g., institutional dayrooms) are already open in their physical design. An open program may be implemented with few, if any, extensive physical modifications to the setting.

A frequent criticism of open environments is greater potential for distractibility, because of increased noise levels and visual distractions. Research in day-care centers has shown that an open environment does not interfere with small group, training, or other activities (e.g., naps) that require minimum distraction (Twardosz, Cataldo & Risley, 1974). Daycare centers for nondisabled infants and toddlers may arguably be different from settings for developmentally disabled individuals but one need only witness feeding time for 20 infants to note the similarities. The same principles and procedures apply. For example, noise levels can be reduced by choosing sound-absorbing furniture, wall, and floor coverings; visual distractability can be minimized by lower ambient lighting and use of spot lighting.

Another frequent criticism of the open design is clients' loss of privacy. In actuality, this may be less of a problem as a result of improved supervision and thus easier detection of privacy violations. Furthermore, we are advocating use of an open environment in designing the living space for clients. Open design may not necessarily apply to clients' private quarters. But even in the living area, it may be desirable to designate a private or quiet area where clients can rest from ongoing activities. This quiet space must be used judiciously, however, so that clients do not spend too much time resting.

A second guiding principle is the use of activity zones. Each zone is a discrete area in which specific activities occur at specific times. We have found activity zones to be the most effective use of space within an open environmental design. As one might expect, the zone approach requires special arrangements of the program as well as physical environment. For example, assigning staff to supervise specific activity zones rather than groups of clients (i.e., zone versus man-to-man staffing) results in less dead time and more active engagement for both clients and caregivers (LeLaurin & Risley, 1972).

It is important to schedule concurrent activity zones whenever possible. Specifically, it is essential to have a centralized holding zone from which clients may move to other activity zones throughout the day. This central activity area is always staffed by at least one caregiver and furnished with an abundance of engaging materials. When clients are not involved in other activity zones (e.g., meals, toieting, training, recreation) they remain in the central activity area, where staff circulate to prompt and reinforce appropriate engagement responses.

When activity zones are established, it is also important that clear boundaries separate concurrent activities. This serves to designate supervision boundaries for staff (i.e., they are responsible for all clients within their zone). Zone boundaries may also be conditioned as discriminative stimuli for clients, signalling the locations in which certain behaviors can and cannot occur (e.g., toileting is only reinforced in the toileting zone).

We have alluded to several advantages in using activity zones. Dead time may be reduced by scheduling a continuous holding activity to occupy clients between other activities. Rules governing appropriate and inappropriate activity in each zone may be established and their enforcement facilitated by clearly defined zone boundaries. The use of zones may also increase the amount of individualized attention clients receive. When staff are responsible for an entire group of clients, as in the man-to-man technique, they may have less time to spend with clients individually. With the zone approach, clients typically arrive at each zone singly, so the caregiver can immediately provide individual attention to engage them in the new activity.

Although the zone approach offers several advantages, there are common criticisms. First, proponents of the man-to-man or family-group approach to activity planning argue that it is preferable because more individualized attention can be given to each client according to his or her needs (Crosby, 1976). In reality, there may be less individualized attention with this approach, since caregivers must continually supervise an entire group of clients. As a result, clients spend considerable time waiting for other group members to complete an activity before the next activity can begin.

It is also assumed that the man-to-man approach permits closer interpersonal relationships between staff and clients. Presumably, clients are contacted by fewer caregivers so closer relationships develop and clients receive more consistent care. It should be noted, however, that a given caregiver, who generally works a 40-hr week, is with clients less than half of the time they are awake. Further, during this time, the caregiver is or should be distributing attention among all clients in the family group. Thus, there is little assurance that clients will receive more consistent care with the man-to-man approach. Alternatively, consistent care can be assured with the zone approach by specifying exactly how staff should conduct zone activities with each client and training all staff to operate the zone accordingly.

A third concern with the zone approach is maintaining zones and ensuring that clients remain in a designated area, participate in prescribed activities, and so on. We have found this to be a common problem in establishing a zone system and may be the major reason the approach is not adopted more readily. However, we have also found that zones can be maintained, if available materials and activities are sufficiently stimulating to maintain clients' interest. The key to maintaining a zone is to ensure that clients' participation is adequately and consistently reinforced either through selection and presentation of reinforcing materials and activities or the use of programmed contingencies.

This point is illustrated by noting procedures used in operating a central activity zone. First, the central activity zone is furnished with a variety of toys and materials that have been empirically selected because they promote high levels of independent engagement (Favell & Cannon. 1977; Jones, Favell, Lattimore & Risley, 1984). If clients are ambulatory, materials may be displayed on open shelves to promote independent selection (Montes & Risley, 1975). Clients are encouraged to select and engage in appropriate activity with materials. This may initially require using reinforcement contingencies whereby clients are rewarded (e.g., with edibles and praise) for any approach and contact with materials. Differential reinforcement may be used to promote client versus staff-initiated engagement. For example, edible reinforcers may be delivered only when clients independently select and play with toys, and social praise may be used to maintain toy play or when a caregiver must initially prompt toy play.

Additional rules may be established for the zone to maintain appropriate engagement. For example, clients may be prevented from taking materials outside of the zone and inappropriate engagement (e.g., throwing objects) may be consequated by requiring clients to leave the zone temporarily. If materials and activities in the zone are truly reinforcing, temporary exclusion from the zone may be effective in supressing disruptive behavior.

A third design principle governs the assignment of staff responsibilities within the treatment environment. It is most effective to prepare staff as generalists who are capable of meeting almost all client needs. The generalist approach ensures that each caregiver is trained in all aspects of client care. This permits smooth and efficient movement from one activity zone to another across the day. In contrast, a specialist approach allows less flexibility in scheduling, since paraprofessionals are hired, trained, and supervised by independent disciplines (e.g., physical therapy, nursing, special education) to provide a specific type of care. Paraprofessionals (e.g., nursing or special education aides) are responsible to different supervisors. This makes it difficult to identify any one person responsible for overall services. The quality of care received with specialist caregivers depends upon the ability of each separate supervisor to select, train, supervise, and coordinate services without confusing or omitting responsibilities between specialties.

In a generalist approach, multidisciplinary treatment components of care are disseminated through a single responsible supervisor. A generalist approach maximizes accountability for quality of care, allows more flexibility in time and personnel for scheduling services, and provides an on-site supervisor. A specialist approach results in service disruptions when a specialist is unavailable (e.g., sickness or bad weather) or when conflicts arise between specialists' schedules. Finally, the generalist approach enhances implementation and integration of multidisciplinary services across zones, since all caregivers are capable of providing all aspects of care.

In the generalist model, professional staff function primarily as consultants. They prescribe services and design specific programs for clients, provide training and follow-up to caregivers, and when more sophisticated treatment is required, provide therapy directly to clients. Freed from the responsibility of supervision, they can practice the skills for which they were trained.

The simplified management structure also serves to buffer caregivers from concurrent demands by various professionals. Input from each discipline is directed to the program supervisor, who in turn assigns work responsibilities to caregivers. As a result, greater integration of services is achieved.

Steps in Planning Activity Zones

Our experience suggests that it is best to implement changes in one activity at a time but with minimal delay between activities. Steps in programming an activity zone are described below.

Activities that will occur in the setting should be identified and priorities set for establishing necessary zones. First, identify those activities that must occur each day. These will be determined, in part, by the purpose and nature of a particular program. For example, residential programs must be concerned with health care activities, whereas a day treatment program will be concerned more with training activities. Activities will also be determined largely by clients' needs. Programs for clients with severe, multiple handicaps may require a greater emphasis on health and medical care. For higher functioning clients, training and other activities to promote independent responding may have greater emphasis. In addition to client-related activities, consideration must also be given to environmental maintenance activities. Time and space must be programmed for housekeeping, material preparation and storage, equipment maintenance, and so forth.

Once activities have been identified, priorities should be set for implementing zones. The first priority should usually be setting up a central activity zone, since this activity typically does not exist in most programs and because it will serve as the geographic and organizational hub for all other activities. Second priority typically goes to reprogramming health care activities, followed by training and other special activity zones, and finally, environmental maintenance.

The first step in implementing a given activity zone is to determine the environmental requirements for the activity. These include physical features of the environment, such as (1) floor space; (2) spatial arrangement to maximize client engagement and staff efficiency; (3) delineation of zone boundaries; (4) lighting, acoustic, and ventilation requirements; (5) equipment and material selection; and (6) signage. We have already noted several considerations in establishing boundaries between zones, control of lighting and noise, and material selection and presentation. Additional suggestions for programming the physical environment are provided below.

Floor-space requirements will depend on the type of activity, number of occupants in a zone at once, equipment required for the activity, and type of clients served (e.g., clients in wheelchairs may require more or less space for certain activities than ambulatory clients). Floor space for each zone will also be determined by the space available in the setting and the number of zones operating concurrently. The spatial relationship between zones should also be considered in planning floor space for a zone. The central activity zone should be the geographic center for all other zones. Zones that operate concurrently should be set up in close proximity to each other, if clients will be moving between zones.

Zones should be spatially arranged to maximize clients' independent engagement. Where desirable, zones should be accessible so clients can move freely among activities. Independent engagement may also be enhanced by arrangement of materials and equipment (e.g., displaying toys on open shelves to prompt independent selection). Where appropriate, seating should be arranged to promote social interaction; chairs should be arranged facing each other or clustered around tables rather than lined up side by side or classroom style (Sommer, 1969).

Space should also be arranged to maximize staff efficiency. There are a number of assessment techniques, derived from the field of human factors engineering, for determining the most efficient work setting arrangement. One technique is the trip frequency diagram (Krick, 1962) that can be used to analyze—and reduce—movements between work centers within a zone. The technique involves observing a work activity over a period of time and recording the number of trips made between work centers.

One final consideration in the physical design of an activity zone is signage to convey necessary treatment information to staff. This is especially important with a generalist staffing approach, where all staff will conduct all activities with all clients. We have found two types of sign boards to be effective. One is an activity board that lists general and client-specific information explaining how the activity should be conducted. This includes the sequence in which clients will participate in the activity, health and training information, positioning considerations, preferred reinforcers, prosthetic equipment needs, and so on. Typically, the activity board lists all clients down the left-hand side with specific instructions provided beside each client's name. The Master Schedule Board lists in half-hour blocks the scheduled activity for each client. This board should be located over the central activity zone to prompt staff to prepare clients for activities.

The second step in implementing an activity zone is to determine program requirements for the activity. The exact work method and time allocated for conducting the activity should be determined. The work method may be determined by first listing all of the important steps involved in conducting the activity. To accomplish this, we have found it useful to conceptualize each activity as three distinct subroutines, and list the important components of each.

The first subroutine is setup for the activity that involves gathering and preparing all necessary equipment, materials, and so forth for the activity. It is important that set-up procedures are completed before the first client enters the zone. This ensures that a caregiver does not have to interrupt the activity or leave a client unattended to locate materials. We have found it useful to complete many of the setup procedures for an activity a day in advance. Thus, setup for the next day's activity is often the last step in completing the activity. It is also useful to arrange all materials for an activity on an activity cart. The cart is brought out to conduct the activity, then restocked and stored for the next day.

The second subroutine is actually conduciing the activity. All essential steps in conducting the activity are specified in sequential order. Arriving at the optimal sequence of steps involves conducting the activity as desired and making note of each specifiable step. In most cases, there are several correct ways to conduct an activity. Selection of the best alternative should be based on two general criteria: (1) which alternative comes closest to serving the clients' best interest (i.e., which results in greatest client engagement), and (2) which alternative is least aversive to staff (i.e., is most likely to be conducted by staff as specified).

In specifying the method for conducting the activity, it is essential that specific engagement opportunities be included. Two types of opportunities should be specified. First, staff should be instructed to prompt client participation at each step in the activity that involves the client. In bathing, for example, staff should prompt the client to independently complete as much of each step (e.g., undressing, washing, rinsing, drying) as possible. The degree of independence will vary from client to client, but the important point is that independent responding is maximized for each client. Second, specific learning or practice opportunities should be programmed for each client in accordance with his or her habilitation goals. For example, a client who is working on language development should have specific opportunities for language production (e.g., prompting and reinforcing naming of body parts) included as part of the activity.

Finally, procedures should be specified for cleaning up after the activity is completed. As noted, it may be most efficient to replenish all materials and make as many preparations as possible for conducting the activity again the next day.

Once the work method has been specified, optimal time requirements for completing the activity should be determined. Knowledge of time requirements is important so that sufficient time can be scheduled for each activity zone. It is also important to ensure that adequate time is spent with each client. Improving efficiency of work methods is not intended to reduce the time needed to complete activities but rather to remove time-wasting aspects of the activity so that more time can be spent prompting client engagement in the activity.

Traditional time-study methods (Krick, 1962) can be used to determine time requirements for each activity. Briefly, these methods involve observing a well-trained caregiver conduct the activity and timing each subroutine in the activity. Ideally, a time study should be conducted for each client in each activity. Alternatively, representative samples can be taken and an average time requirement calculated for each activity.

The third step in programming an activity zone is to specify the rules for participation in the activity. As noted rules are important to maintain appropriate client engagement and to operate the zone in general. Rules for participation also provide staff with an effective, consistent method for dealing with problem behaviors when they occur. These rules are actually specification of social contingencies that should be used to consequate client behavior.

Several techniques are effective for maintaining appropriate engagement and dealing with problem behaviors. First, positive reinforcement is provided contingent on being engaged. As staff contact clients in a zone, they systematically reinforce clients who are appropriately engaged in the prescribed activity and withhold reinforcement from those who are not engaged. Second, staff use prompting procedures to initiate engagement in those clients who are not participating and to encourage more diverse forms of engagement in those who are participating (e.g., prompt a more elaborate use of a material). Third, staff use incidental teaching procedures (Hart & Risley, 1976) to promote client-initiated learning. The technique involves staff responding to client-initiated interactions by prompting a more detailed client response. For example, if a client approaches the caregiver extending a toy as if to prompt a toy play interaction, the caregiver responds by praising the client for initiating the request and then prompts the client to explain what he or she wants, to name the toy, to show how the toy is used, and so on.

Often, programming a highly reinforcing activity zone is sufficient to control clients' disruptive behavior. It is, nonetheless, important to specify rules for dealing with disruptive behavior should it occur. First, behaviors that will not be permitted in an activity zone should be specified. These should include general behaviors that are not allowed (e.g., inappropriate use of materials, aggression toward other clients) and specific problem behaviors for individual clients (e.g., SIB). These behaviors must be clearly specified so that all staff who operate the activity zone know the behaviors that should be consistently consequated for each client. This information may be conveyed by signs posted in each zone. The procedure used for dealing with clients' inappropriate engagement is contingent observation (Porterfield, Herbert-Jackson & Risley, 1976). With this procedure, caregivers respond to each instance of disruptive behavior in the following manner:

1. Interrupt the behavior, briefly describe to the client the form and inappropriateness of the behavior, and briefly explain what would be appropriate behavior in the situation.
2. Escort the client to the periphery of the activity, require him or her to sit, and instruct him or her to observe the appropriate engagement of other clients.
3. Once the client has been watching quietly for a brief period (usually less than 1 min), the caregiver asks the client if he or she is ready to rejoin the activity and engage in appropriate behavior.
4. When the client returns to the activity, the caregiver makes a point of providing positive attention for the next appropriate engagement response emitted.

The effectiveness of contingent observation, in which the client becomes an observer rather than a participant, relies on a reinforcing setting. Temporary removal of the client from the activity will be effective in reducing problem behavior only if the activity is sufficiently attractive to the client. For some clients, this mild procedure may not be sufficient, even when highly reinforcing activities and materials are available. More aversive procedures such as exclusionary time out may be required. It cannot be overemphasized, however, that the effectiveness of more aversive procedures also relies on the availability of a reinforcing environment.

CONCLUSION

The importance of an engaging environment to maintain clients' appropriate engagement and, consequently, to promote development has been emphasized. On the basis of our own research and experience in designing living environments, we have provided a number of suggestions for programming an engaging environment. Inherent in this approach is the premise that behavior is controlled by the environment in which it occurs and may be modified by systematically manipulating environmental determinants.

Development of more effective treatment techniques and settings requires that we gain a better understanding of the environment's influence on behavior. Better understanding will result only from systematic analyses of environment–behavior relationships—analyses of the sort described here and elsewhere (e.g., Iwata, Dorsey, Slifer, Bauman & Richman, 1982; Jones, Risley & Favell, 1984).

Ideally, data from these analyses will lead to a taxonomy of environmental requirements by behavior deficits. Such a taxonomy would aid in the prescriptive placement of developmentally disabled individuals in the most suitable treatment environment for their particular type and severity of disability. It should be emphasized, however, that the client's needs will change over time and features constituting the optimal environment will change accordingly. As clients exhibit more developmentally advanced engagement, the environment must offer more sophisticated—and typically, more demanding—engagement opportunities.

REFERENCES

Bijou, S. W., & Dunitz-Johnson, E. (1981). Inter-behavioral analysis of developmental retardation. *The Psychological Record, 31,* 305–29.

Crosby, K. G. (1976). Essentials of active programming. *Mental Retardation. 14*(2), 3–9.

Favell, J. E., & Cannon, P. R. (1977). Evaluation of entertainment materials for severely retarded persons. *American Journal of Mental Deficiency, 81*(4), 357–61.

Hart, B. M., & Risley, T. R. (1975). Incidental teaching of language in the preschool. *Journal of Applied Behavior Analysis, 8,* 411–20.

Iwata, B., Dorsey M., Slifer, K., Bauman K., & Richman, G. (1982). Toward a functional analysis of self-injury. *Analysis and Intervention in Developmental Disabilities, 2,* 3–20.

Jones, M. L., Favell, J. E., & Risley, T. R. (1983). Socioecological programming. In J. Matson & F. Andrasik (Eds.) *Treatment issues and innovations in mental retardation.* New York: Plenum.

Jones, M. L., Favell, J. E., Lattimore, J., & Risley, T. R. (1984). Improving independent engagement of nonambulatory multihandicapped persons through the systematic analysis of leisure materials. *Analysis and Intervention in Developmental Disabilities. 4,* 313–32.

Jones, M. L., Risley, T. R., & Favell, J. E. (1984). Ecological patterns: An ecobehavioral perspective in assessment. In J. L. Matson & S. Breuning (Eds.), *Assessing the mentally retarded.* New York: Grune & Stratton.

Jones, M. L., & Risley, T. R. (1984). *Procedures for the MANIFEST Observation System.* Lawrence, KS: Living Environments Group.

Jones, M. L., Lattimore, J., Ulicny, G. R., & Risley, T. R. (1986). Programming for engagement; Environmental design to control behavior disorders. In R. P. Barret (Ed.), *Treatment of severe behavior disorders: Contemporary approaches with the mentally retarded* (pp. 123–55). New York: Plenum.

Klesges, R. D., Woolfrey, J., & Vollmer, J. (1985). Am evaluation of the reliability of time sampling versus continuous observation data collection. *Journal of Behavior Therapy and Experimental Psychiatry, 16,* 303–8.

Krick, E. V. (1962). *Methods engineering.* New York: Wiley.

LeLaurin, K., & Risley, T. R. (1972). The organization of day-care environments: "Zone" verses "man-to-man" staff assignments. *Journal of Applied Behavior Analysis, 5,* 225–32.

Montes, F., & Risley, T. R. (1975). Evaluating traditional day care practices: An empirical approach. *Child Care Quarterly, 4,* 208–15.

McWilliam, R. A., Trivette, C. M., & Dunst, C. J. (1985). Behavior engagement as a measure of the efficacy of early intervention. *Analysis and Intervention in Developmental Disabilities, 5,* 33–45.

Porterfield, J. K., Herbert-Jackson, E., & Risley, T. R. (1976). Contingent observation: An effective and acceptable procedure for reducing disruptive behaviors of young children in group settings. *Journal of Applied Behavior Analysis, 9,* 55–64.

Sommer, R. (1969). *Personal space: The behavioral basis of design.* Englewood Cliffs, NJ: Prentice-hall.

Twardosz, S., Cataldo, M., & Risley, T. (1974). Open environment design for infant and toddler day care. *Journal of Applied Behavior Analysis, 7,* 529–46.

13

Family Assessment in Autism

SANDRA HARRIS

INTRODUCTION

Living in a family is not easy. Living in a family with a handicapped child, especially a child with a disability as serious as autism, is even tougher. It is not surprising that the stress of raising an autistic child manifests itself in the relationships among family members (Harris & Powers, 1984). Sometimes, however, we may be at risk of assuming that problems that arise in a family with a handicapped child are primarily a product of the child's special needs; we fail to appreciate the extent to which other factors may influence on the family as well.

Because multiple factors may converge to create stress, it is important to assess all the relevant sources of stress that act on a family. This chapter describes a framework for family assessment that is sensitive to the impact of the child's handicap on the family, while acknowledging that the family's discomfort may arise from problems independent of the child's disability and that in turn influence how they perceive the child.

It is impossible to do a complete assessment of a family with an autistic child without a careful study of the child's behavior. However, the concern of the present chapter is the family as an interactive unit and so the focus is on that larger group. It is assumed that the reader has a basic understanding of assessing the child's functioning and the relationship between that assessment process and treatment planning, or will seek that knowledge elsewhere in the present volume or other sources (e.g., Newsom & Rincover, 1981).

Difficult as it is to properly assess an individual, the assessment of the nuclear family, or subunits of that family such as the marriage, the sibling group, or the relationship between parent and child are even more complex. It is here that the chapter places most of its emphasis, offering the reader a framework for understanding the kinds of stressors that impact on families and how these normal stressors may be intensified by the presence of a child with autism. This chapter aims to inform the clinical activities of therapists from a variety of theoretical perspectives and therefore focuses more on the problems confronting the family than on a theoretical delineation of the family's maladaptive mode of problem solving. It also considers the nuclear family in its broader context—that of the extended family and the community. The relationships among members of the extended family as well

SANDRA HARRIS • Applied and Professional Psychology, Rutgers University, Piscataway, New Jersey 08854.

as the resources made available by the wider society can have a substantial impact on the handicapped child and the family as whole.

A FRAMEWORK FOR FAMILY ASSESSMENT

Families bring with them to each new problem the individual resources and needs of the members, their collective history of strategies for problem solving and relating, and their ties to the extended family and community. According to McCubbin and Patterson (1983), there are three kinds of resources that influence the family's ability to adapt to a crisis. These include the individual resources of each family member, the family system's internal resources, and available social support. Within the broad category of personal resources, McCubbin and Patterson (1983) identify four subcategories: financial resources, educational attainment, physical and emotional health, and psychological characteristics. Within the domain of family system resources, McCubbin and Patterson (1983) refer to such factors as family cohesion and adaptability as contributing to the family's capacity for flexible problem solving. Social support includes available help from one's extended family, neighbors, and community.

Doing a meaningful assessment for intervention requires an understanding of these variables as well as the nature of the current stressful event. What is the problem this family is trying to solve? What individual, collective, and community resources are available to them? What historical experiences shape their perceptions of this problem and their ability to solve it? Knowing the answers to questions of this kind, which address both the nature of the current problem and the ongoing functioning of the family, may enable the clinician to generate preliminary treatment hypotheses.

Although this chapter separates assessment from treatment for heuristic purposes, in practice these processes are frequently tightly interwoven, with the child's or family's response being the primary guide to whether one is on the right diagnostic track. Depending on the presenting problem and the severity and subtlety of the problems presented the clinician may spend a few minutes, several hours, or a sustained period of time at any level of this assessment process, including child assessment, individual family member evaluations, examination of the internal resources of the family, and evaluation of social support.

Choosing the proper focus for an in-depth assessment can have important implications in terms of both credibility with the family and efficient use of the clinician's time. If a family with an autistic child were to consult me concerning their child's tantrums and mentioned a problem with alcohol abuse on the part of one of the parents, I would not abandon the assessment of the child, but I would also expand to include a detailed assessment of family members and the family as a unit. By contrast, if a family with a history of stable and effective functioning were to consult me concerning a behavior management problem with their autistic child, my primary focus would be on the child's behavior and only secondarily on the individual family members and the resources of the family system.

INTERVIEWING THE FAMILY

Volumes have been written about interviewing families (e.g., Bowen, 1978; Minuchin, 1974; Stierlin, Rucker-Embden, Wetzel & Wirsching, 1980). Each approach to family treatment is guided by its own view of what constitutes vital treatment data. Rather than competing with that extensive literature, the present chapter focuses on a question of special concern when meeting a family with an autistic child. That is, to what extent should the autistic child be involved when one is evaluating and treating the family as a functioning unit?

In my experience, it is important to include the child in some but not all family interviews. The child should be included so that the clinician can understand the child's behavior, observe how the family copes with the child's needs, and how they present the child to someone from outside the family. The child may be excluded from at least some of the interviews, so that the rest of the family will have the opportunity to share their feelings without the constant interuptions often created by the autistic child. It is difficult to reflect on one's feelings and provide a coherent narrative to the clinician when a child is banging his head, tearing down the drapes, or urinating in the corner. (It is also a substantial challenge to the clinician!) Not having the child present during part of the assessment process may also communicate to the family that it is not essential for everything they do to revolve around the child. In some families, this may be an important step in enabling them to change dysfunctional patterns that have limited the family's ability to grow in diverging directions.

The clinician may also find it useful to observe the child in school, and the family at home in order to understand the naturalistic context in which they live. For the behavior therapist, this is an opportunity to collect systematic data about the child's behavior and the interactions among family members. For the family therapist, it is an opportunity to observe patterns of interaction in the natural habitat.

Although the primary vehicle for family assessment is the interview, other techniques can be useful as well. Systematic behavioral observation, particularly of the parent–child dyad, is a well-developed approach to assessment. Some paper and pencil questionnaires are useful in the assessment of the participants' perceptions of the dyadic and family relationships. Detailed descriptions of a few test instruments and observation systems are provided in the pages that follow.

THE FAMILY–CHILD INTERACTION

When a family is concerned about the management of their autistic child or with difficulties created in their lives by the child's disability, the clinician's first step in the assessment process is to seek a comprehensive picture of the child's functioning. How severe is the handicap? What resources does the family have available to cope with the child's needs? How would an intervention aimed specifically at the child affect the family as a whole? For example, Koegel, Schreibman, Johnson, O'Neill, and Dunlap (1984) report that training parents in behavior modification techniques not only improves the child's behavior, but gives the family more time for leisure and recreational activities thus suggesting that child focused interventions benefit family functioning as well. On the other hand, one must be aware of the risks entailed in a total focus on the child's needs to the exclusion of the rest of the family (Harris, 1984).

Measuring Parent–Child Interactions

If one wants to assess how parents cope with the management problems posed by their autistic child, and how the child responds to parental efforts, there are a number of systems for data collection. Behavior therapists and developmental psychologists have created a variety of coding systems for describing specific interactions between developmentally dis-abled children and their parents including teaching techniques (e.g., Koegel, Glahn & Nieminen, 1978; Weitz, 1982), parent and child language exchanges (e.g., Harris, 1983), and play and social interchanges (e.g., Mash, Terdal & Anderson, 1973; Stoneman, Brody & Abbott, 1983).

Using either standarized codes or versions simplified for clinical purposes it is possible to assess the interaction between adult and child, using these data to help the parents modify their interactions with the child. Assessment and intervention at this level is often a fairly straightforward process because we have a useful social learning theory framework in which to analyze the interactions and a substantial body of data concerning training parents and siblings to be behavior managers (e.g., Harris, 1983; Koegel, Schreibman, Britten, Burke & O'Neill, 1982; Schopler & Reichler, 1971).

Treatment Planning

If the assessment suggests that treatment should be aimed at the child the clinician would provide appropriate services or make suitable referrals and then evaluate the child's and the family's response to intervention. If the difficulties are brought under control by parent training in behavior modification, placement in a suitable school, or the design of a program to deal with a particular skill deficit, the intervention efforts would terminate at this point. If this intervention is not effective, or if the preliminary assessment suggests that the problem does not lie primarily in issues concerning the child, the assessment progresses to the next step, that of assessing the individuals within the family and the family as unit.

One example of the need to continue the assessment process would be the family who seem unwilling or unable to master or apply systematic management techniques with their child. Another would be the family who are responsive to the interventions, but who raise new problems when the child's behavior is brought under effective control.

The movement from the assessment of the child to in–depth consideration of the other members of the family and their functioning as a unit can take either a few minutes or many sessions. Even after identifying the presence of significant problems in individual or family functioning it may be necessary to do sustained work with the child alone, until there is sufficient family trust to address issues of a broader nature. Ongoing consultation about child management may occur in conjunction with any of the other interventions described below. The therapist can never afford to ignore the compelling realities of the child's behavior regardless of what other issues may arise. The therapist who is not skilled in providing this level of assessment and treatment should ensure that these services are being made available to the family by someone else.

ASSESSMENT OF INDIVIDUAL FUNCTIONING

As noted above, personal resources can be important factors in determining how a family copes with the stress of raising an handicapped child (McCubbin & Patterson, 1983). A great deal has been written about techniques for assessing individuals, and this chapter does not linger on those issues. Such individually determined variables as earned income, parental educational attainment and physical health can be important factors in enabling a family to respond effectively to the needs of their handicapped member. Having enough money to buy assistance with child care, having the educational skills to facilitate one's activities as an advocate for the child, knowing how to communicate effectively with service delivery agencies, and having the physical stamina to sustain one's efforts all constitute the kinds of personal resources that enable family members to cope more effectively with the child's needs. Parents who have limited incomes, are physically ill, or not well educated are thus at a decided disadvantage in meeting the needs of their autistic child. They may well require greater social support to compensate for a lack of individual resources.

One's personal and emotional functioning must also be considered as variables in assessing how the individual family member responds to the stress of raising a handicapped child. Although there are no persuasive data suggesting that the members of families of children with autism experience more serious psychopathology than other families (e.g., Koegel, Schreibman, O'Neill & Burke, 1983), neither is there any reason to expect that this population is not part of the normal distribution of psychological difficulties.

Some parents of children with autism have previous histories of substance abuse, depression, anxiety, psychosis, and the myriad of other forms of psychologically maladaptive behavior that present themselves in any clinical setting. In our emphasis on appreciating the essentially normal functioning of most families of autistic children we must not fail to recognize that subsample of families whose maladaptive responses would have posed difficulties, even in the absence of a handicapped child.

Treatment Planning

Psychopathology of a longstanding or severe nature typically requires intensive family and/or individual treatment. In some cases, it may be necessary to refer the family to specialized resources such as a drug or alcohol rehabilitation program, inpatient psychiatric care, and so forth. Impoverishment of individual resources may also require a greater reliance on social support.

ASSESSMENT OF THE FAMILY SYSTEM

Although there are a number of different perspectives from which to view the development and functioning of internal family resources, we have previously discussed the notion of the life cycle of the family (Harris & Powers, 1984) as a helpful framework for understanding the normal stresses and coping responses that occur in families. Because families with autistic children are for the most part "ordinary" families to whom an extraordinary thing has happened, it is useful to think about their experiences from a perspective that appreciates the normal context in which they live as well as the extraordinary stress created by their child's handicapping condition.

The Family Life-Cycle

A family life-cycle approach to understanding the stress in families places an emphasis on appreciating the demands that are imposed on families as they encounter normal transitional challenges (Carter & McGoldrick, 1980a; Figley & McCubbin, 1983; McCubbin & Figley, 1983). This includes the difficulties faced by a newly married couple in adapting to each other's expectations, families, and traditions (Boss, 1983; McGoldrick, 1980) or the period of stress after a baby is born when the family changes to accomodate a new member (Bradt, 1980). Other typical transitional events include the child's starting school (Bradt, 1980), entry into adolescence (Ackerman, 1980; Kidwell, Fischer, Dunham & Baranowski, 1983), and leaving home (McCullough, 1980), the aging and death of one's parents, and the death of one's spouse (Walsh, 1980). These are all "normal" but stressful events that may be accompanied by a period of intense discomfort and even maladaptive behavior before the family finds a solution and restablizes its functioning. Because most of these events occur within the life of a family that includes an autistic child and have an interactive effect with the chronic stress of raising that child, assessment of the family's developmental status may yield important data about the context in which they are functioning.

For the family for whom a transitional event occurs out of sequence the stress may be even greater than when the transition is an expected one (Burton & Bengston, 1985; Carter & McGoldrick, 1980b). For example, a family with young children may be far more disrupted by the death of a parent than a family with grown children (Crosby & Jose, 1983; Herz, 1980). An unmarried teenage couple faces more stress with the birth of a child than does an older married couple. Were the child autistic in either of these situations, the demands on the family might be so intense as to require considerable support from the extended family, the community, or both.

The comprehensive assessment of the internal resources of the family with an autistic child includes a consideration of the position of the family as a developmental unit within the life cycle framework. How does the family's developmental status affect their ability to deal with the child? Conversely, how does the chronic stress of raising a handicapped child influence the family's response to a developmental crisis? The interaction between these two sources of stress will become evident to the alert clinician. For example, a teacher might request consultation when a previously responsive family fails to carry through with home programming and one or both parents seem sad or distracted. The assessment might indicate that an older child in the family is leaving for college and the family as a unit is struggling with this separation. Although there might be secondary concerns about the autistic child, the focus of the family's discomfort might well be this normal separation process.

Special Vulnerability

The family with an autistic child faces many of the same life-cycle challenges as other families, but the demands may be intensified by the additional stress of a child with a handicap. For example, chronic sorrow about the child's handicap may be reactivated by life cycle events which constitute real or symbolic transition points to the family (Wikler, Wasow & Hatfield, 1981). These added stresses may prolong or intensify the family's response to life problems, making an effective resolution more difficult. Thus, integrating a baby into family routines always demands some degree of accomodation and change, but integrating an autistic child may pose extraordinary challenges because of the pain of learning about the diagnosis, the need to meet intensive demands for special management, and so forth (Harris & Powers, 1984).

It is useful to think about family vulnerability to dysfunction in terms of accumulating demands (McCubbin & Patterson, 1983; Patterson & McCubbin, 1983). Although the family of an autistic child may be as capable of coping with normative demands as any other family, adding to that the need to cope with the child's extraordinary needs may push the family to at least temporary, and sometimes sustained, periods of maladaptive responding. In recognition of the interactive effect between normative demands and the child's needs, assessment of the family with an autistic child should aim at understanding the position of the family in the life cycle; the child's handicap; how the special needs of the child may influence the ability of the family to resolve problems created by a normative transition; and how the transitional crisis may affect the family's way of coping with the child's needs.

Some families are more resiliant to stress than others. As Bristol (1984) makes clear, it is not that some families of autistic children are exempt from the pain and sadness of living with the child's disability, but that they seem able to recover more rapidly from periods of stress. Bristol (1984) studied resilient families and points to successful adaptation as related to the degree of family cohesion, expressiveness, and active recreational orientation. Less resilient families may be those coping with a higher level of chronic stress for whom the addition of one more stressor disrupts a delicate balance. The family that is disengaged, emotionally constricted, or involved in few if any leisure activities may need help in changing these patterns to create a broader base of support and flexible problem solving (McCubbin & Patterson, 1983).

Measuring Marital and Family Responses

Although not yet as precise as some of the observation codes for interactions between parents and their developmentally disabled children, attempts are being made to allow detailed descriptions of the interactions that occur between spouses (e.g., Baucom, 1982; Jacobson, 1977, 1978, 1979) and between parents and their adolescent, non-developmentally disordered children (e.g., Alexander, Barton, Schiavo, & Parsons, 1976; Robin, 1981). Much of this work has been innovative and important in allowing us to take a more refined look at helping families solve serious problems. Although it has not yet been shown directly applicable to the family with an autistic child, there is little reason to expect this research would be not be valid with that population.

There are also some paper-and-pencil measures useful for understanding how individual family members are adapting to stress, how they view specific dyads such as the parent–child or marital relationship, and how they view the family as a unit. For example, the Questionnaire on Resources and Stress (Holroyd, 1974; Holroyd, Brown, Wikler & Simmons, 1975; Holroyd & McArthur, 1976) was designed for families having a handicapped member and has been researched with parents of autistic children. The scale taps a variety of areas, including perceived time demands, attitude toward child, and felt lack of social support.

The Parenting Stress Index (Abidin, 1983) was designed to identify parent–child dyads under stress. The questionnaire yields a profile of subscales within three broad domains: Parent Domain, Child Domain, and Situational/Demographic Domain. Chavkin (1986) found that the responses of mothers of school-age autistic children differed from those of mothers of spina bifida and normal children matched for chronological age, on the Child Domain dimensions of adaptability of child, child demandingness, child distractibility, and acceptability of child.

Another example of the contribution of paper and pencil instruments to assessment of the family is found in research on the relationship between marital satisfaction as measured by the Dyadic Adjustment Scale (Spanier, 1976) and a newly developed measure of parental distribution of child care responsibilities (Boyle & Harris, 1986). Parents of autistic children who described higher marital satisfaction also reported a more equitable distribution of child care activities than did parents with a lesser degree of marital satisfaction (Boyle & Harris, 1986). Although this correlational finding does not permit cause-and-effect conclusions, it does highlight the interaction between two areas of family life and the need to be sensitive to these interactive effects.

Moos (1975) designed the Family Environment Scale to describe the family in terms of 10 dimensions, such as cohesion, conflict, organization, and control. Britsol (1984) used this scale to discriminate families of autistic children from a control group of families with nonhandicapped children and found the families of autistic children had a higher moral–religious emphasis and lower level of reported participation in social and recreational activities.

These paper-and-pencil measures, although potentially useful for clinical assessment, are currently better proven for making discriminations among research groups than facilitating decision making for individual families. It may nonetheless be helpful to use scales of this kind to highlight areas of family or individual functioning that merit attention through interviews and direct observation.

Treatment Planning

The clinician is always weighing the relative contributions of the child's handicap versus other family factors to the functioning of the family. Some crises are created more by the child's disability than by other issues facing the family and intervention needs to be targeted to that level of disruption. When there is an interactive process between the child's disability and the family's developmental needs, a combination of services to help the family meet the needs of the child while also improving the functioning of the family as a unit is appropriate. In the event that this intervention does not prove effective or the initial assessment suggests the presence of a chronic or severe form of family and/or individual dysfunction, the family and its members should be assessed carefully for indications of more serious psychological problems.

When issues of a life cycle nature are the primary focus of the family's discomfort, supportive counseling and problem solving may enable them to resolve these normative issues. It must once again be emphasized that family therapy aimed at helping the family strengthen their internal resources, or at remediating long standing maladaptive patterns must be conducted in an atmosphere that recognizes and respects the very real demands imposed on the family by the autistic child's special needs.

ASSESSING SOCIAL SUPPORT

Although addressing issues of individual adjustment or strengthening the internal resources of the family system may be critically important to some families, others may need enhanced formal and informal social support to sustain their efforts with their child. Social support is identified by Bristol (1984) as an important factor in how families cope with their autistic child's handicap. She reports that families who cope effectively are more likely to have better support from the extended family and from other parents of handicapped children.

This finding highlights the importance of ensuring that one's assessment of the family includes a consideration of the extended family and the contributions relatives make to the nuclear family. Grandparents, especially maternal grandmothers, can be a valuable source of ongoing emotional, physical, and financial support (Gath, 1978; Harris, Handleman & Palmer, 1985). Single parent families and those living far from their extended family may be at special risk for a lack of informal social support.

In addition to being a valued resource, family ties can be a source of stress for the nuclear family and may be a factor contributing to heightened vulnerability. Parents who have never successfully dealt with issues of separation from their own families of origin can bring those issues to their family of procreation and manifest the unresolved struggles in that new unit (e.g., Minuchin, 1974).

Because we carry our family history with us where ever we go, the assessment must ask not only about the positive contributions the extended family makes, but the negative factors that may arise from these relationships as well. Rejecting or critical responses about the handicapped grandchild or the parents' management of the child may intensify the parents' distress and increase their sense of isolation. Such negative reactions may reflect longstanding patterns of family interaction. For some extended families the child's disability may have particular meaning within the family's history. An exploration of issues of this sort may help free the entire family from needless burdens of historical baggage and allow the adults to unite in meeting the child's special needs.

In addition to a good informal support network, Bristol (1984) reports that less stressed families of autistic children enjoy better formal support services than do more stressed families. Having one's child enrolled in a good school, the availability of respite services, a caring pediatrician, a full-year school calendar, vocational training programs, group homes, and other basic services necessary for the education, training, and ongoing support of the autistic person and the family can substantially reduce family stress.

Treatment Planning

The identification of defects in formal support services points to an important area for intervention. When the formal support network is inadequate the clinician should determine whether the problem lies primarily in the failure of the community to provide services, or a lack of skill on the part of parents in using available resources. Intervention may include providing parents with support and guidance in dealing with service delivery systems. In many communities, it may also require the clinician to join the parents in active advocacy for suitable services.

Deficits in informal support may sometimes be addressed through family sessions aimed at understanding the relationships among members of the extended family and finding ways to encourage their participation. Parents may need help in learning how to approach family and friends for the support they need.

SUMMARY

Although raising an autistic child is difficult for any family, some families seem more able to cope than others. When a family seeks help in dealing with an autistic child or with other issues in the family, it is useful to consider both the impact of the child's handicap on the family and how the family's developmental status within the life cycle may influence their ability to cope with the child's handicap.

The assessment model presented in this chapter includes assessment of the autistic child, an evaluation of the parent–child interaction, examination of individual resources of family members, consideration of the internal resources of the family system, and assessment of the services and support network available from the extended family and community.

Interviewing the family, systematic observation of the child and various subgroups of the family as well as the family as a unit, as well as paper-and-pencil tests may all contribute to the clinician's systematic assessment. In practice, assessment and intervention are often tightly interwoven activities with the family's response to treatment guiding the next phase of assessment.

REFERENCES

Abidin, R. R. (1983). *Parenting stress index—Manual (PSI).* Charlottesville, VA: Pediatric Psychology Press.

Ackerman, N. J. (1980). The family with adolescents. In E. A. Carter & M. McGoldrick (Eds.), *The family life cycle: A framework for family therapy* (pp. 147–69). New York: Gardner.

Alexander, J. F., Barton, C., Schiavo, R. S., & Parsons, B. V. (1976). Systems-behavioral intervention with families of delinquents: Therapist characteristics, family behavior, and outcome. *Journal of Consulting and Clinical Psychology, 44,* 656–64.

Baucom, D. H. (1982). A comparison of behavioral contracting and problem-solving/communications training in behavioral marital therapy. *Behavior Therapy, 13,* 162–74.

Boss, P. G. (1983). The marital relationship: Boundries and ambiguities. In H. I. McCubbin & C. R. Figley (Eds.), *Stress and the family. Vol. I: Coping with normative transitions* (pp. 26–40). New York: Brunner/Mazel.

Bowen, M. (1978). *Family therapy in clinical practice.* New York: Jason Aronson.

Boyle, T. D., & Harris, S. L. (1986). The relationship between marital satisfaction and the distribution of parent involvement with developmentally disabled children. Manuscript submitted for publication.

Brandt, J. O. (1980). The family with young children. In E. A. Carter & M. McGoldrick (Eds.), *The family life cycle: A framework for family therapy* (pp. 121–146). New York: Gardner.

Bristol, M. M. (1984). Family resources and successful adaptation to autistic children. In E. Schopler & G. B. Mesibov (Eds.), *Issues in Autism. Vol. III. The effects of autism on the family* (pp. 289–310). New York: Plenum.

Burton, L. M., & Bengtson, V. L. (1985). Black grandmothers. Issues of timing and continuity of roles. In V. L. Bentson & J. F. Robertson (Eds.), *Grandparenthood* (pp. 61–77). Beverly Hills, CA: Sage Publications.

Carter, E. A., & McGoldrick, M. (Eds.). (1980a). *The family life cycle. A framework for family therapy.* New York: Gardner.

Carter, E. A., & McGoldrick, M. (1980b). The family life cycle and family therapy: An overview. In E. A. Carter & M. McGoldrick (Eds.), *The family life cycle: A framework for family therapy* (pp.3–20). New York: Gardner.

Chavkin, D. (1986). Stress in mothers of eight to twelve year old autistic and spina bifida children. Unpublished doctoral dissertation, Rutgers State University, Piscataway, NJ.

Crosby, J. F., & Jose, N. L. (1983). Death: Family adjustment to loss. In C. R. Figley & H. I. McCubbin (Eds.), *Stress and the family. Vol II. Coping with catastrophe* (pp. 76–89). New York: Brunner/Mazel.

Figley, C. R., & McCubbin, H. I. (Eds.). (1983). *Stress and the family. Vol. II. Coping with catastrophe.* New York: Brunner/Mazel.

Gath, A. (1978). *Down's syndrome and the family—The early years.* London: Academic.

Harris, S. L. (1983). *Families of the developmentally disabled: A guide to behavioral intervention.* Elmsford, NY: Pergamon.

Harris, S. L. (1984). The family and the autistic child: A behavioral perspective. *Family Relations, 33,* 127–34.

Harris, S. L., Handleman, J. S. & Palmer. C. (1985). Parents and grandparents view the autistic child. *Journal of Autism and Developmental Disorder, 15,* 127–37.

Harris, S. L., & Powers, M. (1984). Behavior therapists look at the impact of the family system. In E. Schopler & G. B. Mesibov (Eds.), *Issues in autism, Vol. III: The effects of autism on the family* (pp. 207–24). New York: Plenum.

Herz, F. (1980). The impact of death and serious illness on the family life cycle. In E. A. Carter & M. McGoldrick (Eds.), *The family life cycle: A framework for family therapy* (pp. 223–40). New York: Gardner.

Holroyd, J. (1974). The questionnaire on resources and stress: An instrument to measure family response to a handicapped member. *Journal of Community Psychology, 2,* 92–4.

Holroyd, J., Brown, N., Wikler, L., & Simmons, J. (1975). Stress in the families of institutionalized and non-institutionalized autistic children. *Journal of Community Psychology, 3,* 26–31.

Holroyd, J., & McArthur, D. (1976). Mental retardation and stress on the parents: A contrast between Down's syndrome and childhood autism. *American Journal of Mental Deficiency, 80,* 431–6.

Jacobson, N. S. (1977). Problem solving and contingency contracting in the treatment of marital discord. *Journal of Consulting and Clinical Psychology, 45,* 92–100.

Jacobson, N. S. (1978). Specific and nonspecific factors in the effectiveness of a behavioral approach to the treatment of marital discord. *Journal of Consulting and Clinical Psychology, 46,* 442–52.

Jacobson, N. S. (1979). Increasing positive behavior in severely distressed marital relationships: The effects of problem solving training. *Behavior Therapy, 10,* 311–26.

Kidwell, J., Fisher, J. L., Dunham, R. M., & Baranowski, M. (1983). Parents and adolescents: Push and pull of change. In H. I. McCubbin & C. R. Figley (Eds.), *Stress and the family. Vol. I: Coping with normative transitions.* (pp. 74–89). New York: Brunner/Mazel.

Koegel, R. L., Glahn, T. J., & Nieminen, G. S. (1978). Generalization of parent-training results. *Journal of Applied Behavior Analysis, 11,* 95–109.

Koegel, R. L., Schreibman, L., Britten, K. R., Burke, J. C., & O'Neill, R. E. (1982). A comparison of parent training to direct child treatment. In R. L. Koegel, A. Rincover, & A. L. Egel (Eds.), *Educating and understanding autistic children* (pp. 260–79). San Diego, CA: College Hill.

Koegel, R. L., Schreibman, L., O'Neill, R. E., & Burke, J. C. (1983). The personality and family-interaction characteristics of parents of autistic children. *Journal of Consulting and Clinical Psychology, 51,* 683–92.

Koegel, R. L., Schreibman, L., Johnson, J., O'Neill, R. E., & Dunlap, G. (1984). Collateral effects of parent training on families with autistic children. In R. F. Dangel & R. A. Polster (Eds.), *Parent training: Foundations of research and practice* (pp. 358–78). New York: Guilford.

Mash, E. J., Terdal, L., & Anderson, K. (1973). The response-class matrix: A procedure for recording parent-child interactions. *Journal of Consulting and Clinical Psychology, 40,* 163–4.

McGoldrick, M. (1980). The joining of families through marriage: The new couple. In E. A. Carter & M. McGoldrick (Eds.), *The family life cycle: A framework for family therapy* (pp. 93–119). New York: Gardner.

McCubbin, H. I., & Figley, C. R. (Eds.). (1983). *Stress and the family. Vol. I: Coping with normative transitions.* New York: Brunner/Mazel.

McCubbin, J. I., & Patterson, J. M. (1983). Family transitions: Adaptation to stress. In H. I. McCubbin & C. R. Figley (Eds.), *Stress and the family. Vol. I: Coping with normative transitions* (pp. 5–25). New York: Brunner/Mazel.

McCullough, P. (1980). Launching children and moving on. In E. A. Carter & M. Goldrick (Eds.), *The family life cycle: A framework for family therapy* (pp. 171–95). New York: Gardner.

Minuchin, S. (1974). *Families and family therapy*. Cambridge: Harvard University Press.

Moos, R. H. (1975). *Evaluating correctional and community settings*. New York: Wiley.

Newsom, C., & Rincover, A. (1981). Autism. In E. J. Mash & L. G. Terdal (Eds.), *Behavioral assessment of childhood disorders* (pp. 397–439). New York: Guilford.

Patterson, J. M., & McCubbin, H. I. (1983). The impact of family life events and changes on the health of a chronically ill child. *Family Relations, 32,* 255–64.

Robin, A. L. (1981). Controlled evaluation of problem-solving communication training with parent–adolescent conflict. *Behavior Therapy, 12,* 593–609.

Schopler, E., & Reichler, R. (1971). Parents as co-therapists in the treatment of psychotic children. *Journal of Autism and Childhood Schizophrenia, 1,* 87–102.

Spanier, G. B. (1976). Measuring dyadic adjustment: New scales for assessing the quality of the marriage and similar dyads. *Journal of Marriage and the Family, 38,* 15–28.

Stierlin, H., Rucker-Embden, I., Wetzel, N., & Wirsching, M. (1980). *The first interview with the family*. New York: Brunner/Mazel.

Stoneman, Z., Brody, G. H., & Abbott, D., (1983). In-home observations of young Down syndrome children and their mothers and fathers. *American Journal of Mental Deficiency, 87,* 591–600.

Walsh, F. (1980). The family in later life. In E. A. Carter & M. McGoldrick (Eds.), *The family life cycle: A framework for family therapy* (pp. 197–220). New York: Gardner.

Weitz, S. (1982). A code for assessing teaching skills of parents of developmentally disabled children. *Journal of Autism and Developmental Disorders, 12,* 13–24.

Wikler, L., Wasow, M., & Hatfield, E. (1981). Chronic sorrow revisited: Parent vs. professional depiction of the adjustment of parents of mentally retarded children. *American Journal of Orthopsychiatry, 51,* 63–70.

14

Nutrition and Developmental Disabilities
Clinical Assessment

DANIEL J. RAITEN

INTRODUCTION

Autistic children grow up to be autistic adults. Until proved otherwise, autistic children have the same nutritional requirements for growth and development as nondisabled children. These two facts are generally ignored when considering the relationship between nutrition and autism/pervasive developmental disability (PDD). Although there has been considerable debate about the potential role of nutritional factors in autism, there is little concrete evidence to support either an etiologic link or nutritionally based treatment modality (Raiten & Massaro, 1986). The medical attention given to autistic children is usually centered around behavioral symptomatology rather than growth and development. Consequently, those individuals who have focused on nutrition have emphasized the potential for nutritional interventions as treatments rather than health maintenance regimens (Raiten & Massaro, in press).

This chapter focuses on available methodologies for the identification of a nutritional problem. The discussion on assessment presents a brief overview of the nutrition and autism relationship, with an example of the kinds of thought processes that have linked specific nutrients such as vitamins to the disorder.

Background: Nutrition, Biochemistry, and Metabolic Correlates

Several researchers have proposed the existence of either specific biochemical (Rimland, 1973), or metabolic (Coleman, 1985) anomalies with nutritional components that when corrected may ameliorate some or all of the behavioral sequelae associated with autism. Evidence linking biochemical or metabolic problems with autism is tentative. The bulk of the work regarding metabolic correlates of autism has been done by Coleman (1976), who has suggested that autism is actually a "constellation of symptoms, i.e., a syndrome." She also

DANIEL J. RAITEN • Department of Behavioral Medicine, Children's Hospital, National Medical Center, Washington, D.C. 20010.

suggested that there may be subgroups within this syndrome, a notion that has been supported by the bulk of the studies that have examined either the biochemical or neurophysiologic aspects of autism (Piggott, 1979). While many of the reported metabolic errors may be coincidently associated with the autistic pattern, several may represent potential classes within the autistic syndrome, where the metabolic error is responsible for the clinical outcome and may also have a nutritional component.

The various theories regarding neurochemical differences among subgroups of autistic children has been recently reviewed (Anderson & Hoshino, 1986). Some researchers have attempted to link neurochemical theory with nutrition science. The most prominent example is a group of French researchers who made a concerted effort to correlate catecholamine metabolism with vitamin B_6 (pyridoxine) (Lelord, Muh, Barthelemy, Martineau, Garreau & Callaway, 1981; Martineau, Barthelemy, Garreau & Lelord, 1985). In light of the inextricable role played by pyridoxine in the biosynthetic pathways for the catecholamines (Dakshinamurti, 1977), speculation about its therapeutic efficacy are understandable. Unfortunately, design limitations and a lack of control for confounding variables such as nutritional status or concurrent drug therapies have prevented the evolution of any insight into the proposed link between pyridoxine and autism.

Case Study: Evolution of a Hypothesis

Coleman and Blass (1985) cited several examples of autistic children with lactic acidosis who may represent a nutritionally compromised metabolic subgroup. Among several possibilities, lactic acidosis may be related to nutritionally mediated clinical situations, including thiamine deficiency (Campbell, 1984). Thiamine (vitamin B_1) is active in several intermediary enzyme systems essential to nervous system metabolism as well as in the synthesis of such neurotransmitters as the catecholamines, dopamine and norepinephrine, and acetylcholine (ACh) (Pike & Brown, 1984). Hakim used a thiamin-deficient diet to produce a reversible cerebral acidosis. Several other workers have correlated thiamine deficiency with such disorders as depression and schizophrenia (Carney, Ravindran, Rinsler & Williams, 1982), and neurologic disorders associated with malabsorption syndromes and liver failure (Langohr, Petruch & Schoth, 1981). Raiten, Massaro, and Zuckerman (1984) found a large percentage (23%) of a sample of autistic children at risk of thiamine deficiency despite adequate intakes. Conclusions drawn about the relevency of the later findings were tempered by findings of similarly high percentages of at risk children in comparison groups of learning disabled and control subjects.

The possible role of thiamine in developmental disorders such as autism becomes more plausible within the framework of an early insult paradigm. There is evidence, supported by a substantial body of literature, that lactic acid accumulates in discrete areas of the mammalian brain as a consequence of thiamine deficiency. One possible scenario could involve a susceptible child with a defect in a thiamine-dependent enzyme exposed to a marginal level of thiamine or, who as a result of the defect, requires more thiamine. In light of the profound effects on memory and behavior seen in the alcohol-induced thiamine deficiency syndrome, Wernicke's encephalopathy, a similar insult to the developing nervous system might be catastrophic.

Speculation similar to the above thiamine hypothesis has been the impetus behind a major move within the field of child psychiatry. Orthomolecular psychiatry or the "megavitamin" approach to the treatment of developmental disorders such as autism, like the above thiamine theory, is based on well-established principals about the role of nutrition in the functional integrity of the nervous system. In fact, there is ample historical precedent for the medical use of vitamins not only for the treatment and prevention of the classical deficiency syndromes, but also for the treatment and prevention of the now well recognized vitamin responsive inborn errors of metabolism (Fernhoff, Danner & Elsas, 1981). Moreover, evidence for the intimate role that nutrition and specific nutrients play in the function and integrity of the nervous system is well couched in a substantial body of literature (Dakshinamurti, 1977). Unfortunately, while the megavitamin approach may be well founded in scientific theory, its clinical utility or validity has not been effectively demonstrated within the framework of sound scientific methodology (Raiten & Massaro, 1986).

NUTRITIONAL ASSESSMENT: RATIONALE

The preponderance of research to date connecting nutrition and autism has concentrated on issues related to either etiology or potential treatment modalities. There is no evidence of increased requirement for specific nutrients in autistic children. Conversely, little attention has been paid to nutrition in the broader sense as an integral component in the health of the autistic child (Raiten, in press). This observation can in part explain why the studies linking nutrition to autism have been flawed. Without an appreciation of the processes of nutrition, which include ingestion, digestion, absorption, metabolism, and eventual utilization of nutrients, little valid information can be garnered regarding any postulated relationship between either general nutrition or specific nutrients and autism.

Aside from the biologic aspects of nutrition, there is a complex array of sociocultural–behavioral factors that affect a child's eating habits and consequent nutritional status. Autistic children have been described as having bizarre eating habits (Wing, 1979; Raiten & Massaro, 1986). The potential for behavior affecting nutrition is at least as great as the potential for nutrition to affect behavior. Yet, because of the desire to find a nutritionally related etiologic or treatment connection, such factors as eating idiosyncracies or drugs affecting nutritional adequacy and, therefore, general health have been largely ignored in this population (Raiten, in press).

It is conceivable, and perhaps likely, that there is a subgroup of autistic children that has a metabolic defect resulting in an increased requirement for one or more nutrients in order to enhance the activity of specific enzyme systems. However, it must also be recognized that problems associated with nutritional factors may exist that are unrelated to the primary or secondary disorder (Table I). In 1977, a committee under the auspices of the National Academy of Sciences identified five domains of functional competence that may be compromised in a nutritional deficiency. These areas are: cognitive ability, disease response (immunity), reproductive competence, physical activity and work performance, and social/ behavioral performance. Examples of functional changes associated with specific nutritional deficiencies are listed in Table I. In a normal population, detection of changes in any of these parameters is problematic. In an already compromised group, such as autistic children, deficits in such domains as cognitive performance or social/behavioral competence could easily blend into the preexsisting symptomatology and thereby, be attributed to the primary disorder. Therefore, in these children the approach must include sensitivity to the possibility of a nutritional problem and the willingness to take the appropriate steps nessessary for its identification.

The ability to select appropriate assessment techniques stems in part from an apprecia-

Table 1. Neurological and Behavioral Effects of Some Vitamin Deficiencies[a]

Vitamin	Neurological	Behavioral
Thiamine (B1)	Wernicke's encephalopathy, peripheral neuropathy, polyneuritis	Mental depression, apathy, anxiety, irritability, korsakoff's psychosis
Riboflavin (B2)	EEG abnormalities, peripheral neuropathy	Depression, anxiety, personality disorders
Niacin, nicotinic acid, niacinamide, (B3)	Neurological degeneration, tremor, spasticity, loss of position sense, exaggerated tendon reflexes, progressive paralysis of lips, tongue, mouth, pharynx, and larynx, abnormally increased skin sensitivity, abnormal sensations such as burning of prickling	Associated with pellagra: apathy, anxiety, mania, hyperirritability, memory deficits, delirium, organic dementia, emotional lability
Pyridoxine, pyridoxal, puradoxamine (B6)	Lack of muscle coordination, convulsions, EEG changes hyperacousia	Depression, nervous irritability
Pantothenic acid	Neuritis, lack of motor coordination, staggering gait, numbness, paresthesia	Restlessness, fatigue, irritability, depression
Biotin	Abnormally increased skin sensitivity	Depression, extreme lassitude, somnolence
Cyanocobalamin (B12)	Combined systems diseases: diminished vibratory and position sense, abnormal EEG, motor weakness	No specific behavioral effects reported. Symptoms may occur as with other deficiency states: irritability, depression, confusion, paranoia, delusions, memory loss, hallucinations
Folic acid, folacin, pteroylglutamic acid	No CNS symptoms reported after 2nd year of life, In infants: mental retardation, lack of muscle coordination, continuing writhing movements	Forgetfulness, Apathy, insomnia, irritability, depression, psychosis, delirium, dementia
Vitamin C (Ascorbic acid)	No CNS symptoms reported	Lassitude, personality changes such as those occurring in physically ill persons, such as hypochondriasis, depression and hysteria

[a]Adapted from Lipton, Mailman, and Nemeroff, 1979.

tion of the kinds of changes that occur during the course of a nutritional deficiency. Brin (1978) listed five stages of a nutritional deficiency. According to Brin's scheme, the development of a nutrient deficiency progresses from such generalized symptoms as weight loss or lethargy, to specific biochemical and anatomic lesions and eventual death. Consequently, clinical assessment should progress from general nonspecific indicators of overall intake and status to specific biochemical measures.

Table II is a representation of a hierarchy of decision-making for the identification of potential nutritional problems in autistic children. It is based on the theory that nutritional assessment should precede from general assessment of factors that would have an impact on intake, to evaluation of potential specific problems.

Risk Assessment: Screening

Routine screening methods must be comprehensive and sensitive, yet uncomplicated so that untrained personnel and caregivers can administer them. The first step could be incorporated into the routine history taken for all clients upon entrance into a new program or during the initial diagnostic interview. A detailed nutritional history taken either during an interview or by questionnaire should be similar in scope to those used by Kalisz and Ekvall (1984) or Raiten and Massaro (1986). Integral components of a nutritional history would be infant feeding practices, timing of introduction of solid foods, parental observations about food acceptance and preferences, eating idiocyncracies, sensitivities or allergies, and any other anecdotal information about eating behavior or response to foods. In addition, there should be information about the family's health history, the child's drug history, and past or present nutritional supplementation practices. Information about current status would include an

Table 2. Flow Chart of Decision Making

I. Initial intake

   A. Family health history, individual health (drugs)

   B. Nutritional history—preferences, infant feeding, allergies/sensitivities, dietary restrictions

   C. Food Frequency Questionnaire, 24-hour dietary recall

   D. Clinical exam—anthropometrics (growth history), height, weight, body composition (skinfold thickness, triceps and subscapular)

If indicated by anything in the intial history, proceed to II.

II. Further assessment of dietary intake and biochemistry.

   A. Three-day diet records

   B. Clinical exam—specifically designed to reveal early stages of specific lesion (ex: visual acuity, presence of skin lesions, immunocompetence, neurological exam). Biochemistry tests to be chosen based on dietary information that may reveal potential deficiencies in specific nutrients.

If specific nutritional problems are revealed, proceed to III.

III: Intervention

   A. Supplementation with specific nutrient to be followed by:

   B. Clinical biochemical and exam using same protocols in II

   C. Continuous periodic follow-up including an effective education and counseling program and random urinalysis to document compliance.

appraisal of current feeding skills, and some measure of current intake. Kalisz and Ekvall (1984) suggested that if the dietary intake measure or clinical examination (including anthropometric measures of height, weight, and body composition) taken during the initial history indicated a problem, the next step should be to get a more accurate reflection of intake and some measure of activity.

Several red flags would warrant further follow-up evaluation of a given child. Among those items garnered from the history that would indicate nutritional risk are a current or long-term drug history (Raiten, in press), unusual eating habits, history of food allergy or sensitivity, or indications that the caregiver is currently manipulating the diet in order to alleviate a perceived nutritional problem. Problems included in the latter case would be an elimination diet such as the Feingold Diet (Feingold, 1975), or the elimination of foods that would be due to perceived or diagnosed food allergies. Unsupervised elimination diets can be potentially harmful when foods supplying essential nutrients are eliminated without substitution of alternative nutrient sources (David, Waddington & Stanton, 1984).

Nutrition and Growth: The Clinical Examination

Warning signs may become evident during the initial clinical examination. Willard (1982) gives an excellent outline for administration and interpretation of a routine clinical examination. Included in his presentation is a list of the most commonly used anthropometric methods as well as the most common types of errors.

Anthropometric measures (i.e., height, weight, skinfold thickness) are sensitive measures of a child's response to their environment. Standards such as those compiled and prepared by the National Center for Health Statistics (NCHS), enable the clinician to track any changes in the growth of their patients. There are limitations to the use of these standards. For instance, normal standards bare little relevance to certain groups of disabled children such as severely brain-damaged children or subgroups of children with cerebral palsy. In those situations in which the primary disorder results in severely dimished growth potential, comparisons with normal growth charts provide little relevant information about nutritional status. It is not known what is normal for such severely compromised children; serial measures of growth for each child over time must be relied on. When considering the applicablity of normal standards for autistic children, recent studies compared samples of autistic children to normal subjects and found no differene between the study samples, but a nonsignificant trend toward shorter stature in autistic children when compared with expected norms (Raiten et al., 1984).

Changes in growth rate, height, and weight may be indicative of a number of clinical problems. Poor intake over the short term will cause weight loss. The long-term impact of insufficient intake will include changes in growth rate. Height and weight should be followed routinely. On the other end of the malnutrition spectrum, obesity will be reflected in such measures as weight for height and skinfold thickness. Obesity may result simply from overeating, a situation that while easily diagnosed, is not so easily ameliorated in an autistic child. Another contributing factor to obesity is psychopharmacology. There are several plausible explanations for obesity associated with drugs and among them are fluid retention, fat redistribution, glucose insensitivity, and decreased activity (Awad, 1984). Irrespective of the cause, obesity in autistic children is associated with the same risk factors for chronic diseases as in normal children and should be dealt with appropriately.

However, these measures are often used improperly or are not taken at all. The measures have no diagnostic validity by themselves. Preferably, a child should be followed serially and compared with national norms for growth. For example, if a child is small in stature at the initial screening, one cannot necessarily conclude that the child's growth has been stunted unless previous measurements reveal a change in the child's growth pattern. Similarly, a child may be in the upper percentiles for weight, yet without some reflection of body composition one cannot conclude based solely on weight that the child is obese. As with any phase in the flowchart of nutritional assessment, the interpretation of anthropometric data must be supplemented with reliable corroborative data.

DIETARY ASSESSMENT: ISSUES

Corroborative evidence for a potential nutritional problem revealed by a clinical exam is most likely to be found in a detailed nutritional history that contains some measure of normal intake. While measures of nutrient intake do not always correlate with physiology, i.e., circulating levels of specific nutrients, they do enable the clinician to further refine their diagnostic accuity.

There are several methods for the collection of intake data. Each has its own inherent strengths and weaknesses. The choice of assessment technique should be based on the needs that must be met. Several universal problems are associated with the collection of accurate intake data. First, the mere knowledge of the collection procedure will influence the response of the caregiver/client. An awareness that someone is evaluating the child's diet along with speculation about the clinician's expectations can to varying degrees influence the outcome of an interview, recall, or diet record. The second issue involves the constraints imposed by the lack of complete and accurate food composition tables. The technology for accurate analysis of individual foods exists, and the computer software for itemized diet analysis is available. The problem is that there is a lag in the ability to evaluate and list all the possible individual and combined food items. Finally, most methods of collection of intake data, short of keeping individuals in a controlled environment, rely on either the memory or record keeping ability (or both) of the caregiver client, neither of which are always reliable.

To a large extent, the first and third problems can be overcome by a conscientious effort by the clinician to inform, support, and assuage the client about the record procedure during the initial interview or training session. When conducting a dietary interview or training session, one should avoid questions that suggest the correct answers such as: "Did you have a dark green or deep yellow vegetable today?" More importantly, the interviewer should avoid expressions or indications of judgment about the foods reported. The goal is to gather as much unbiased and accurate information about intake as possible. Judgments about adequacy can be made only after collection and analysis of good data. If the interviewer believes that there have been omissions, they can ask open-ended nonjudgmental questions to generate more information, such as: "What did you drink with your lunch?" or "What did you put on your sandwich?"

In the individual case, the objective is to further corroborate the existence of a possible nutritional problem. In general, the available software used for these types of evaluations contain data bases that are essentially sufficient when employed by someone trained in their use. However, there should be an awareness of the limitations of a given data base. Most of the existing computer software programs rely on the USDA Handbook #8-Composition of Foods (1980) data base. This particular source contains many foods that have not been analyzed for specific nutrients or contains outdated information based on inaccurate assay procedures. In the case of vitamin B_6, many diets, when analyzed, will appear deficient when in fact it is the lack of complete data for the vitamin B_6 content of many foods. Consequently, when a diet is analyzed by someone naive to these limitations, a child could be inaccurately diagnosed as being at risk for a nutritional deficiency. The existence of these types of limitations further strengthens the case for as many corroborative sources as possible before drawing conclusions about either individual or group nutritional status.

Methods

There are three general categories of methods used for dietary assessment: interview, recall, and diet records or diaries. The interview can contain a 24-hr recall and/or food frequency, or these latter two methods can be done by the client and brought back at the next follow-up meeting, whereas the diet record can only be kept at the residence by the caregiver. The dietary history should contain all the items discussed earlier (i.e., health history, eating habits, concurrent or past drug usage), in addition to the diet recall and food frequency records. By utilizing both the 24-hr recall and the food frequency inventory, the clinician eliminates many of the pitfalls found when these methods are used separately. For instance, the major limitations of the 24-hr recall are associated with its reliance on the client's memory. It requires a trained interviewer to elicit a reasonable representation of the diet consumed. Moreover, by limiting the analysis to one day there is the risk that that particular day may not be representative of normal intake (e.g., a weekend or holiday). The addition of the food frequency inventory, in which information is collected about how often certain foods are eaten over a given time period, can support or refute the validity and reliability of the recall. Again, the major shortcomings of these two methods are their lack of precision and reliability.

Diet records kept by the client/caregiver avoid some of the problems of the recall or frequency methods. This approach involves a conscientious effort by the client/caregiver to accurately record all foods eaten. Generally, records are kept over 1-, 3-, or 7-day periods. The 24-hr record is subject to the same problems as the 24-hr recall, i.e. 1 day may not be a representative reflection of normal intakes. The 7-day record is probably the most representative reflection of intake (Stuff, Garza, O'Brian-Smith, Nichols & Montandon, 1983). The major problem associated with the 7-day record is related to the length of time. Keeping an accurate record of food intake for a week can be tedious and oppressive for some caregivers. The 3-day diet record is a valid measure of both quantity and quality of normal intake. Gersovitz, Madden, and Smiciklas-Wright (1978) found that diet records of up to 4 days were resistant to the so-called flat slope syndrome, i.e., over reporting of small intake and under-reporting of large intake. Perhaps more importantly, this recording procedure is less invasive and tedious.

The most obvious limitation to the analysis of diets from records are the variations in an individual's estimates of the amount of food eaten and his/her failure to describe the food in sufficient detail. This problem may be overcome by effective and explicit instruction and the use of food models for visual representation of actual portion sizes.

One final note about requesting extensive diet records particularly in this population. Record keeping is a lot to ask of a caregiver of a normal child. One must be sensitive to the problems that a parent or caregiver of an autistic child has in normal daily routine when imposing the added burden of recording intake. For this reason, the recommendation of Kalisz and Ekvall (1984), that diet records be requested only after evidence of dietary problems is found in the initial history and recall, is especially pertinent to this group.

BIOCHEMICAL ASSESSMENT: ISSUES

Biochemical testing for individual nutrients may be done routinely, however, because they are inherently invasive, specific tests are probably best used only when there are clear indications from clinical screening that they are warranted. Cases for which specific testing might be warranted would include suspected dietary inadequacies or children receiving various medications (e.g., anticonvulsants). The discussion of biochemical tests of nutrient status will not include normal clinical screening techniques, e.g., liver enzyme studies or CBC.

The most fundamental questions that can be asked about any assessment procedure is "what does it measure?" In the case of a given assessment test of nutritional status, there are several concerns. Does the test measure long-term or short-term status? In other words, is the test measuring today's breakfast or does it reflect long-term intake patterns? Related to this issue are the concepts of specificity and sensitivity. Solomons and Allen (1983) defined sensitivity as the probability that a given test for a specific nutrient will be positive in a malnourished individual whereas specificity is the probability that a test will be negative in a well nourished individual. In addition, it is crucial to have some reflection of what a given assessment means to the individual at a given point in time. This latter issue of functionality has been addressed by Solomons and Allen (1983). Within the context of Brin's scheme (1978), an assessment procedure should reflect early changes in the function of a particular nutrient dependant system, Solomons and Allen (1983) used a systems classification scheme to categorize potential functional indices of nutrient status. Unfortunately at this time, many of the tests suggested lack specificity and therefore require backup indications of specific nutrient deficiencies. For instance, changes in nerve function; e.g., electroencephalography cannot be attributed to a particular deficiency without prior indications via intake records and/or biochemistry.

In general, when considering which test to use for a particular nutrient, the assay must be considered for its sensitivity to detect early stages of a problem and its specificity to avoid the possibility of a false-positive result. It is equally important that the test be a reflection of the functional status of the nutrient rather than a random measurement of the level of the nutrient. The most critical feature of the functionality issue is the provision of information about the processes of nutrition as they relate to the nutrient, and how the nutrient is performing within its own biologic context. In addition, functional tests will be more indicative of long term intake patterns rather than transient changes in diet. For example, the assessment of vitamin B_1 (thiamine) status can be accomplished by the measurement of thiamine in the blood or by measuring the activity of the thiamine-dependent enzyme, transketolase (Sauberlich & Dowdy, 1974). The former method will provide information about current intake that may or may not be adequate. The latter will also provide data about absorption and intake but will also provide indications about activation and conversion of thiamine into its active coenzyme form as well as how it is performing in a dependent enzyme system. While *in vitro* tests of *in vivo* function such as the transketolase assay may or may not be direct reflections of the changes in performance predicted by the NAS committee, they are better indicators of the process of nutrition than a simple static measurement. Furthermore, they will supply evidence of marginal or subclinical deficiency before the outward manifestations of a clinical lesion appear.

As with any of the other stages of nutritional assessment, it is preferable to have two biochemical indicators of specific nutrient status along with diet records, but if time or other constraints are present, the test most reflective of the normal function of the nutrient should be chosen.

Methods

A partial list of current laboratory tests for the assessment of nutritional status is given in Table III. A more complete review of available chemical tests is given by Sauberlich (1984). Several of the vitamins listed only have static or point indices of status available, e.g. biotin, pantothenic acid. Some have indirect measures of adequate nurtiture, e.g., vitamin A and vitamin B_{12}, that do not reflect function but do reflect certain aspects of nutrition, i.e., intake, absorption and transport. The assessment of several vitamins rely on the use of loading tests which may be viewed as indicators of several processes of nutrition, intake, absorption, and utilization in dependent systems. The load is a reasonably sensitive test of functionality that relies on the administration of a substance that requires a vitamin for its normal metabolism. In the tryptophan load test, a deficiency of vitamin B_6 will result in the elevation of the metabolite xanthurenic acid produced in the conversion of tryptophan to

Table 3. Biochemical Tests of Vitamin Status

Vitamin	Assay
Vitamin A	Retinol binding protein
	Serum retinol
	Serum ascorbic acid
	Leukocyte ascorbic acid
	Tyrosine load test
Vitamin C	Serum ascorbic acid
	Leukocyte ascorbic acid
	Tyrosine load test
Thiamin (B1)	Urinary thiamine
	Erythrocyte transketolase stimulation test
Riboflavin (B2)	Urinary thiamine
	Erythrocyte glutathione reductase stim-ulation test
Niacin (B3)	Urinary 2 pyridone/N-methyl-nicotinamide ratio
Pyridoxine (B6)	Erythrocyte alanine (ALT) or aspartate (AST) aminotransferase stimulation test
	Plasma pyridoxal phosphate levels
	Tryptophan load test
	Urinary 4 pyridoxic acid
Pantothenic acid	Urinary or blood pantothenate
Biotin	Urinary or blood biotin
Vitamin D	Serum 25-hydroxycholecalciferol
	Serum 1,25-dihydroxycholecalciferol
	Serum calcium
	Serum phosphorus
	Bone density
Vitamin E	Erythrocyte fragility test
	Serum vitamin E
Folic acid	Erythrocyte folate
	Deoxyuridine suppression test
Vitamin B12	Serum B12
	Schilling test (for intrinsic factor)
Vitamin K	Prothrombin test

niacin. The major flaw in this test is that it lacks specificity in that several other factors, i.e., riboflavin status or estrogen therapy may influence the pathway.

The most commonly used functional tests are the enzyme stimulation assays. In these tests, an enzyme that requires a specific nutrient (e.g., thiamine) is isolated from tissue (e.g., red blood cells). The activity of the enzyme is measured *in vitro* before and after the addition of the coenzyme or vitamin. Increases in the activity of the enzyme beyond a designated cutoff is indicative of a potential deficiency. When backed up by sufficient intake data and corroborative biochemistry (e.g., urinary excretion), these meet the criteria of sensitivity, specificity, and functionality to make them reliable indices of vitamin nutriture. Additionally, because the tissue sample is usually erythrocytes with life expectancy of approximately 120 days, these stimulation tests also reflect long-term intake patterns.

One area of clinical assessment that has received considerable attention and been given unwarranted credibility as a useful tool for nutritional assessment is hair analysis. Within the context of the issues discussed above (i.e., sensitivity, specificity, and functionality), these methods warrant some coverage. Hair analysis for the assessment of essential trace minerals, e.g., zinc (Gibson, 1979), copper, and exposure to heavy metals such as lead (Capel, Pinnock, Darrell, Williams & Grant, 1981) has gained increasing popularity in recent years, especially in the field of childhood psychiatric disorders (Massaro, Raiten & Zuckerman, 1983). More importantly, there is a large industry that has been created that utilizes hair analysis as the integral component for nutritional assessment. The proposed virtues of hair analysis include ease of sampling, lack of invasiveness, and relative ease of storage and transportation. There are no scientifically verified studies to support the validity of hair analysis for the assessment of minerals and heavy metals, although many studies rely on hair analysis for the assessment of minerals and heavy metals. Unfortunately, one of the major drawbacks against hair analysis stems from the involvement of many different laboratories. There is no standard protocol that is followed by all laboratories for the processing and analysis of hair. Consequently, the standards from each laboratory lack any reasonable semblance of reliability. Any two laboratories could take the same sample and arrive at different conclusions about an individual's mineral status. Due to the lack of a normalized standard data base, both laboratories could be wrong.

The processing of hair is a critical step for analysis as many of the elements being assessed are ubiquitous in the environment. The limitations in current processing procedures were clearly demonstrated by Buckley and Dreosti (1984), who found that standard washing procedures were ineffective and could not remove exogenous mineral without affecting endogenous levels. The validity of hair analysis is further drawn into question in the study by DeAntonio, Katz, Scheiner, and Wood (1982), in which no correlation could be found between samples of scalp hair and pubic hair from the same individuals. Hambidge (1982) presented a list of the major limitations of hair analysis and concluded that hair analysis had limited values. Massaro *et al.* (1983) found that hair analysis was unreliable owing to extreme variability in and between samples taken from autistic, learning-disabled, and normal children. Factors such as environmental contamination, sex, age, race, rate of hair growth, and geographic location all contribute to render hair analysis useless as a sole clinical indicator of nutritional status in the individual.

CONCLUSIONS

This chapter was intended to provide basic information with which to initiate an evaluation of the nutritional status of an autistic child. While the dialectical progression of ideas about nosology and etiology of autism/PDD must and will continue, we must not lose sight of the basic needs of these children for growth and health. Clinicians and caregivers must be vigilant and cognizant of changes in their children that may be indicative of a nutritional problem and take the appropriate steps for its identification and resolution. It is hoped that a similar protocol as that delineated in Table II could be implemented in any program designed to monitor and enhance the quality of life of these special individuals.

REFERENCES

Awad, A. G. (1984). Diet and drug interactions in the treatment of mental illness—A Review. *Can. J. Psychiat. 29,* 609–13.

Bender, D. A. (1983). Effects of estradiol and Vitamin B6 on tryptophan metabolism in the rat: Implications for the interpretation of the tryptophan load test for Vitamin B6 nutritional status. *British Journal of Nutrition, 50,* 33–42.

Brin, M. (1978). Drugs and environmental chemicals in relation to vitamin needs. In J. N. Hathcock & J. Coon (Eds.), *Nutrition and Drug Interrelations.* New York: Academic.

Buckley, R. A., & Dreosti, I. E. (1984). Radioisotope studies concerning the efficacy of standard washing procedures for the cleansing of hair before zinc analysis. *American Journal of Clinical Nutrition, 40,* 840–6.

Capel, D., Pinnock, M. H., Darrell, H. M., Williams, D. C., & Grant, E. C. G. (1981). Comparisons of concentrations of some trace, bulk, and toxic metals in the hair of normal and dyslexic children. *Clinical Chemistry, 27,* 875–81.

Carney, M. W. P., Ravindran, A., Rinsler, M. G., & Williams, D. G. (1982). Thiamine, riboflavin, and pyidoxine deficiency in psychiatric in-patients. *British Journal of Psychiatry, 141,* 271–2.

Coleman, M. (1976). Introduction. In M. Coleman (Ed.), *The Autistic Syndrome.* New York: North-Holland.

Coleman, M., & Blass, J. P. (1985). Autism and lactic acidosis. *Journal of Autism and Developmental Disorders, 15,* 1–8.

Dakshinamurti, K. (1977). B vitamins and nervous system function. In R. J. Wurtman & J. J. Wurtman (Eds.), *Nutrition and the Brain, 1,* New York: Raven.

David, T. J., Waddington, E., & Stanton, R. H. J. (1984). Nutritional hazards of elimination diets in children with atopic eczema. *Archives of Disease in Childhood, 59,* 323–5.

DeAntonio, S. M., Katz, S. A., Scheiner, D. M., & Wood, J. D. (1982). Anatomically-related variations in trace metal concentrations in hair. *Clinical Chemistry, 18,* 2411–13.

Gibson, R. S., & DeWolfe, M. S. (1979). Copper, zinc, manganese, vanadium, and iodine concentraitons in the hair of Canadian low birth weight neonates. *American Journal of Clinical Nutrition, 32,* 1728–33.

Hakim, A. M. (1984). The induction and reversibility of cerebral acidosis in thiamine deficiency. *Annals of Neurology, 16,* 673–9.

Feingold, B. F. (1975). Hyperkinesis and learning disabilities linked to artificial food flavors and colors. *American Journal of Nursing, 75,* 797–803.

Fernhoff, P. M., Danner, D. J., & Elsas, L. J. (1982). Vitamin-responsive disorders, In P. J. Ganz & V. S. Marcum (Eds.), *Human nutrition—Clinical and biochemical aspects.* Washington, D. C.: American Association of Clinical Chemistry.

Gersovitz, M., Madden, J. P., & Smiciklas-Wright, H. (1978). Validity of the 24-hour dietary recall and seven-day record for group comparisons. *Journal of the American Dietary Association, 73,* 48–55.

Kanner, L. (1943). Autistic disturbances of affective contact. *Nervous Children, 2,* 217–50.

Langohr, H. D., Petruch, F., & Schroth, G. (1981). Vitamin B_1, B_2, and B_6 deficiency in neurological disorders. *Journal of Neurology, 225,* 95–108.

Lipton, M. A., Mailman, R. B., & Nemeroff, C. B. (1979). Vitamins, megavitamin therapy, and the nervous system. In R. J. Wurtman & J. J. Wurtman (Eds.), *Nutrition and the Brain (Vol. 3).* New York: Raven.

Massaro, T. F., Raiten, D. J., & C. H. Zuckerman. (1983). Trace element concentrations and behavior:

Clinical utility in the assessment of developmental disabilities. *Topics in Early Childhood Special Education, 3,* 55–61.

National Academy of Sciences. (1977). *Report of study team. IX. World food and nutrition study.* Washington, D. C.: National Academy of Sciences.

National Center for Health Statistics (NCHS). (1900). *Growth charts.* Washington, D. C.: Department of Health, Education and Welfare Public Health Service, National Center For Health Statistics Growth Charts.

Piggot, L. R. (1979). Overview of selected basic research in autism. *Journal of Autism and Developmental Disabilities, 9,* 199–218.

Raiten, D. J., & Massaro, T. F. (1985). Perspective in the nutritional ecology of autistic children. *Journal of Autism and Developmental Disabilities.*

Raiten, D. J., & Massaro, T. F. (1986). Nutrition and developmental disabilities: an examination of the orthomolecular hypothesis. In D. J. Cohen, A. Donnellan, & R. Paul (Eds.), *Handbook of Autism and Disorders of Atypical Development.* New York: Wiley.

Raiten, D. J., Massaro, T. F., & Zuckerman, C. H. (1984). Vitamin and trace element assessment of autistic and learning disabled children. *Nutrition and Behavior, 2,* 9–17.

Rimland, B. (1973). High dosage levels of certain vitamins in the treatment of children with severe mental disorders. In D. Hawkins & L. Pauling (Eds.), *Orthomolecular Psychiatry.* (pp. 513–39). San Fransisco: W. H. Freeman.

Sauberlich, H. E. (1980). Interactions of thiamine, riboflavin, and other B vitamins. *Annals of the New York Academy of Sciences, 355,* 80–97.

Solomons, N. W., & Allen, L. H. (1983). The functional assessment of nutritional status: Principles, practice, and potential. *Nutrition Review, 41,* 33–50.

Stuff, J. E., Garza, D., O'Brian-Smith, E., Nichols, B. L., & Montandon, C. M. (1983). A comparison of dietary methods in nutritional studies, *American Journal of Clinical Nutrition, 37,* 300–6.

Willard, M. D. (1982). *Nutrition for the Practicing Physician.* Menlo Park, CA: Addison-Wesley.

Wing, L. (1979). *Children apart.* Washington, D. C.: National Society for Autistic Children.

IV

Special Issues

15

Diagnosis and Assessment of Autistic Adolescents and Adults

GARY B. MESIBOV

INTRODUCTION

In 1983, Dr. Eric Schopler asked whether an adolescent or adult could have autism. Following that question he wrote:

> When that question was asked one or two decades ago, most people familiar with the term 'autism' would have said 'Certainly not.' They had heard of Leo Kanner's work (Kanner, 1943). He had used the term 'infantile autism.' It meant a psychiatric disorder of early childhood including severe disturbances of human relationships, speech, communication, and cognitive functions. It also involved all kinds of behavior problems, including repetitive behaviors and resistance to their change.
>
> According to that definition the only way the diagnosis could be made for an adult was retroactively, from a person's early history. But if you met an adult whose early history you did not know, most people had no idea what characteristics and current behaviors might be expected to make up the diagnosis of autism.

Schopler's remarks emphasize the major diagnostic problem confronting those working with autistic adolescents and adults. In addition to the problem of appropriate diagnosis, researchers and clinicians have been hampered by the lack of assessment instruments designed to assist in the development of individualized teaching programs for autistic adolescents and adults. Most existing instruments in the field of autism are designed for younger children and do not provide adequate information on the vocational, leisure, and social skills that become more important as these children grow into adolescence. Existing assessment instruments for severely handicapped adolescents and young adults were not designed with autistic individuals in mind and so do not have the essential components for adequate assessment of an autistic person's skills and abilities.

Because of the important increase in interest in adolescents and adults with autism (Schopler & Mesibov, 1983) and the lack of appropriate diagnostic criteria and assessment instruments, the TEACCH Program has been working on these problems in recent years. We

GARY B. MESIBOV • Division TEACCH, The University of North Carolina at Chapel Hill, Chapel Hill, North Carolina 27599-7180.

have also been examining other ways of facilitating the work of parents and professionals with this population. The purpose of this chapter is to describe the work we are doing and the instruments being developed.

DIAGNOSIS

The TEACCH program has consistently distinguished between diagnosis and assessment in the following way: Diagnosis is the process of determining whether an individual is appropriately classified as autistic. The diagnostic process emphasizes characteristics autistic people have in common. Assessment is used for evaluating all the person's characteristics and traits, not only those that are part of the autism definition, and is essential for individualized education and management. The assessment process emphasizes unique characteristics of individuals and how they differ from one another.

Diagnostic Clarity and Consistency

While it is assessment rather than diagnosis that gives the information crucial for developing individualized education and treatment programs, the diagnostic process does serve some important functions. The first is for research consistency and generalizability. Many advancements in treatment and education of autistic people have come from current research ideas and innovations. Interpretation and replication of these findings require compatibility among the research subjects in different parts of the world. This is possible only if investigators use consistent diagnostic characteristics for classification purposes. Diagnostic clarity and consistency are also crucial for following autistic people as they grow up to understand better the normal developmental milestones associated with this disability.

Diagnostic clarity and consistency also have important treatment implications. Although autistic individuals differ greatly from one another, there are some common characteristics which distinguish them from others diagnosed with mental retardation without autism or schizophrenia. The main treatment implication is that those diagnosed as autistic generally do best in structured, individualized, and psychoeducationally oriented environments. Professionals trained to deal with autistic people better understand their communication and interpersonal needs. On the other hand, clients receiving a different diagnosis often receive programs that are more verbally oriented and assume certain social and interpersonal skills (e.g., imitation, responsiveness to social reinforcement). Although these treatments will generally be effective with these other populations, they can cause considerable problems for those with autism. Drug-treatment strategies are also quite different for those with autistic characteristics and the accompanying neurological difficulties.

Finally, there are some political realities which make it important to accurately classify autistic individuals. Because of the severity of their handicap and their need for individualized educational programs, autistic individuals require intensive and somewhat expensive programs and services. Although these costs are justified financially because appropriate programming can reduce long-term costs by improving their prognosis (Schopler & Mesibov, 1983), visibility and political efforts to obtain adequately funded services are essential. Without appropriate diagnoses and understandings of their children's difficulties and needs, families of autistic children would not have the leverage and visibility that are essential for the development of adequately funded programs.

Diagnostic Developments at TEACCH

In order to meet these research, treatment. and political needs, the TEACCH Program has been working to develop reliable and valid diagnostic criteria for adolescents and adults with autism. In working with these clients, our first assumption is that anyone diagnosed as autistic in childhood retains that diagnosis as an adult, even though considerable changes and improvement may occur. This assumption is consistent both with most definitions of autism as pervasive and lifelong and with the extensive outcome literature suggesting that these clients do improve but are rarely cured (Lotter, 1978). This assumption also acknowledges that autism is easiest to diagnose in younger children because the characteristics of the syndrome become more variable as autistic children grow older.

Childhood Autism Rating Scale

The major diagnostic instrument within the TEACCH Program over the past decade has beeh the Childhood Autism Rating Scale (CARS) (Schopler, Reichler, DeVellis & Daly, 1980). This instrument was recently revised (Schopler, Reichler & Renner, 1986) and contains data from autistic children from the TEACCH program over the past ten years. When it was originally developed in the 1970s, the CARS represented a major advance in the diagnosis of autism because of its sound theoretical basis. The selection of items on this 15 point rating scale was based on the major diagnostic systems and rating scales of the time including Kanner (1943), Creak (1963), and Rimland (1964). As with the original instrument, the revised CARS is a rating scale of autistic characteristics which has demonstrated exemplary reliability and validity. For anyone familiar with autism, it is easy to administer after minimal training. Items rated on the new CARS include Relating to People; Imitation; Emotional Response; Body Use; Object Use; Adaptation to Change; Visual Response; Listening Response; Taste, Smell, Touch Response and Use; Fear or Nervousness; Verbal Communication; Nonverbal Communication; Activity Level; Consistency of Intellectual Response; and General Impressions.

Use of CARS with Adolescents and Adults

Our recent efforts have been designed to adapt this instrument for use with adolescents and adults. As stated earlier, in adapting the CARS for adolescents and adults, our first assumption was that any child diagnosed as autistic retains that diagnosis for life. A problem arises when it is necessary to decide about an adolescent or adult who did not have an earlier diagnosis of autism. To evaluate the effectiveness of the CARS with this group, we examined CARS data for autistic youngsters who had been diagnosed before age 10 and reevaluated after age 13. We were able to locate 59 such children in our program. The mean difference between their CARS scores before age 10 and after age 13 was 2, suggesting that autistic characteristics decrease over time for children in our program. We then adjusted the CARS cutoff from 30 to 28 for the adolescent administration. Using this new cutoff of 28, 92% of those youngsters would still be diagnosed as autistic, whereas only 8% would be misdiagnosed. This finding suggests that, with a slight modification of the cutoff score, the CARS is a reasonable diagnostic instrument for autistic adolescents and adults.

Changes in Autism with Maturity

Using the same sample of 59 autistic youngsters, we then examined changes in the 15 CARS items to see how the characteristics of autism change over time. Table I shows significant changes in many of the CARS items from the initial administration to the administration after adolescence. Significant decreases occur on the following items: Imitation, Body Use, Object Use, Adaptation to Change, Visual Response, Taste and Touch Response and Use, Verbal Communication, Nonverbal Communication, Activity Level, and Global Impression. With the exception of Global Impression, all of the significant changes indicated decreases in autistic characteristics over time.

Because so many of the individual CARS items decreased, reflecting improvements over time, we also found it instructive to examine those items that did not change. The most surprising result was that Relating to People did not show any change because that is one of the best-documented improvements that occurs in autistic people during adolescence (Mesibov, 1983; Rutter, 1983; Schopler & Mesibov, 1983). However, when the data were examined according to intellectual level, an interesting trend was observed. Using an IQ cutoff of 43 (median score), those in the higher range showed significant improvement and those in the lower range did not. Therefore, the increase in sociability in our sample came mainly from the higher-functioning individuals.

Emotional Response showed no significant change over time and this was true at all intellectual levels. Some have suggested that the neurologic basis of autism involves brain areas determining emotional response (Rutter, 1983), which might make this difficulty less amenable to intervention efforts. This finding is also consistent with clinical observations of autistic adults whose affect and emotional relatedness remain bland and relatively flat (Mesibov, 1983).

Fear or Nervousness was the third category showing little change over time. The

Table I. Mean Ratings for Autistic Group ($N = 59$) on Individual CARS Items
before Age 10 and after Age 13

Item	Rating prior to age 10	Rating after age 13	Difference
1. Relating to People	2.71	2.74	−.03
2. Imitation	2.85	2.29	.56[a]
3. Emotional Response	2.75	2.81	−.06
4. Body Use	2.71	2.52	.19[a]
5. Object Use	2.58	2.29	.29[a]
6. Adaptation to Change	2.47	2.10	.37[a]
7. Visual Response	2.45	2.47	−.02
8. Listening Response	2.58	2.28	.30[a]
9. Taste, Smell, Touch Response and Use	2.33	2.05	.28[a]
10. Fear or Nervousness	2.08	1.90	.18
11. Verbal Communication	3.13	2.84	.29[a]
12. Nonverbal Communication	2.42	2.12	.30[a]
13. Activity Level	2.28	1.95	.33[a]
14. Consistency of Intellectual Response	2.55	2.38	.17
15. General Impression	2.58	2.81	−.23[a]

[a]Significant at $p < .05$ level.

problems of understanding a most confusing world combined with the neurologic and/or biochemical difficulties that make autistic people more easily agitated seem to be fundamentally related to the autism syndrome and not amenable to much change over time. Clinical experience with the older population suggests that anxiety itself is not always the best target for intervention. Instead, when one assists autistic individuals in developing more efficient coping strategies (Campbell, Perry, Small & Green, 1987), their anxiety levels often decrease.

Intellectual Functioning was the final item showing no change over time. The wide scatter of skills and abilities has always fascinated investigators with this population (Kanner, 1943), and seems no less pronounced with adults than with younger children. This suggests that the general strategy of building strengths while also adapting the environment to minimize deficits is reasonable and likely to be most productive (Schopler, Reichler & Lansing, 1980). It also suggests that efforts to bring deficits up to the level of strengths might be overly optimistic and a less useful strategy in the long run.

Finally, it was somewhat perplexing that even though most individual CARS items show a decrease over time, the General Impression scores increased. Any explanation of this finding is speculative at best. However, this appears to reflect our growing understanding of autism. When the initial CARS ratings were made, the narrower classic Kanner definition of autism was in use. As our sophistication with this population has grown, we have come to understand that a broader range of behaviors can still be consistent with a diagnsis of autism (Wing, 1981). This broader interpretation of the autism syndrome is likely to be reflected in giving higher ratings to the General Impression item, which allows the examiner to give a subjective impression.

Administration of the CARS

Our research on the CARS has also investigated administration techniques. When we began our work with younger children, our ratings were made while observing psychoeducational testing. We have since found that the CARS can be administered reliably in a variety of different ways without changing the results (Schopler *et al.*, 1986). More recently the CARS has been reliably administered while observing psychoeducational testing, as well as based on direct observations in less standardized settings. We have also obtained reliable scores based on parental report or a client's history in a comprehensive chart. An important advantage of the CARS is its convenience and ability to provide reliable information in a variety of settings.

In summary, the CARS was initially developed to facilitate the diagnosis of autism, based on the behavioral characteristics included in the current definitions of the autism syndrome. Although initially used with younger children, current research suggests that it is equally reliable and valid with adolescents and adults, although the cutoff scores for the older group should be adjusted to account for developmental improvements (Garfin, McCallon & Cox, in press). Our research also indicated which characteristics (e.g., Imitation) showed the greatest improvement over time and which ones were most resistant to change (e.g. Emotional Response).

ASSESSMENT

The purpose of an assessment is to facilitate the development of individualized educational and behavior management programs. In contrast to a diagnosis, which examines common characteristics in autistic individuals, assessments look at the unique aspects of individuals in order to develop the appropriate individualized plans which are so essential for working with autistic youngsters. Before describing our adolescent and adult assessment research, a brief discussion about the assessment process might help clarify some common misconceptions.

In general, those working with autistic youngsters are involved with several kinds of assessments. Our TEACCH clinics do more formal assessments. These occur during the initial diagnosis and then from 1 to 5 years afterward, depending on the needs of the child and his/her family. These formal assessments help with placement decisions and also in generating appropriate individualized education and behavior management systems.

In addition to these clinic-based assessments, teachers in our classrooms are assessing their children and educational programs daily. Because of the behavioral fluctuations we observe in autistic children and their difficulties in generalizing across situations, it is unreasonable to assume that a single plan, however well conceived, can endure without modifications for 1–5 years. We only expect our formal assessment to provide a general outline along with some specific strategies for beginning the work with a child and his/her family. However, these strategies must be assessed and modified on the basis of a teacher's or therapist's day-to-day experience with the youngster. Therefore, the assessment process can be seen as divided into two parts: longer-term, clinic-based (formal) assessments and the day-to-day assessments that occur in the classroom. Each of these parts plays an important role and, in a good situation, they complement one another. Here we will deal with longer-term, clinic-based assessment as it relates to adolescents and adults with autism, while Chapter 18 deals with the day-to-day classroom assessment.

Purposes of Clinic-Based Assessments

The Initial Assessment

The more formal clinic-based assessments are usually done at the initial diagnosis and then during regular follow-up visits. These assessments can serve several important functions. During an initial diagnosis, the clinic-based assessment provides a starting point for the understanding of how to work with an autistic youngster. Therefore it is essential that this assessment provide a comprehensive and broad-based picture of the child. It is also important for concrete and appropriate recommendations to be generated from this initial assessment so that the autistic child, his/her family, and others working with them will experience some early success.

The Reevaluation Assessment

When a clinic-based assessment is part of a 1- to 5-year reevaluation, its purpose is slightly different. Obviously those working with the autistic youngster already should have established a starting place and achieved some early results so these will not be the issues. However, a comprehensive reevaluation can be helpful in objectively highlighting which areas have shown improvement and what the nature of that improvement has been. This can be extremely important when working with a group of youngsters who frequently improve so slowly. It is very helpful for those working with these youngsters on a day-to-day basis to have areas of improvement identified and highlighted.

A reevaluation is also helpful to assure that long-range goals are kept in focus and that a balanced program is in place. For example, those working with a youngster on a day-to-day basis might not realize that their work is so strongly geared toward communication skills that the self-help and gross motor areas are being neglected. A comprehensive clinic-based assessment can help point out such an imbalance.

Another purpose of a clinic-based assessment is to provide a framework and philosophical statement concerning what should be done for a particular child. The structure of an assessment instrument greatly influences what will be discussed during an evaluation and the areas from which recommendations will be generated. Therefore, because the structures and categories of an assessment instrument have such an influential role, it is essential that they represent the areas considered most important and productive.

Assessment of Strengths

Related to the issue of specific categories and structures is the TEACCH Program's emphasis on a positive approach and the development of strengths and skills. Because of this emphasis and the fact that many parents and/or teachers observe our assessments, it is extremely important that our instruments tap areas of strength so that these might be recognized and highlighted. An important goal of our assessment day in the clinic is for the autistic child to come away feeling good about about him or herself and for the family and teachers to discover new strengths and abilities in the child. The identification of strengths is also important for our intervention approach which emphasizes using strengths to help minimize the effects of deficits in autistic clients.

With these thoughts guiding our efforts, the TEACCH Program developed the Psychoeducational Profile (PEP) in our early work with autistic children (Schopler & Reichler, 1979). Because this instrument is discussed elsewhere (Chapter 1), it will not be described in this chapter. However, the PEP was originally developed for children described by others as untestable and has been extremely effective in generating long-term goals as well as individual, concrete objectives. It also nicely structures our assessment efforts around developmental levels and important skills such as imitation, communication, cognitive skills, and motor abilities. Moreover, the attractive materials and appropriate expectations maximize the chances that autistic children, even those with severe handicaps, will be able to demonstrate their strengths and abilities.

The Adolescent and Adult Psychoeducational Profile

Over the years, it has become apparent to us that autistic children change quite dramatically as they go through puberty, as do nonhandicapped children. As the implications of these changes became clear, we realized that a new assessment instrument was necessary for us to accomplish our goals. Although these adolescent changes required some important modifications in our assessment instrument, there were also many strategies from the PEP that still seemed useful for the older age group. Therefore, several aspects of our assessment instrument for autistic adolescents and adults (AAPEP) remained quite similar to our original PEP (Mesibov, Schopler, Schaffer & Landrus, 1988).

AAPEP Structure

First, the AAPEP continues the use of a pass–emerge–fail scoring system. The emerging score is the critical one for programming because it suggests that a child has some knowledge of what is required but lacks the skill necessary for complete understanding and satisfactory task performance. Directing examiners to focus on emerging skills enables them to identify those areas that are likely to benefit most from intensive instructional efforts.

The AAPEP is also similar to the PEP in giving examiners the flexibility that is essential to accurately assess autistic students. This flexibility enables examiners to teach new skills and adjust the materials and presentation techniques as necessary. In this way examiners receive the information about the skill acquisition process that is so crucial if one is to make recommendations appropriate for autistic youngsters.

Third, the amount of language is minimized and there is little emphasis placed on speech. As with the PEP, these modifications are designed to make the testing situation as conducive as possible to the identification of skills in these youngsters who have so much difficulty with verbal language and the concept of speed. By minimizing the use of verbal instructions and providing numerous opportunities to model and observe visual cues for most of the items, the AAPEP ensures that autistic children will have ample opportunities to demonstrate their strengths and skills.

Finally, like the PEP this test is geared to the lower functioning, less verbally oriented autistic population. These more severely handicapped clients are the ones most difficult to assess and for whom other instruments are not available. Those higher-functioning clients who have too many skills for this assessment instrument will generally be able to use tests designed for a broader population.

Although we have tried to develop an assessment instrument that would be as consistent with the original PEP as possible, there are several important ways in which the PEP and AAPEP are different. The primary reasons for these changes were to incorporate new ideas learned from our extensive experience with the PEP and to adapt the instrument to the needs and philosophical orientations associated with adolescent and adult autistic clients.

First, our AAPEP is not as strongly developmental as the PEP. While developmental concepts and notions are extremely important for working with younger children, they do not have the same meaning as clients grow older. A 25-year-old person with an MA of 4 is different from a 10-year-old with the same MA. For example, we have noted that our older clients become much more interested in things like contemporary music and members of the opposite sex. The AAPEP has been adapted to better examine these new interests and accompanying skills. Experience with older clients has also suggested that vocational, interpersonal, leisure, and community integration skills require more emphasis than the developmental levels that are so important for effective work with younger children. We have therefore structured this adolescent and adult test around these areas.

Another change resulted from our Program's experiences since the PEP was developed. It is obvious to most investigators that autistic clients demonstrate different skills in different environments (e.g., home, school, clinic). Therefore, in order to assess skills accurately, it is important for an assessment instrument to look at behavior in each of these relevant settings. We have always done this less formally by interviewing parents and teachers as part of the assessment process. However, in developing the AAPEP, we incorporated all these aspects into one instrument. The AAPEP accomplishes this by directly assessing the autistic client's skills in a clinic as is done with the PEP and most other assessment instruments. However, the AAPEP has additional home and school/work scales that are administered to the major person in each setting. For example, the home scale is filled out from an interview with the parents or group home manager, depending on where the child resides. Similarly, a school or work scale is based on an interview with the teacher or supervisor in that setting. This three-part assessment allows the examiner to systematically obtain information about the autistic child's functioning in his/her most common environments.

By having three assessments (direct, home, school/work) of each skill area (e.g., vocational skills, interpersonal skills), the AAPEP enables one to obtain a comprehensive picture of a child's functioning with a single instrument. For example, within an area such as interpersonal relationships, this instrument allows the examiner to obtain a direct assessment of the client's skills based upon direct interactions with him/her, perceptions of the parents, and observations of the teacher. This provides an integrated picture, resulting in appropriate and potentially effective teaching plans for each individual client.

The other important difference between the PEP and AAPEP is in the actual skills that are measured. The main reason for developing the AAPEP was because the skills we emphasize with older children are quite different from the developmental levels that are most productive in working with preadolescents. For the AAPEP we have selected skills that are most important for the older age group to maximize their possibilities for meaningful and productive community integration. These include vocational skills, independent functioning, leisure skills, vocational behavior, functional communication, and interpersonal skills.

AAPEP Reliability

The AAPEP has evolved over several years. Extensive feedback from our five clinics has been incorporated into the present version.

Following this pilot-testing process, a research project to assess the reliability and validity of the AAPEP was conducted involving 60 adolescents and adults with developmental disabilities functioning in the moderate to severe range of mental retardation. The average age of the participants was 20 years, 4 months, and the average IQ was 41.2. The average age and IQ did not differ between the autistic and nonautistic participants. As expected, the only significant difference between these two groups was in their CARS scores measuring autistic characteristics. The autistic group averaged 31.6 on the CARS; the nonautistic group averaged 19.7.

Interrater reliability was determined by having a research assistant observe 25% of the assessments and score them along with the examiner. The percentage of agreement on each individual item constituted the reliability score. Table II illustrates the overall reliability on the AAPEP as well as the reliability for each scale on each of the three tests (direct, home, school/work). Overall reliabilities are quite high with few exceptions. The only significant problem seems to be for Interpersonal Behavior on the Direct Observation Scale. Consequently, the problematic items have been reworded to help eliminate those difficulties.

AAPEP Validity

Validity is a more difficult attribute to measure, especially on an assessment instrument of this nature dealing with a low incidence disability. In general, validity refers to a test's ability to measure what it was designed to measure. With psychological assessment instru-

Table II. AAPEP Reliability Data

	Autistic (r)	Control (r)	Total (r)
AAPEP	.845	.872	.865
Direct Obs	.844	.931	.879
Voc Skill	.809	.917	.851
Ind Func	.950	.955	.952
Leisure Skill	.896	.899	.897
Voc Beh	.783	1.000	.855
Func Comm	.851	.850	.873
Int Beh	.438	.920	.679
Home	.820	.817	.843
Voc Skill	.884	.751	.855
Ind Func	.898	.875	.910
Leisure Skill	.670	.749	.740
Voc Beh	.854	.879	.875
Func Comm	.719	.930	.840
Int Beh	.754	.793	.799
School/Work	.831	.882	.862
Voc Skill	.981	.881	.939
Ind Func	.762	.892	.822
Leisure Skill	.800	.844	.850
Voc Beh	.786	1.000	.856
Func Comm	.929	.905	.927
Int Beh	.583	.921	.738

ments, validity is most frequently determined by correlations between the new test and other assessment instruments most commonly used. The problem with determining the validity of the AAPEP is that there are no available tests measuring anything similar.

Therefore, it was decided to determine the validity of this test by going back to its original purpose. The main goal of the AAPEP is to generate recommendations that will be helpful for individual adolescents and adults with autism. Although there are no assessment instruments designed for this purpose, the most common source of recommendations for these clients are in their individualized education programs (IEPs) or individualized habilitation programs (IHPs) for adults who have aged out of public schools. The validity of the AAPEP was established by determining whether the recommendations generated from this assessment instrument were able to improve upon the IEPs or IHPs.

To accomplish this, a summary paragraph was written for each of the 60 clients. Following the paragraph was a list of 10 recommendations—five from the IEPs or IHPs of these clients, and five generated from the AAPEP. The recommendations were randomly mixed together in no established order. Each set of 10 recommendations was then presented to two professionals with extensive experience with adolescents and adults in community-based programs. One of these professionals was from the TEACCH Program and worked primarily with autistic and communications handicapped children. The other professional was from an adult program working primarily with mentally retarded people without autism. Raters were blind as to the source of each recommendation (IEP, IHP, or AAPEP). For each client, each rater rank ordered the 10 recommendations in terms of their helpfulness.

The results of this study are listed in Table III. There was a significant main effect of recommendation and a group by recommendation interaction. These results suggest that the AAPEP recommendations were viewed as significantly more helpful than those already in the client's IEPs and IHPs. Although there were no significant differences in the helpfulness of these recommendations for autistic as compared with nonautistic clients, the significant interaction suggests that group differences are somewhat greater for the autistic clients. Therefore, the AAPEP recommendations were seen as quite helpful for autistic as well as nonautistic clients and seemed to improve upon what was already available for them. Although more helpful for both groups, the trend was strongest for clients with autism.

In summary, we have found the AAPEP to be a reliable and valid assessment instrument for severely handicapped adolescents and adults with autism as well as for those with moderate to severe mental retardation without autism. Reliability measures indicate that the scoring criteria are clear and that experienced examiners will be able to generate consistent results. This is an important criterion for any assessment instrument.

However, probably the most impressive aspect of this instrument involves the validity measures. The data clearly demonstrate that the AAPEP generates useful recommendations that are not available through existing mechanisms. The fact that this test generates recommendations that blind raters found more helpful than those already in the clients' files makes the AAPEP unique among assessment instruments for handicapped clients. Few existing instruments have proved effective using such a stringent validity criteria.

The other important finding is that the test is equally useful for moderately and severely retarded adolescents and adults without autism. Although it has been suggested that the best practices used with autistic clients will be helpful for other developmentally handicapped populations as well, there have been few empirical studies to document this assumption. Our work has been able to demonstrate this assumption with the AAPEP.

SUMMARY AND CONCLUSIONS

We have come a long way since Leo Kanner first coined the term *infantile autism* (1943). We have learned that autism is not a disability associated only with childhood but rather a lifelong, chronic handicap (Schopler & Mesibov, 1983). We have also learned that developmental changes associated with nonhandicapped adolescents also occur in autistic people, although the manifestations of these changes vary with language ability and developmental levels (Mesibov, 1983). This chapter describes the current work of Division TEACCH that has advanced our understanding of these adolescents and young adults through our program's diagnostic and assessment instruments refined to meet the unique needs and

Table III. Mean Ratings of Helpfulness of
AAPEP versus IEP or IHP Recommendations
for Autistic and Nonautistic Clients

Group	AAPEP	IEP or IHP	Total
Autistic	10.67	7.64	9.22
Nonautistic	10.09	8.23	9.16
Total	10.38	7.95	—

challenges of this older age group. We believe this work will continue to add to our understanding of the developmental changes that occur as autistic people grow older and to their
ongoing education and treatment.

REFERENCES

Campbell, M., Perry, R., Small, A. M., & Green, W. H. (1987). Overview of drug treatment in autism.
    In E. Schopler & G. B. Mesibov (Eds.), *Neurobiological issues in autism* (pp. 341–356). New
    York: Plenum.
Creak, E. M. (1963). Childhood psychosis: A review of 100 cases. *British Journal of Psychiatry, 109,*
    84–89.
Garfin, D. G., McCallon, D., & Cox, R. (in press). Validity of the Childhood Autism Rating Scale with
    autistic adolescents. *Journal of Autism and Developmental Disorders.*
Kanner, L. (1943). Autistic disturbance of affective contact. *Nervous Child, 2,* 217–250.
Lotter, V. (1978). Follow-up studies. In M. Rutter & E. Schopler (Eds.), *Autism: A reappraisal of
    concepts and treatment* (pp. 475–495). New York: Plenum.
Mesibov, G. B. (1983). Current perspectives and issues in autism and adolescence. In E. Schopler & G.
    B. Mesibov (Eds.), *Autism in adolescents and adults* (pp. 37–53). New York: Plenum.
Mesibov, G. B., Schopler, E., Schaffer, B., & Landrus, R. (1988). *Individualized assessment and
    treatment for autistic and developmentally disabled children. Vol. 4. Adolescent and adult psycho-
    educational profile (AAPEP).* Austin, TX: Pro-Ed.
Rimland, B. (1964). *Infantile autism.* New York: Appleton-Century-Crofts.
Rutter, M. (1983). Cognitive deficits in the pathogenesis of autism. *Journal of Child Psychology and
    Psychiatry, 24,* 513–531.
Schopler, E. (1983). Introduction: Can an adolescent or adult have autism? In E. Schopler & G. B.
    Mesibov (Eds.), *Autism in adolescents and adults* (pp. 3–10). New York: Plenum Press.
Schopler, E., & Mesibov, G. B. (Eds.). (1983). *Autism in adolescents and adults.* New York: Plenum.
Schopler, E., & Reichler, R. J. (1979). *Individualized assessment and treatment of autistic and develop-
    mentally disabled children. Vol. 1. Psychoeducational profile (2nd ed.).* Austin, TX: Pro-Ed.
Schopler, E., Reichler, R. J., DeVellis, R. F., & Daly, K. (1980). Toward objective classification of
    childhood autism: Childhood autism rating scale (CARS). *Journal of Autism and Developmental
    Disorders, 10,* 91–103.
Schopler, E., Reichler, R. J., & Lansing, M. (1980). *Individualized assessment and treatment for
    autistic and developmentally disabled children. Vol. 2. Teaching strategies for parents and profes-
    sionals.* Dallas, TX: Pro-Ed.
Schopler, E., Reichler, R. J., & Renner, B. R. (1986). *The childhood autism rating scale (CARS).* New
    York: Irvington.
Wing, L. (1981). Language, social, and cognitive impairments in autism and severe mental retardation.
    Journal of Autism and Developmental Disorders, 11, 31–44.

16

Diagnosis and Subclassification of Autism
Concepts and Instrument Development

MICHAEL RUTTER, ANN LeCOUTEUR, CATHERINE LORD,
HOPE MACDONALD, PATRICIA RIOS, and SUSAN FOLSTEIN

INTRODUCTION

Since Kanner first described the syndrome of autism in 1943, there has been substantial progress in the diagnosis and classification of the disorder (see chapter by Rutter and Schopler, this volume). As a result, both ICD-9 (World Health Organization, 1978) and DSM-III (American Psychiatric Association, 1980), the two major systems of psychiatric classification, broadly agree on the main features to be taken into account in diagnosis. In essence, the main weight is placed on a particular type of deviance in language, a particular type of deviance in social relationships, and particular patterns of repetitive and stereotyped behaviour, together with developmental abnormalities that have been evident from before the age of 30 months. The recently published guidelines for DSM-III-R (American Psychiatric Association, 1987) and the draft guidelines for ICD-10 (World Health Organization, 1987) follow the same general principles, although both have attempted to provide somewhat greater specification on the patterns of abnormality in these areas that are thought to be most characteristic of autism. In addition, because of practical difficulties in the application of the 30-month cutoff for developmental abnormalities, this has been raised to 3 years of age. Most of the published interview, questionnaire, and observational methods of assessment (see Rutter and Schopler, Chapter 2, this volume) have focused similarly on these diagnostic features, although they differ somewhat in their emphasis. Most have been primarily concerned with the diagnosis of autism in mentally handicapped children, as the majority of autistic individuals show some degree of mental retardation. The instruments have been developed with the main aim of making diagnoses for treatment purposes or for decisions on

MICHAEL RUTTER, ANN LeCOUTEUR, HOPE MACDONALD, and PATRICIA RIOS • Department of Child and Adolescent Psychiatry, Institute of Psychiatry, University of London, London SE5 8AF, England.   CATHERINE LORD • Department of Pediatrics, University of Alberta, and Department of Psychology, Glenrose Rehabilitation Hospital, Edmonton, Alberta T5G 0B7, Canada.   SUSAN FOLSTEIN • Department of Psychiatry and Behavioral Science, Johns Hopkins University, School of Medicine, Baltimore, Maryland 21205.

placement in different service facilities. The instruments work reasonably well in meeting these objectives, but there are now new purposes that require some modification in methods of assessment. This chapter describes some measures developed to meet these emerging needs.

Inevitably in medicine we have to start with diagnostic criteria for a clinical picture that seems to represent a common set of problems. That is exactly what was done with autism and the procedure has worked well. As outlined in the chapter by Rutter and Schopler, autism has been found to differ substantially from the four main groups of disorders with which it has been compared; namely, general mental retardation, specific developmental disorders of language, schizophrenia, and the common types of emotional and conduct disturbances in childhood. Nevertheless, research has shown that the clinical syndrome of autism, as usually defined, is not synonymous with the disorder as genetically transmitted. Thus, Folstein and Rutter (1977) found that the concordance rate for autism in monozygotic pairs was only 36% (compared with zero% in dizygotic pairs) but the concordance rate rose to 82% when a broader pattern of cognitive and language disabilities was considered. Concordance for this broader pattern was only 10% in dizygotic pairs, suggesting that what was inherited was a broader pattern of cognitive deficits that included, but was not restricted to, autism. A recent follow-up of the same set of twin pairs by A. Le Couteur (personal communication) has shown that this pattern continues as the individuals reach adult life. The discordant monozygotic co-twins, when seen in adult life, still showed a variety of problems (with social difficulties rather more apparent than when they were young) but, yet, their disorders do not meet the criteria for autism. Family studies have given rise to a similar set of conclusions (August et al., 1981). The siblings of autistic individuals were found to show a 15% rate of a mixed bag of cognitive and language difficulties, a rate some five times that in the siblings in the Down's syndrome control group. The twin study, however, makes clear that these associated problems are not just cognitive disabilities but, rather, they include quite marked (albeit subtle) social deficits as well. There is a need for discriminating assessment instruments that can pick up these important autism-related disabilities in persons of normal or near-normal intelligence. At present, we have to discuss the problems as autism-related, but the genetic evidence indicates that, in reality, they concern the same condition as autism, genetically speaking. That these autism-related conditions often do indeed reflect the same genotype is shown by the findings from monozygotic twin pairs discordant for autism (LeCouteur, Rutter, Summers, & Butler, in press) and from family studies (Bolton, personal communication), both of which have shown that the fragile-X chromosomal anomaly is associated with them as well as with autism. The limitation at the moment is that we lack the knowledge on precisely how to diagnose and define these "lesser variants" of autism.

It has been a common experience in medicine to find that clinical conditions that were once thought to be homogeneous ultimately turn out to be heterogeneous once knowledge on etiology becomes available. The same is happening in the field of autism. It has long been known that occasional cases of autism are attributable to specific medical conditions, such as phenylketonuria, tuberous sclerosis, and congenital rubella (Folstein & Rutter, 1987, Reiss, Feinstein & Rosenbaum, 1986). Unfortunately, the clinical study of such cases leaves a lot to be desired by modern standards and it is not at all clear whether the picture of autism in these cases due to specific causes is the same or different from that found in the larger group of autistic disorders where the etiology is unknown. During the past few years, two other specific etiologic groups have become identified. First, there is Rett's syndrome (Hagberg et al., 1983). This condition has so far been exclusively found in girls and the clinical picture is somewhat different from autism in that there is an intellectual decline during the preschool years together with neurologic abnormalities, particularly involving abnormalities in purposive movements. The social and behavioral abnormalities, too, are not quite the same as those in autism (Olsson & Rett, 1985), but it is apparent that in the past many girls with Rett's syndrome were misdiagnosed as suffering from autism (Witt-Engerstrom & Gillberg, 1987). Unfortunately, a lack of adequately discriminating measures of social behavior has meant that the differences and similarities between Rett's syndrome and autism have yet to be fully charted.

Second, it has been found that some 5–10% of autistic individuals suffer from the fragile-X anomaly (Bregman et al., 1987; Brown et al., 1985). There is continuing controversy on the question of whether or not the association with fragile-X is more strongly associated with autism than with mental handicap more generally, but this chromosomal abnormality clearly accounts for a higher proportion of cases of autism than any other previously identified etiology. Again, the literature is contradictory on whether or not cases of autism due to the fragile-X anomaly are clinically similar to, or different from, other cases of autism and, equally, there is disagreement on the extent to which children with the fragile-X who do not meet the usual criteria for the syndrome of autism nevertheless show autisticlike features. Once more, more discriminating clinical measures are required.

Third, interest has come to be paid to Asperger's syndrome (Wing, 1981) and schizoid disorder of childhood (Wolff & Barlow, 1979; Wolff & Chick, 1980). Both terms have been applied to individuals who seem to show socioemotional deficits and circumscribed interest patterns similar to those seen in autism, but who have now shown the language retardation usually found in autism and who often (perhaps always) show the additional feature of marked clumsiness. It remains to be established whether these represent distinct clinical entities. Some investigators have been skeptical as to whether they do (Schopler, 1985), many have seen the conditions as variants of autism (Gillberg, 1985; Wing, 1981), but some have considered that, although similar in some ways, the conditions are distinct from autism (Wolff & Barlow, 1979; Szatmari et al., 1986). The data are not yet available to decide between these competing views but the necessary evidence will depend in part on adequate clinical assessments in individuals of normal intelligence, who do not show any marked retardation in language, and many of whom are of adult age. Some of the instruments described in this chapter seek to fill that gap.

Finally, attention during recent years has turned to the crucial, but difficult, issue of which abnormal psychological processes might underlie the syndrome of autism. Table I outlines the various steps involved in this search for the identity of the basic disordered psychological process. Thus, in the field of language, the first step was to show by various group comparisons, in which there was adequate control for general level of intellectual and behavioural functioning, that autistic children tended to be more impaired in their language than in other aspects of cognition (Lockyer & Rutter, 1969; Hermelin & O'Connor, 1970). The next step was to determine if the pattern of language deficit associated with autism was in any way distinctive and different from that found in other conditions. Research findings shows that it was (Bartak et al., 1975; Hermelin & O'Conner, 1970). Autistic children tended to show a deficit that involved conceptual and thought processes as well as a wide range of language impairment across various modalities. The third step required an identification of the features of language that were unimpaired, together with those that were specifically deviant. A variety of studies produced consistent findings indicating that autistic individuals were not particularly impaired with respect to either phonology or syntax, and possibly also not in semantics, although the evidence on this latter feature is not wholly unambiguous. The

Table I. Search for a Specific Underlying Psychological Deficit

Step 1	Identification of area of functioning in which abnormalities of some type differentiate individuals with autism from those with other forms of handicap (behavioral or developmental)
Step 2	Delineation of pattern of functioning in that area that differentiates individuals with autism from those with other handicaps
Step 3	Demonstration that there is not impairment in those aspects of functioning in that area that are not included in the supposedly characteristic pattern
Step 4	Inference regarding a possible specific psychological deficit pathognomonic of autism
Step 5	Demonstration through study of individuals chosen on the basis of this deficit that it is regularly associated with the autistic behavioral syndrome
Step 6	Redefinition of autism in terms of the presence of specific psychological deficit
Step 7	Demonstration that the deficit is associated with a specific etiology or etiologies

specific deviant feature seemed to lie within the area of pragmatics (Cromer, 1987). The fourth step involved an extrapolation from this pattern of strengths and weaknesses to an inference on what might be the key abnormality, i.e., what psychological process or mechanism might be involved. This research chain has lead to a shift of emphasis from language to socialization. The research findings to date do not, as yet, lead to a precise delineation of the abnormal process, but they have taken us much closer to that highly desirable goal.

Thus, Attwood (1986) showed that autistic individuals were impaired in their use of gesture but only in those that were concerned with the transmission of emotional meaning. Hobson (1986) showed that autistic children differed from mental age-matched normal children and mentally handicapped children with respect to their ability to appreciate the meaning of either still photographs or videotaped sequences, but this deficit only applied when the pictures involved socioemotional cues. Autistic children were poor at making differentiations according to age and gender (Hobson, 1983) and also according to different types of emotional expression (Hobson, 1986).

An earlier study by Hobson (1984) showed that autistic children were not specifically impaired in their ability to appreciate the visuospacial perspective of others but, more recently, Baron-Cohen et al. (1985) showed that they were impaired when the perspectives were conceptual rather than perceptual. A further study by the same investigators (Baron-Cohen et al., 1986) showed that autistic children were also impaired in their understanding of sequences that told a story but that this disability seemed to be restricted to sequences involving an understanding of the intentions or beliefs of other people. On the basis of these findings, Hobson (1988) proposed that the basic deficit in autism may concern a lack of empathic understanding for social and emotional aspects of interpersonal communication. He has suggested that this social deficit may be responsible for the language abnormalities that are so characteristic of autism. Conversely, Baron-Cohen (1988) argued that the deficit is cognitive rather than social, and that autistic children, in effect, lack a "theory of mind" so that they are unable to appreciate other people's intentions and expectations. He suggests that it is this deficit that underlies the social abnormalities, as well as the linguistic ones.

Much further experimental work is needed in order to delineate the precise qualities of the basic disordered psychological process in autism. Of course, it may well turn out that there is not one abnormal process but several. Nevertheless, the ultimate goal would be to delineate these processes in order to redefine the syndrome in terms of those who do and those who do not show the specific basic psychological deficit. The expectation then is that this psychological deficit may be shown to be associated with one or more specific etiologies. This has been the traditional way in medicine with laboratory findings (the equivalent of the psychological deficit) coming to replace clinical signs and symptoms as diagnostic criteria when the abnormal process becomes better understood. As the basic biologic disorder is identified, so the clinical diagnostic criteria become both sharpened and redefined. It is obvious that there is a good way yet to go before anything as precise as that is achieved in the field of autism. Nevertheless, in addition to the further experimental work that is required, it seems desirable that the clinical instruments should seek to incorporate those phenomena that appear closer to the postulated psychological abnormalities.

NEW DIAGNOSTIC INSTRUMENTS

Three different types of instruments have been developed by us: those based on interviews with key informants (the autistic diagnostic interview, ADI, and the interview to assess socioemotional functioning, SEF), an interview/observational assessment procedure to be used with the individuals themselves (autistic diagnostic observation schedule—ADOS together with a subject version of the SEF interview), and a set of psychometric tasks designed to tap the individual's skills in the production and discrimination of emotions in the visual and auditory modalities.

Autistic Diagnostic Interview

The autistic diagnostic interview, (ADI) (LeCouteur *et al.*, in press) provides a detailed coverage of three main areas of functioning during the first 5 years of life: (1) language and communication; (2) social development; and (3) development of play. In each case, an account is obtained of the course of the development with particular attention to the child's functioning at 30 months and 36 months (in order to obtain the information needed to decide whether development was abnormal before this age). These same three areas are then covered systematically with respect to the subject's current behavior, with questioning to determine whether any of the key features were abnormal at any age between 5 years and the time of interview. The coverage of behaviors is extensive and includes all features necessary to meet the diagnostic criteria in ICD-10 and DSM-III-R.

The interview has four main features that differentiate it from most other interview-based diagnostic instruments in the field of autism. First, it is an investigator-based interview rather than a respondent-based interview. Many of the structured interviews that are currently available in psychiatry and psychology take the latter form. That is, the questions are predetermined and carefully standardized, with codings based on whether the respondent says "yes" or "no" to the behaviours in question. Inevitably, such respondent-based interviews necessarily rely on all informants interpreting the questions in the same way and all informants having the necessary conceptual understanding to make the distinctions necessary for the coding of each behavior. When dealing with subtle differentiations in the field of communication, social relationships, and play this is a very dubious assumption. Accordingly, an investigator-based approach has been chosen instead. In this style of interview, the structuring lies in the details of the coding for each behaviour. Because this is not based on an affirmative or negative answer to a closed question, it is possible to be both more detailed and more structured in the criteria for each behavior to be assessed. The responsibility is placed on the investigator to obtain all necessary information in order to make each rating. There are a variety of specified screening questions, but their purpose is not to obtain an affirmative or negative response from the informant but rather to guide the interviewer on the nature of the information to be obtained. A variety of further probes are suggested for each item but the detailed specification is provided in the operational definition for each rating. Such an interview style is heavily reliant on skilled interviewers who have been trained in detail on the specific interview. That is, the training involves not only general interviewing skills but also training on the conceptual distinctions involved in each and every one of the ratings in the interview schedule, together with training on how to question for each one. Such training takes, on average, some 2 months or so, with variation dependent not only on people's interviewing skills but, more especially, on their clinical experience and familiarity with autism. This style of interviewing is one that has been widely used in British clinical epidemiology, and it has been shown that ratings using this style can be made both reliable and valid with appropriate training (Brown & Rutter, 1966; Graham & Rutter, 1968; Quinton *et al.*, 1976; Rutter & Brown, 1966).

The second key feature is the heavy emphasis on the need to obtain detailed descriptions of actual behavior. General statements are not acceptable. Rather, informants are asked to give a sequential account of the subject's behavior in actual incidents or episodes. These descriptions provide not only a means for checking on the comparability across interviewers and on the extent to which ratings adhere to the structured criteria given, but also the raw material for a reassessment of particular behaviors if subsequent knowledge indicates that further distinctions have to be made.

Third, the codings have been focused with attention to a careful delineation of the particular patterns of deviance supposedly specifically associated with autism. This is associated with the fourth key feature, i.e., an effort carefully to differentiate delay in the development of particular psychological functions from deviance in the pattern of the behaviors in question. Some impression of the style of the rating may best be given by a few examples. Thus, the rating on amount of social communication, has as its 0 (normal rating) the specification extensive use of language (at whatever capacity obtained) for social interchange; i.e., much chat, comment, and remarks that appear to have social (rather than object getting) intent. The rating of 2 (definitely abnormal) specifies most communication either object-oriented (i.e., to ask for things), or response to questions, or echolalic, or concerned with partiular preoccupation; little or no social chat.

The rating of 0 on friendships/peers specifies "one or more relationships with person *in own age group* (approx.) with whom [are shared] activities of a personal (nonstereotyped) variety, seen outside formal group setting (such as club), and with whom there is definite reciprocity and mutual responsiveness." The most abnormal rating of '3' specifies "no peer relationships that involve selectivity and sharing."

The most abnormal rating on unusual sensory interest specifies "preoccupation with unusual sensory interest that takes up a major amount of time or prevents/limits alternative use of that material to the exclusion of other aspects of its ordinary function."

In addition to the range of phenomena in these three main areas of behavior, there is also coverage of a variety of other phenomena that may be of clinical importance, such as self-injury, pica, overactivity, or aggression.

The reliability and validity of the ADI was established through the use of 32 videotapes of interviews with mothers, one half of whom had children clinically diagnosed as autistic and one half clinically diagnosed as mentally handicapped but not autistic. The children were all aged 7–19 years and the groups were equated for IQ with scores in the 30–93 range. One half of the subjects for the study came from Edmonton, Canada (having been under the care of CL) and one half from London, England (having been under the care of MR). Using a balanced incomplete block design (Fleiss, 1986) four raters (two Canadian and two British) each rated a total of 16 tapes, 6 of which were in common with their local colleague and 5 of which were in common with each of their two overseas colleagues. In all cases the raters were kept blind to the clinical diagnosis. The mean percentage agreement on individual behaviors necessary for the diagnosis of autism across all pairs of raters ranges from 81 to 89% and the mean weighted κ (pooling rating pairs) ranged from .55 to .97 across all the specific behaviors used in the diagnosis of autism (see under Algorithm).

The individual behaviors necessary for diagnosing autism were combined in order to create an algorithm to produce a diagnosis of autism according to ICD-10 criteria. Thus, each item was scored 0 (no abnormality of the type specified), 1 (a slight abnormality of the type specified), or 2 (marked abnormality of the specified type). Twelve items were included in a section on abnormalities in communicative behavior, the algorithm requiring a minimum score of 8 in this section for verbal subjects (and 6 for nonverbal subjects); 14 items were included in a section on reciprocal social interaction, the algorithm requiring a minimum

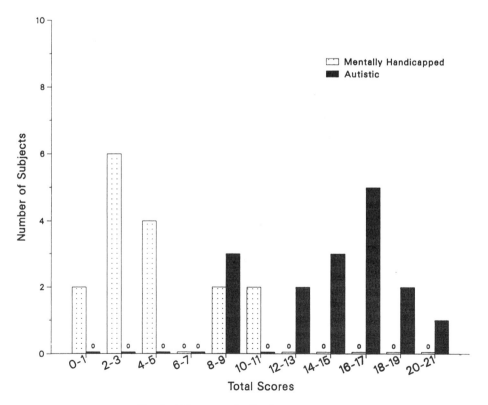

Fig. 1. ADI communication/language score.

score of 10; and a section on repetitive and stereotyped behaviors comprised six items, a minimum score of 4 being required. A fourth section dealt with early development, the codings specifying whether it was delayed or deviant in each of the three key areas of communication, socialization, and play. The algorithm required that development be delayed or deviant at age 3 years in at least one area.

The validity of the ADI algorithm to differentiate autism and mental handicap was examined by comparing the scores for the 16 children in each diagnostic group (i.e., autism and mental handicap), using the ratings made by raters in descending order according to reliability and experience. The findings were analyzed separately according to the three main areas of symptomatology relevant to diagnosis. The differentiation was highly significant in all three areas (Figs 1–3) but with some overlap in the case of language/communication and reciprocal social interaction. However, when the three areas were summated to produce a total score there was no longer any overlap between the groups (Fig. 4). All the autistic subjects met the abnormalities by 36 months criterion; furthermore, all met the separate criteria for each of the three areas of symptomatology, whereas none of the mentally handicapped subjects did so. Two met the criteria for one area, three did so for two areas, but none did so for three areas. We may conclude that the focus on detailed descriptions of the quality of children's behavior in these three areas has paid off in providing a much more satisfactory diagnostic differentiation than that reported for other instruments. However, it should be

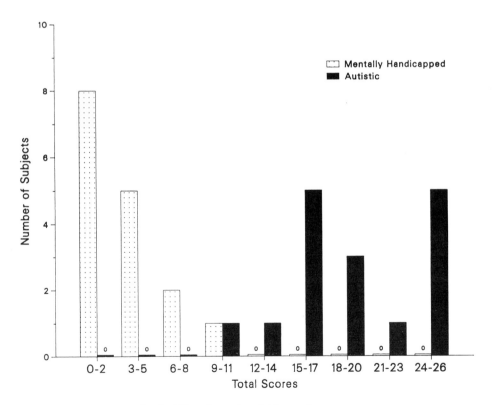

Fig. 2. ADI reciprocal social interaction score.

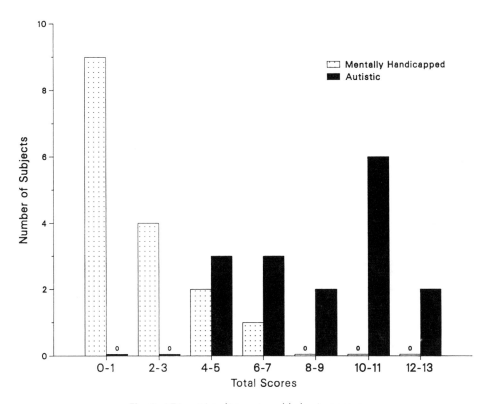

Fig. 3. ADI restricted/stereotyped behaviors score.

noted that these findings apply to a group that excludes preschool children and those who show the most severe forms of mental handicap. Clinical experience suggests that the differentiation may well be much more difficult in those with a mental age below, say, 3 years.

Socioemotional Functioning Interview

The ADI has proved an effective diagnostic instrument for autism as diagnosed according to DSM-III-R or ICD-10 criteria. However, the phenotype for autism appears to extend rather more broadly than this. In her follow-up of the discordant monozygotic co-twins in the Folstein and Rutter (1977) study, ALC has shown that the nonautistic co-twins, although not fulfilling the criteria for autism, nevertheless show a variety of socioemotional problems (Le Couteur, personal communication). The family studies also suggest that social difficulties may occur in family members with language and cognitive disabilities but without autism as traditionally diagnosed. The socioemotional functioning interview is designed to pick up these more subtle social problems found in individuals without gross handicap. The general style of the interview is closely similar to that employed with the ADI but differs in that it has both a subject and informant version. The interview covers the subject's level of independence (as indicated by the ability to travel independently, to arrange their own holidays, and

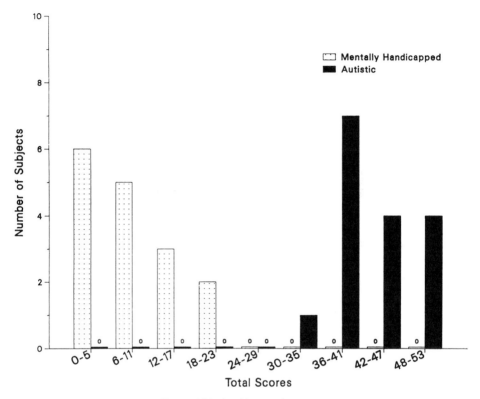

Fig. 4. ADI algorithm total score.

to plan their own leisure activities). Thus, the leisure activity rating specifies for the 0 rating that the child has a range of interests (e.g., cinema, music, sport) and at least fortnightly engages in one of them (on own or with others, but on own initiative). The 2 rating specifies few spontaneous adult/type interests, although the child may go to public places alone (e.g., railway stations to take train numbers, football clubs, special social group). The more severe 3 rating specifies leisure activities usually arranged by others.

The interview also covers various types of interpersonal difficulties. For example, there is a coding of the person's perception of other's annoyance. The 0 coding specifies appropriately picks up minor cues before problems arise, and the 3 rating specifies only aware if strictly disciplined/threatened with dismissal/exclusion.

The third section of the interview deals with friendships and social relationships. This section deals with both casual, and also more intimate relationships. For example, the coding on acquaintances specifies as 0 normal range of casual social contacts, able to make social relations at clubs, social gatherings, in shops, and so forth. The 2 coding specifies little or no making of acquaintances. As with a number of other social features, it is necessary to have a means of dealing with autisticlike abnormalities that do not come within the main dimension of the rating. Thus, with acquaintances, there is a special coding to deal with this situation, specifying large range of acquaintances with whom interactions are unusual in quality (e.g., makes extensive contacts with shopkeepers, bus drivers, librarians). Some of the ratings deal with concepts within the social arena, such as the concept of marriage. The 0 rating specifies some indication of special qualities of marriage (e.g., commitment, involvement, responsibility). The quality of the language or the description is irrelevant as long as the required components are present in some form. The abnormal 2 rating specifies description of personal or egocentric aspects of marriage relevant only to self (e.g., get a day off).

Other ratings deal with the intensity and emotional quality of relationships. For example, the love relationship rating specifies for the 0 coding definite emotionally intense heterosexual relationship (current or in past) with evidence of both strongly positive emotion in presence of other person and definite missing/pining/longing/preoccupied thinking when apart. Finally, there are sections dealing with fantasies and dreams, in view of the suggestion that these may be diminished or absent in autistic individuals (Bemporad, 1979), and self-image, with questions designed to determine whether a person thinks of him/herself as different from other people in any way and whether (s)he is aware of how other people view him or her. The data on reliability and validity of this measure are not yet available, but it is clear that the areas covered by this interview constitute an essential component of the overall assessment of social features associated with autism.

Autistic Diagnostic Observation Schedule

The ADOS instrument (Lord, Rutter, Goode, Heemsbergen, Jordan, Mawhood, and Schopler, in press) provides a standardized interview/observation assessment lasting about half an hour, that aims to tap social, communicative, and language behaviours thought to be diagnostic of the syndrome of autism. It is based on a social communicative sequence that combines a series of unstructured and structured situations that serve to provide a set of "presses" for particular kinds of social and communicative behavior. Some of the situations aim to provide a relaxed informal and unstructured social setting in which the subject has to take the initiative for social overtures, the aim being to determine how well (s)he is able to sustain the social interaction in situations with a minimum of structural direction. Others are deliberately structured so that the examiner provides a standardized social-communicative task designed to determine how the subject responds to, and builds on, specific social stimuli and demands. In short, it is intended to provide a standardized set of opportunities in which to observe the social and communicative behaviors exhibited by autistic persons. Although it is known that autistic individuals often produce fewer spontaneous social and communicative behaviors than do other people, one of the assumptions behind the ADOS is that it is the quality of these social behaviors that is particularly crucial to the diagnosis of autism. Thus, the ratings evaluate the quality of social behavior, as well as the occurrence or absence of particular items of social behavior.

Another assumption basic to the instrument is that social behavior necessarily involves more than one person. In effect, the examiner is a kind of confederate in a social experiment. (S)he follows a set protocol that provides particular social and contextual presses. The presses are derived from the nature of the tasks or materials or the examiner's behaviour, so creating situations designed to elicit key behaviors.

There are nine components to the observational assessment (after an introductory period):

1. In a puzzle-type construction task, the purpose is to observe the subject's interactive behavior and to elicit whether and how the subject asks for help (the task being engineered so that this is necessary).

2. In an unstructured task, the individual is given a set of toy objects that provide the opportunity for make-believe play.

3. The examiner seeks to engage the subject in joint interactive play, again using miniature materials suitable for make-believe situations. The key aim here is to determine how far the subject shows reciprocity in interactive play and the ability to develop the interaction and show initiative in extending it.

4. A drawing game taps the subject's turn taking ability.

5. A demonstration task requires the subject to communicate a familiar series of actions using gestural mime (e.g., the procedure of brushing teeth from the moment of going to the bathroom to putting the toothpaste away). The task assesses not only miming skills, but also the socioemotional interactions that go along with demonstrating a familiar behavior to a stranger.

6. The child is presented with a large poster picture of a complex scene with several different activities, the child being required to describe the activities in the picture.

7. The child is presented with a picture book without words in which the pictures tell a sequential story. The child is asked to convey the story in the pictures.

8. The experimenter seeks to engage the subject in a conversation, the aim being to tap various aspects of conversational skills.

9. There is a phase of questioning that aims to assess the subjects' ability to describe

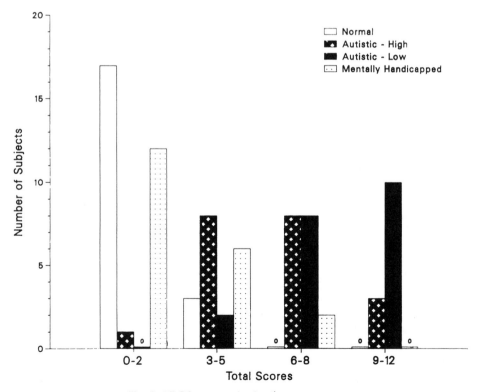

Fig. 5. ADOS communication/language score.

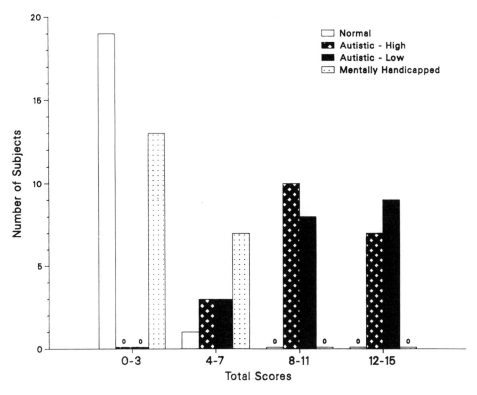

Fig. 6. ADOS reciprocal social interaction score.

social and emotional qualities, together with the objective of providing a verbal context in which to express emotions, exhibit empathy, and show social awareness.

Each of the tasks gives rise to a series of specific ratings on behaviors shown during the task, but the whole of the assessment session is used to provide a series of ratings on operationalized scales dealing with social, communicative, and repetitive or stereotyped behaviors. It is these latter ratings that provide the main data for diagnosis.

The assessment is designed as a social interaction in which the examiner is expected to show varying degrees of initiative and responsivity in order to tap different aspects of the child's functioning. It is necessarily dependent on the clinical skills of the examiner, and training is required for the administration and scoring of the ADOS. The protocol for the examiner is complicated because it consists of a hierarchy ranging from the provision of an open-ended opportunity for spontaneous behavior to requirements that the subject be directed to structure their behavior in quite specific ways. Clinical skills are required in order to achieve the appropriate balance between provoking or eliciting some behaviour from the subject and at the same time not overcueing or directing the particular type of behavior to be elicited.

The ADOS is standardized for subjects with an estimated mental age of 3 years or greater. The reliability and validity data, however, are available only for subjects who have some limited language, and whose estimated level of expressive language as well as nonverbal performance ability is 3 years or greater. Suggestions for using the ADOS with lower-functioning children are available, but reliability and validity for this group has yet to be established. The assessment procedure can be used not only for children but for adolescents and young adults.

The reliability of the ADOS was established through the use of 40 videotapes of interviews with children and adolescents who had been clinically diagnosed as autistic and half clinically diagnosed as mentally handicapped but not autistic. The children were all aged between 6 and 18 years and the groups were equated for IQ with scores in the mildly mentally handicapped range. Approximately two thirds of the subjects for the study came from the United States or Canada (having been known to CL) and one third from London (having been under the care of MR). Four raters (two Canadian and two from England) each rated a total of 16–20 tapes with 6–8 tapes in common with each colleague. In addition, a fifth rater scored four tapes with each other rater. In all cases, the raters were kept blind to the clinical diagnosis. The mean percentage agreement for individual rating across all pairs of raters ranges from 58% to 86% and the mean weighted κ (pooling rating pairs) ranged from .58 to .84 across all the specific behaviors used in the algorithm for the diagnosis of autism.

It is has been found that the ADOS provides an effective means of tapping both social

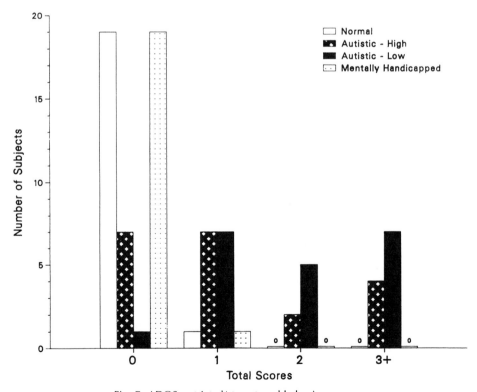

Fig. 7. ADOS restricted/stereotyped behaviors score.

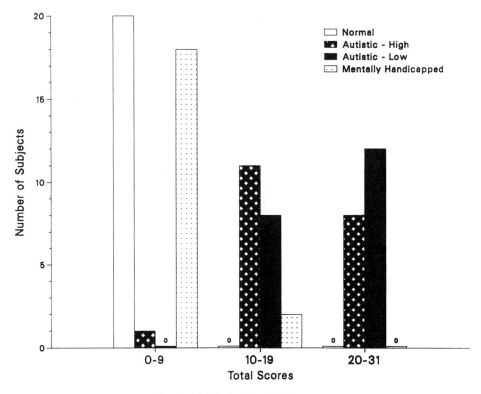

Fig. 8. ADOS algorithm total score.

and communicative behaviors, but the time period and the setting are not optimal for documenting repetitive or ritualistic behaviors other than in the more seriously disturbed individuals.

The validity of the instrument was tested by comparing four groups of 20 individuals matched on sex and chronologic age. First, autistic individuals were contrasted with mildly mentally handicapped subjects included in the reliability study who were of comparable chronologic and mental age. Second, autistic individuals with a normal nonverbal intelligence were compared with normal controls. Figures 5–7 provide the summary data for the algorithm scores based for each of the three main domains of behavior used in diagnosis: language/communication, social and repetitive behaviors. The differentiation is highly significant when each is considered separately, but the separation of groups is cleaner when the three are combined (Fig. 8). As already noted, repetitive and stereotyped behaviors were not prominent during the observation session; nevertheless they were present to some degree in 13 out of the 20 higher functioning autistic subjects (compared with just one normal control) and 19 out of 20 mentally handicapped subjects (compared with only one mentally retarded subject). Of the 20 higher-functioning autistic individuals, 17 met the algorithm criteria for both language/communication and social behaviors, as against none of the controls. The comparable figures for the mentally retarded autistic subjects was 20 out of 20 versus two of the nonautistic mentally retarded subjects.

THE RECOGNITION AND EXPRESSION OF SOCIOEMOTIONAL CUES

The experimental work with autistic individuals, noted above, has indicated that they have problems in both the expression and appreciation of socioemotional cues. These tasks (MacDonald, Rutter, Howlin, Rios, LeCouteur & Evered, in press) were designed to tap these areas of functioning in ways that would be applicable to higher functioning subjects. The need here, particularly, is to be able to identify specifically autistic-type deficits in individuals, where the nature of the social abnormalities is in some doubt. This applies particularly in the range of disorders that may be considered "lesser variants" of autism.

The first test is designed to assess the subject's ability to recognize emotional speech. The instrument consists of an audio-recorded series of sentences read by an actor who varied his emotional expression to suit one of four basic emotions: happiness, anger, fear, and sadness. The order of these emotions, and that of a fifth unemotional or neutral type of speech, is randomized across test trials. Within the instrument, two different methods are used to control verbal emotional content. In the first block of 18 trials, the meaning is affectively neutral, e.g., "the library books are on the table." In two further blocks, each with 18 sentences, electronic filtering was used to eliminate critical bands of frequencies so that the words are unintelligible (although the emotional intonations remain). On each trial, the subject is asked to make a multiple-choice judgment about the nature of the intended emotion.

The second test is designed to assess the person's ability to recognize emotions as portrayed in photographs. This is done by means of a task in which the subject is required to match faces selected from the Ekman and Friesen (1976) set of photographs of facial affect with photographs of a context designed to elicit a particular emotion. Thus, 20 photographs each portraying a context (such as a birthday celebration) designed to provoke one of five emotional states (happiness, anger, fear, sadness, or no emotion) are presented individually. The subject is asked to match the context with one facial expression from a five-photograph array of an actor depicting the four basic emotions and the neutral state. Four such arrays are used, each comprising photographs of a different actor, with the position of the correct match being randomized across both arrays and test trials.

The third task assesses the subject's ability to portray particular emotions in facial expression. Subjects are photographed while conveying, via facial expressions, one of the five states (the same five as used in the other tasks). Each emotional expression is attempted and photographed three times. Before attempting each expression, the subject listens to a short description of a situation in which the particular emotion might typically be experienced. The order in which the 15 exressions are photographed is varied randomly among the subjects. The head-and-shoulders photographs in the reliability assessment were rated by five independent judges (lay persons who were naive regarding the task), who individually made multiple-choice responses to each photo. Judges' correct responses (i.e., responses that matched the intended emotion) were summed such that each subject could receive a maximum possible score of 75. There was a statistically significant degree of association between the five judges' accuracy scores for each subject (Kendall's $W = .74$ $p < .001$).

The fourth task assesses the subject's ability to portray emotions in vocal expression. In this task, the subject is audio-recorded while varying the intended emotion of an affectively neutral sentence. The testing procedure was similar to that used for facial expression. The subject listens to a warmup story before each trial, and the order of the 15 expressions was varied randomly among the subjects. In the reliability study, edited audio recordings were presented to five independent judges (again, lay persons naive regarding the task), with the rating and scoring procedures identical to those described for the previous task. Kendall's W for the judges ratings for 30 subjects was .79 ($p < .001$). The validity of this set of tests was determined by comparing 10 autistic males, all of whom met DSM-III and ICD-10 criteria for autism with 10 normal males. The mean age of the two groups was closely comparable (27 years for the autistic group and 26 for the normals) and the groups were also closely matched on Raven's IQ (118 for the autistic subjects and 120 for the normals). However, as would be expected, the normals had superior scores on the British Picture Vocabulary test (mean of 109 versus 84).

The autistic subjects scored worse than the normals on all four tests, the between-group differences being statistically significant for all tests except the vocal expression of emotion. There was considerable overlap between groups when the four tests were considered separately but much less overlap when the four tests were combined. Figure 9 shows the classification of autistic and normal subjects according to the number of tasks on which the score was below the normal mean by more than 1 SD. Figure 10 presents an alternative way of scoring in which the groups are compared on a composite score made up of the scores on the

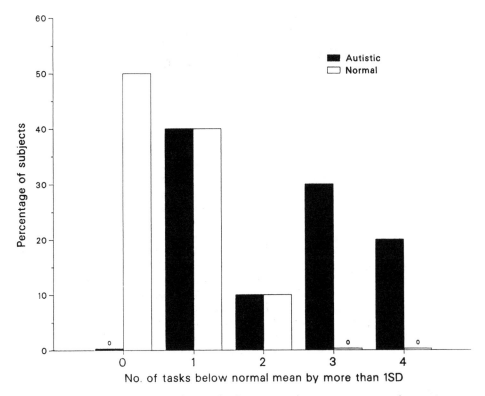

Fig. 9. Classification of autistic and normal subjects according to scores across four socioemotional tasks.

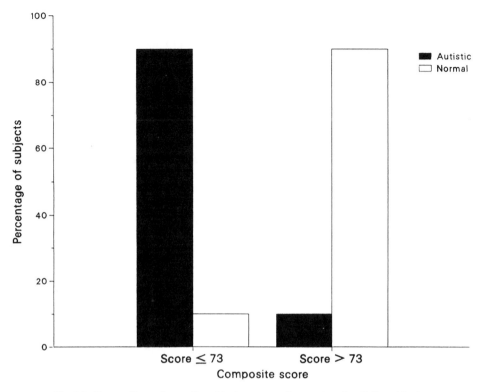

Fig. 10. Composite socioemotional tasks scores of normal and autistic subjects.

four tasks. In the latter comparison, 9 out of 10 normally intelligent autistic subjects obtained abnormal scores compared with only 1 normal subject. It is apparent that there is quite good differentiation of the groups when the tasks are pooled in this way. The overlap on each of the individual tasks is a function of occasional low scores by normal subjects as well as scores within the normal range for some autistic individuals. However, scarcely any normal subjects obtained poor scores on more than one of the four tests whereas all of the autistic subjects scored poorly on at least one. Nevertheless, the fact that autistic subjects sometimes scored quite well is a reflection of the fact that, as a function of trying to focus each task on specific aspects of emotion, the task was necessarily made a non-natural one with much of the social component removed. Autistic individuals still scored somewhat poorly in this situation, but their performance was higher than it might be otherwise because it is clear that quite often they use nonsocioemotional cues in order to make the necessary discriminations. In short, the tasks add to the assessment of socioemotional functioning in autistic individuals of normal intelligence but still they fail to tap all adequate aspects of the socioemotional deficit.

CONCLUSIONS

In this chapter we have described the development of four new diagnostic instruments: two investigator-based standardized interviews (the ADI and SEF), an observation scheme

(ADOS) and a set of experimental tasks. Their purpose is to provide detailed and discriminating measures of the quality of those communicative, social, and play behaviors thought to be characteristic of autism. There has been a deliberate heavy emphasis on the use of clinical skills for the differentiation between key behaviours, because parents cannot be expected to appreciate the crucial diagnostic distinctions. This is especially so in the case of communicative and interactive social behaviors, in which many of the concepts used in diagnosis do not form part of general knowledge. Particular attention has been paid to making the measures appropriate for older autistic individuals and for those of normal intelligence. The instruments that we have developed have been shown to be reliable and to have good discriminative validity and we may conclude that their main purpose has been achieved.

Both the ADI and the ADOS (together with the SEF, if it successfully meets the reliability and validity tests that are underway) may be recommended for clinical use when detailed assessments of specific behaviors are required. The ADI focuses attention on the particular features of communication, social relationships and play behavior that are of diagnostic interest and it it likely that this focus will be of value for training purposes. The ADOS has the merit of providing an appropriate structure for eliciting social and communicative behaviours and the findings make it evident that it does this well. The experimental socioemotional tasks have also been shown to differentiate autistic individuals (in this case those of normal intelligence from normal controls), but their usage remains in the research arena at the moment. It is highly desirable to have available standard tasks that may provide quantitative measures of different aspects of socioemotional skills, both receptive and expressive. However, it cannot be claimed as yet that there is a battery at a stage of development when it can be recommended for ordinary clinical use.

Traditionally, psychiatric diagnosis follows a categorical format, a format followed by both DSM-IIIR and ICD-10. We have shown that the measures may be adapted to produce an algorithm that represents ICD-10 criteria and that its use effectively separates autistic subjects from nonautistic mentally retarded ones. For many purposes, this categorical approach constitutes a practicable and appropriate way of proceeding. Moreover, because the instruments are based on individual behaviors, and not on any particular classification scheme, it should be a straightforward matter to produce further algorithms for different sets of diagnostic criteria when that seems necessary. However, it should not necessarily be assumed that a categorical approach is always the best. There are many circumstances in which there is real doubt as to how and where the lines of demarcation should be drawn. This is so, for example, in the case of severely retarded children many of whom show some autistic features, although they do not meet the standard criteria for the diagnosis of autism (Wing & Gould, 1979). It is also so at the other end of the intellectual spectrum in the gray area between autism and Asperger's syndrome (Wing, 1981) or schizoid disorder of childhood (Wolff & Barlow, 1979). Similar issues arise with the behavioral characteristics of children with the fragile-X anomaly (Bregman et al., 1987). Most strikingly, the categorical approach seems to fall down in the case of monozygotic twin pairs discordant for autism but concordant for a broader range of cognitive/language/social deficits; the same problem occurs in the familial aggregation of these deficits with autism.

It may well be that the difficulties in all these instances lie, not in the categorical approach as such, but rather in the inadequate conceptualization of the categories used. A crucial aim of these instruments is the provision of good measures of many different aspects of social, communicative and play behaviors so that the currently available categories may be put to the test and, it is hoped, improved.

However, it is possible that for some purposes dimensional approaches may be preferable. Accordingly, we have shown how the instruments may be employed to provide quantitative measures of the extent to which functioning is deviant in each of the three main domains of behavior that are used in diagnosis. It is desirable to keep the measures of these domains separate in that it is not self-evident that they represent the same concept. For both research and clinical purposes, it is necessary to have measures that can show the extent to which a particular individual shows deviance in each domain. The three domains used are not the only way in which the behaviors may be grouped and subdivided. If subsequent research shows that some other grouping is preferable, the scoring can simply be adjusted to represent the new concept. We are at a stage in which diagnostic distinctions may prove to be of much greater importance than they were in the past because they may reflect different etiologies. It is important that we have diagnostic instruments that are of a kind that allow such distinctions to be made. Those that we have developed have had that purpose very much in mind.

REFERENCES

American Psychiatric Association. (1980). *Diagnostic and Statistical Manual of Mental Disorders—DSM-III* (3rd ed.). Washington, D.C.: American Psychiatric Association.

American Psychiatric Association. (1987). *Diagnostic and Statistical Manual of Mental Disorders—DSM-III* (3rd ed., rev.). Washington, D.C.; American Psychiatric Association.

Attwood, T. (1986). Do autistic children have unique learning problems. *Communication, 20,* 9–11.

August, G. J., Steward, M. A., & Tsai, L. (1981). The incidence of cognitive disabilities in the siblings of autistic children. *British Journal of Psychiatry, 138,* 416–22.

Baron-Cohen, S. (1988). Social and pragmatic deficits in autism. *Journal of Autism and Developmental Disorders.*

Baron-Cohen, S., Leslie, A. M., & Frith, U. (1985). Does the autistic child have a "theory of mind"?. *Cognition, 21,* 37–46.

Baron-Cohen, S., Leslie, A. M. & Frith, U. (1986). Mechanical, behavioral and intentional understanding of picture stories in autistic children. *The British Journal of Developmental Psychology, 4,* 113–25.

Bartak, L., Rutter, M. & Cox, A. (1975). A comparative study of infantile autism and specific developmental receptive language disorder. I. The children. *British Journal of Psychiatry, 126,* 127–42.

Bemporad, J. R. (1979). Adult recollections of a formerly autistic child. *Journal of Autism and Developmental Disorders, 9,* 179–98.

Bregman, J. D., Dykens, E., Watson, M., Ort, S. I., & Leckman, J. F. (1987). Fragile X syndrome: Variability of phenotypic expression. *Journal of the American Academy of Child and Adolescent Psychiatry, 26,* 463–71.

Brown, G. W., & Rutter, M. (1966). The measurement of family activities and relationships: A methodological study. *Human Relations, 19,* 241–63.

Brown, W. T., Jenkins, E. C., Cohen, I. L., Fisch, G. S., Wolf-Schein, E. G., Gross, A., Waterhouse, L., Fein, D., Mason-Brothers, A., Ritvo, E., *et al.* (1985). Fragile X and autism: A multicenter survey. *American Journal of Medical Genetics, 23,* 341–52.

Cromer, R. F. (1987). Language acquisition. In W. Yule & M. Rutter (Eds.), *Language Development and Disorders.* (Clinics in Developmental Medicine, No 101/102). London: MacKeith Press/ Blackwell Scientific.

Ekman, P., & Friesen, W. V. (1976). *Pictures of facial affect.* Palo Alto, CA: Consulting Psychologist Press.

Fleiss, J. L. (1986). *The design and analysis of clinical experiments.* New York: Wiley.

Folstein, S. & Rutter, M. (1977). Infantile autism: A genetic study of 21 twin pairs. *Journal of Child Psychology and Psychiatry, 18,* 297–321.

Folstein, S. & Rutter, M. (1987). Family aggregation and genetic implication. In E. Schopler & G. Mesibov (Eds.), *Neurobiological issues in autism* (pp. 83–105). New York: Plenum.

Gillberg, C. (1985). Asperger's syndrome and recurrent psychosis—A case study. *Journal of Autism and Developmental Disorders, 15,* 389–97.

Graham, P. & Rutter, M. (1968). The reliability and validity of the psychiatric assessment of the child. II. Interview with the parent. *British Journal of Psychiatry, 114,* 581–92.

Hagberg, B., Aicardi, J., Dias, K., & Ramos, O. (1983). A progressive syndrome of autism, dementia, ataxia and loss of purposeful hand use in girls: Rett's syndrome: Report of 35 cases. *Annals of Neurology, 14,* 471–9.

Hermelin, B., & O'Connor, N. (1970). *Psychological experiments with autistic children.* Oxford: Pergamon.

Hobson, R. P. (1983). The autistic child's recognition of age-related features of people, animal and things. *British Journal of Developmental Psychology, 1,* 343–52.

Hobson, R. P. (1984). Early childhood autism and the question of egocentrism. *Journal of Autism and Developmental Disorders, 14,* 85–104.

Hobson, R. P. (1986). The autistic child's appraisal of expressions of emotion. *Journal of Child Psychology and Psychiatry, 27,* 321–42.

Hobson, R. P. (1988). Beyond cognition: A theory of autism. In G. Dawson (Ed.), *New perspectives on diagnosis, nature and treatment.* New York: Guilford.

Le Couteur, A., Rutter, M., Lord, C., Rios, P., Robertson, S., Holdgrafter, M., & McLennen, J. D. (in press). Autism diagnostic interview: A standardized investigator-based instrument. *Journal of Autism and Developmental Disorders.*

Le Couteur, A., Rutter, M., Summers, D., & Butler, L. (in press). Letter: Fragile X in female autistic twins. *Journal of Autism and Developmental Disorders.*

Lockyer, L., & Rutter, M. (1969). A five to fifteen year follow up study of infantile psychosis. IV. Patterns of cognitive ability. *British Journal of Social and Clinical Psychology, 9,* 152–63.

Lord, C., Rutter, M., Goode, S., Heemsbergen, J., Jordan, J., Mawhood, L., & Schopler, E. (in press). Autism diagnostic observation schedule: A standardized observation of communictive and social behaviour. *Journal of Autism and Developmental Disorders.*

Macdonald, H., Rutter, M., Howlin, P., Rios, P., Le Couteur, A., Evered, C., & Folstein, S. (1988). Recognition and expression of emotional cues in autistic and normal adults. Submitted.

Olsson, B., & Rett, A. (1985). Behavioral observations concerning differential diagnosis between the Rett syndrome and autism. *Brain Development, 7,* 281–9.

Quinton, D., Rutter, M., & Rowlands O. (1976). An evaluation of an interview assessment of marriage. *Psychological Medicine, 6,* 577–86.

Reiss, A. L., Feinstein, C., & Rosenbaum, K. N. (1986). Autism and genetic disorders, *Schizophrenia Bulletin, 12,* 724–38.

Rutter, M., & Brown, G. W. (1966). The reliability and validity of measures of family life and relationships in families containing a psychiatric patient, *Social Psychiatry, 1,* 38–53.

Schopler, E. (1985). Editorial: Convergence of learning disability, higher-level autism and Asperger's syndrome. *Journal of Autism and Developmental Disorders, 115,* 359.

Szatmari, P., Bartolucci, G., Finlayson, A., & Krames, L. (1986). A vote for Asperger's syndrome. *Journal of Autism and Developmental Disorders, 16,* 515–17.

Wing, L. (1981). Asperger's syndrome: A clinical account. *Psychological Medicine, 11,* 115–30.

Wing, L., & Gould, J. (1979). Severe impairments of social interaction and associated abnormalities in children: Epidemiology and classification. *Journal of Autism and Developmental Disorders, 9,* 11–30.

Witt-Engerstrom, I., & Gillberg, C. (1987). Rett syndrome in Sweden. *Journal of Autism and Developmental Disorders, 17,* 149–50.

Wolff, S., & Barlow, A. (1979). Schizoid personality in childhood: A comparative study of schizoid, autistic and mentally retarded children. *Journal of Child Psychology and Psychiatry, 20,* 29–46.

Wolff, S., & Chick, J. (1980). Schizoid personality in childhood: A controlled follow-up study. *Psychological Medicine, 10,* 85–100.

World Health Organization. (1978). *International Classification of Diseases* (9th rev.). Geneva: World Health Organization.

World Health Organization. (1987). *ICD-10 1986 Draft of Chapter V: Categories F00–F99 Mental, Behavioural and Developmental Disorders.* Geneva: World Health Organization.

17

Assessment in the Classroom

GARY B. MESIBOV, MARIAN TROXLER, and SUSAN BOSWELL

INTRODUCTION

The assessment of a handicapped child usually consists of a careful examination of individual strengths and weaknesses, with the goal of understanding that particular youngster and developing the most appropriate individualized educational program for him/her. There are many ways of accomplishing this, and a wide variety of assessment instruments have been developed to facilitate the process. Recently, some theorists have begun to question the value of this process and to ask whether assessment is a necessary or even desirable adjuct to providing educational and treatment services to handicapped children and their families.

Prominent operant behavioral theorists have been in the forefront of these debates. For example, Lovass (1977) argues that elaborate assessments of skills and underlying deficits are irrelevant because the emphasis should be on controlling and manipulating the present behavior. An in-depth analysis of the behavior, environment, and eliciting conditions should give one adequate information for appropriate behavioral interventions and make individualized assessments unnecessary.

Functional theorists have also claimed that assessing individual abilities and skills is inappropriate (Brown, Branston, Hamre-Nietupski, Pumpion, Certo & Gruenewald, 1979; Donnellan, 1980). These investigators argue that assessing individual strengths and deficits is often incompatible with a more functional approach because it leads to pursuing irrelevant instructional objectives. They see a direct connection between the assessment of developmental levels and some of the inappropriate classroom activities frequently observed with autistic children such as learning how to touch their noses.

The position of the TEACCH Program is somewhat different (Schopler & Mesibov, 1983; Schopler, Reichler & Lansing, 1980). It differs from the operant behavioral approach in suggesting an emphasis on developing appropriate skills rather than focusing on behaviors, especially inappropriate behaviors. According to the TEACCH view, the problem with

GARY B. MESIBOV • Division TEACCH, University of North Carolina at Chapel Hill, Chapel Hill, North Carolina 27599-7180.   MARIAN TROXLER and SUSAN BOSWELL • Millbrook Elementary School, Raleigh, North Carolina 27609.

eliminating behavior is that, generally, inadequate attention is devoted to developing appropriate alternatives. For example, autistic children's self-stimulatory behaviors are not viewed as the problem, but rather a symptom. The problem is that these youngsters do not have appropriate alternatives, which suggests that interventions should be focused on developing these.

Our approach at Division TEACCH also disputes the functionalists critique of assessment and the resulting developmental programs. While it is true that an emphasis on assessment and an overreliance on developmental norms have led some investigators to pursue irrelevant objectives, this is not an inevitable consequence of this process. In fact, careful assessments and a thorough understanding of developmental levels can improve functioning in all environments. For example, an understanding of individual strengths, interests, and weaknesses does not preclude the class trip to McDonalds, but rather can make it much more interesting and productive for everyone involved. Therefore, not only do we state that careful assessments are important, but we do not see how one can comply with the mandates of P.L. 94-142 for individualized education for handicapped youngsters without them.

The purpose of this chapter is to describe how assessment techniques can facilitate effective interventions in a classroom. The chapter will begin with a discussion of the reasons for, and the importance of, the assessment process and a description of what should be assessed. Discussions of different aspects of the assessment process will follow including an examination of deficits, strengths, interests, long-range needs, and curriculum areas. Specific case studies will be used throughout to highlight the major issues.

WHY ASSESS

Careful assessments are helpful adjuncts to any treatment or educational program because they provide specific information about individual strengths and needs. However, these assessments are especially important and, in fact, indispensable for those working with autistic clients because of their need for individualization. Although everyone obviously benefits from an individualized approach to learning, autistic youngsters are unable to function without it. Therefore, assessments designed to identify idiosyncratic learning styles are essential.

The wide scatter of abilities demonstrated by these youngsters is the first reason why thorough assessments and individualization are important. With most nonhandicapped youngsters or even those with disabilities other than autism, one often can assume a child's level of functioning on one skill from that child's performance in a related area. For example, children who are better readers generally have longer attention spans and are less distractible than those with more limited reading ability. They also tend to perform longer on language tasks. However, related abilities in autistic children are more variable and much less likely to be highly correlated. Knowing that an autistic child reads well often does not tell much about that child's attention span, language skills, or ability to work independently. Therefore, it is essential with these youngsters to assess each specific skill area independently.

A second important reason for thorough assessment and individualization with this population is because the margin of error in teaching them is much smaller. Because of their limited ability to generalize, their high degree of distractibility, and their concreteness, teaching must be precisely geared to each autistic child's individual level of cognitive, social, and language functioning. In addition, teaching approaches must take into account idiosyncratic responses to the environment, other children, noises, visual distractions, and the many other aspects of a classroom environment that might hinder the ability of an autistic child to learn. The best way to take the various learning variables into account and to relate them to each child's special problems is to base instructional planning on careful assessment.

The importance of a careful assessment and individualization is not unique to autistic children. One could argue that all handicapped youngsters, and even those without handicaps, could benefit from this as well. We would certainly not deny this conclusion. However, the difference between autistic and nonautistic youngsters is not in which group will benefit from careful assessments. The difference is in the wide scatter of abilities and the difficulties in generalizing and abstracting that characterize autistic children and make this assessment process essential because they cannot learn without it. Although other youngsters might benefit similarly from careful assessments, their abilities are more closely correlated with one another, and they are better able to tolerate deviations from an ideal teaching strategy. This process is desirable, although not essential for learning to occur in nonautistic youngsters.

WHAT TO ASSESS

Since the beginning of the TEACCH Program the major emphasis has been on assessing both the child's deficits and scattered or emerging skills (Schopler & Reichler, 1979; Schopler, Reichler & Lansing, 1980). The strategy was to identify deficit areas as well as potential strengths and interests showing promise for remediation. Our assessments were designed to identify emerging skills which were existing deficits that showed potential for growth and development. Those deficits showing less potential for remediation were not worked on as directly and we developed the strategy of altering the environment to minimize the detrimental effects of these nonemerging skills.

For example, a child who matches colors inconsistently might be showing an emerging readinesss to learn this concept and the educational program would emphasize various color matching tasks. On the other hand, an extremely visually distractible child with no signs of developing this skill might need an isolated work area in a corner of the room without visual stimuli so as to minimize the effects of this deficit. Tasks for this child would not require any color-matching ability.

Our early approach and collaboration with parents also made us aware that the classroom does not exist in a vacuum. For example, one student in a classroom was developing interactive play skills with an adult while the parents at home were expressing a strong need for quiet solitary play skills so that they could complete their necessary chores and have time with their children. Situations like this helped us to realize the need for a second source of information if we were to program appropriately for our children. This is why our assessment of individual autistic deficits was combined with an assessment of the parents' home needs.

The third element of our program began to emerge after Division TEACCH had been in existence for about a decade. At this point, we began to see changes in the needs of those students who had been quite young when the program began. As these children grew up, we began to see how they functioned as adolescents and adults, giving us important information about the skills we were teaching. For example, for several years we attempted to teach lower-functioning autistic students how to count objects. This was a deficit that seemed amenable to intervention and many families believed that it was very important. However, although we were able to teach many youngsters to count rotely in one-to-one teaching situations, the children were not usually able to generalize this skill to new materials or to a general conceptual understanding. Given the amount of time and effort that had gone into teaching this skill, we were surprised to learn that our lower-functioning clients who were moving into sheltered workshop settings were not required to count at all. We found that they used jigs, which are visual, concrete, and therefore easier for autistic people to understand. Consequently, now we generally use jigs in place of numerical concepts for lower-functioning children in our classrooms.

In summary, assessment is only important as it relates to developing and implementing individualized program objectives. Over the past two decades, Division TEACCH has developed an assessment process that is designed to look at three major sources of information: deficits characteristic of autism as well as individual strengths and interests, the needs of the family, school and/or work setting, and the skills that will be needed to maximize adult functioning. We will now address each of these areas separately.

CHARACTERISTIC DEFICITS, STRENGTHS, AND INTERESTS

Some of the deficits of autism can most clearly be illustrated by describing the behavior of a 12-year-old autistic student. During the afternoon group activity, Tom is playing Bingo with 4th- to 5th-grade nonhandicapped students. Even though the other students are talking and watching each other's progress with interest, Tom's eyes are glued to his own gameboard. After each number is called, he repeats the number with the word "yes" if he has it on his card and "no" if he does not (e.g., "yes B-14") but makes no other comments or conversation. When Tom wins the game the child beside him has to point this out and direct him to say "BINGO."

This typical example shows many of the characteristic deficits of autism. The ability to relate socially to others, which comes so naturally to nonhandicapped children, is totally lacking. This is especially obvious with Tom during the Bingo game because he has trouble focusing on more than one thing at a time. He rigidly adheres to the rules of the game once he is able to understand them, repeating the rote phrases that were used to teach him how to play. He uses no spontaneous or social language. Although able to follow the rules of the game appropriately, Tom does not have an overall concept of the purpose of playing games (e.g., winning, having fun, competing).

Anyone working with autistic clients must look for these and other characteristic deficit areas as well as the uneven pattern across skills. Only a strong assessment component will allow one to observe these facets that are so important if we are to effectively individualize for these students. In discussing the scatter of abilities, many people only emphasize cognitive areas such as strong math skills but weak verbal comprehension. Although it is important to assess these areas and how they differ from one another in autistic children, it is equally important to assess individual and interpersonal characteristics that can often effect the learning process:

1. Poor social relatedness, which affects responsivity to social reinforcement as well as the ability to function in groups and process interpersonal messages.
2. In addition to language difficulties, problems with communication and the social use of language (many autistic children also have difficulty sequencing and understanding the concept of causality).
3. Difficulty forming concepts and understanding abstract ideas.

4. Lack of internal structures, which makes self-direction, self-control, and self-motivation quite difficult (structures must initially be imposed from the outside if autistic people are to learn how to organize themselves).

5. Inability to generalize learned behaviors to new situations (autistic children respond to subtle environmental variations and a concept learned in one setting must frequently be taught in other settings).

6. Inability to process auditory information (autistic people are generally visual learners).

7. Behavior showing little spontaneity, with a strong need for routine and sameness (their behavior is frequently perservative and rote without understanding meanings or functions).

FAMILY NEEDS

The next source of information crucial to a comprehensive assessment is input from the parents. This input may consist of needs within the home or any other information that the parents can provide. Parents are especially good resources for information about children's likes and dislikes. Sometimes the structure of a classroom does not give children enough time, opportunities, or flexibility for the teacher to have a thorough understanding of what they really enjoy. For example, parents are sometimes very helpful in providing information about reinforcers for children who are hard to reward. A parent might know of a fascination with Sesame Street characters, a favorite song, or a preferred activity. Many effective reward systems start with discussing preferred activities in the home.

In working with parents to coordinate needs for their child, there is frequently significant overlap between their needs and what is being done in the classroom. Areas of particular overlap include self-help skills, communication skills, play and leisure skills, and social behavior. Home is the primary setting where skills taught in the classroom are actually used. Therefore, it is crucial that our programming efforts with autistic children accurately reflect family needs. Teachers will be more effective, if they develop systems at school that can also be used at home. This can only be accomplished if there is ongoing and effective communication between the home and the school.

The family can also be of assistance in structuring the environment around the deficits of an autistic child. In our work with these children, we often find that they can improve but that certain fundamental deficits related to the autism syndrome can never be totally eliminated. In these situations, it becomes necessary to reorganize the environment so as to minimize the adverse effects of these fundamental deficits. Parents can be extremely important allies in restructuring environments.

LONG-RANGE NEEDS

The third source of information for appropriate programming with autistic youngsters is the long-range needs of the students. By looking ahead at their potential living and work settings, we are getting direction for realistic functional programming. Because Division TEACCH works with autistic children at all age levels, we continue to follow our youngsters into adulthood and this longitudinal follow-up information helps us to develop functional programs for our younger children. For example, we know of a 22-year-old autistic adult who works in a sheltered workshop. His mother drives him there each morning and picks him up each afternoon. Upon arriving at work, he puts his lunch and coat away, punches in with a timeclock, and gets his pictured work schedule indicating what his tasks for the morning will be (i.e., folding boxes, stuffing pamphlets). While working, he runs out of materials and asks his supervisor for help by showing her a designated picture card. When the bell rings for break time, he puts his work away and heads to the vending machine. He gets money from his wallet (his mother has put in the correct change that morning) and makes his snack selection. For the rest of break time, he entertains himself with a few of his legos. At the next bell, he cleans up and goes back to check his pictured work schedule for his next task.

The above description of Matt at work illustrates the kinds of functional skills and adaptive behaviors autistic students should be learning in the classroom. While years could be spent teaching colors and shapes, it seems more appropriate to look ahead to the skills that will most likely be needed in adult settings. By age 10 or 11, a child's strengths, weak-nessess, skills, and interests in light of future possibilities should suggest appropriate direc-tions for our programming efforts.

Although we cannot be certain of a child's future at age 10, we can identify certain competencies that will be needed in most postschool environments. These include:

1. A communication system that is as universally understandable and accessible as possible
2. The ability to follow some type of schedule or routine independently
3. Appropriate work skills at as high a level as possible
4. As many appropriate social and interpersonal behaviors as possible
5. Independent self-care
6. As many leisure skills for free time as possible

CURRICULUM AREAS

Curriculum areas in the TEACCH Program are consistent with our assessment instru-ments, the PEP (Schopler & Reichler, 1979) and the AAPEP (Mesibov, Schopler, Schaffer & Landrus, 1988). The PEP identifies the most important developmental skills which are the major focus of our parent training intervention efforts with younger children (Schopler & Reichler, 1971). These skills include: Imitation, Perception, Fine Motor Skills, Gross Motor Skills, Eye-Hand Integration, Cognitive Performance Skills, and Cognitive Verbal Skills.

The PEP also helps us to examine deficit areas characteristic of autism such as problems with Affect, Relating, Use of Materials, Sensory Modes, and Language. These deficits are analyzed on the Pathology Scale which is designed to help the examiner identify charac-teristics of autism that are important to understand for developing effective intervention programs.

As autistic children leave their homes and enter public schools, their needs and our priorities start to shift. In addition to traditional topics like arithmetic, reading, spelling, etc., the focus of our intervention efforts at this stage is highlighted by the AAPEP, our assessment instrument for adolescents and adults. The new priorities that are reflected in the AAPEP are designed to help maintain autistic people in community-based programs as adults and include Vocational Skills, Independent Functioning, Leisure Skills, Vocational Behaviors, Functional Communication, and Interpersonal Skills. Within each of these major skill areas, our curriculum content is determined by the deficits of autism, the needs of the family, and our long-range goals based on experiences with autistic people who have grown up.

Our major goals under vocational skills include a variety of work skills (sorting, matching to jigs, using simple tools), fine motor and eye-hand integration skills, functional academics (i.e., recognizing restroom and exit signs), and gross motor skills. Independent functioning skills include locomotion, moving independently within a circumscribed area, and home skills such as vacuuming, washing dishes, and cleaning clothes. Leisure and play skills are appropriate use of materials, ability to entertain oneself independently, and participation in interactive activities. Work behaviors includes understanding task completion, working for tokens or rewards, remaining on task without intensive supervision, and the ability to follow a schedule. Functional communication involves requesting needs, and expressing desires, following simple directions, making concrete choices, asking for help, and indicating task completion. Finally, our interpersonal behaviors include developing social routines, simple greetings and appropriate facial expressions, cooperative behaviors, and the enjoyment of other people.

To this point, we have discussed some of the basics of our assessment philosophy and the areas that are important to assess. Because of the nature of the autistic deficits and our desire to prepare these clients for community-based functioning, the skills we have targeted are very concrete and specific. In addition, they stress functionality, suggesting a particular type of assessment process. These considerations lead us to assess skills in as natural a setting as possible so that we might be able to consider contextual cues and natural consequences. We have found it important to consider environmental cues as carefully as the specific skills under consideration. Learning styles and strategies are also important to note when working with autistic children.

Following our individualized assessments of strengths, interests, and deficits from the perspectives of families and long-range needs, our informal classroom assessments follow two basic strategies: observations in natural settings and task analysis. Through careful observation, one develops a comprehensive understanding of the environment in which a specific behavior normally occurs. An example might be giving a child his or her clothing in the bathroom and seeing what follows. If the child simply remains seated on the floor, the teacher repeats the situation giving more cues. This should not be viewed simply as a pass—fail testing situation but rather as an information-seeking process. The observation is next designed to see if additional cues produce an emerging skill. The next step might be to pick up the shirt and hand it to the student. If the student takes it and lifts it over the child's own head but is unsuccessful in pulling it down, we have then identified an emerging skill and the place to begin our teaching efforts.

Task analysis is the second strategy used as part of our informal classroom assessments. We use this term broadly, considering more than simply a breakdown of skills in particular sequences. The sequences that are developed are used only as guidelines for our observations, designed to pinpoint where problems are occurring and where skills are emerging.

The strategies of naturalistic observations and task analysis are used to form initial classroom objectives. These objectives represent the beginning of a dynamic process. The teacher must continually assess, develop objectives, teach, reassess, and adjust the objectives as needed. With each reassessment parental needs and information must be updated, goals for future placements must be reevaluated, and the child's particular autistic deficits must be considered. The process proceeds indefinitely and is never static.

EXAMPLES

A few examples might help clarify this process. The first is Ted, a high-functioning, verbal, 7-year-old autistic boy, and the curriculum area under consideration is functional academics–writing. Reports from the PEP have provided the teacher with important information relevant to this target area. In the fine-motor and eye-hand integration areas, he demonstrates a mature grasp, cooperative hand use, the ability to copy the numbers 0 and 1, and the emerging ability to copy a triangle and a square. Cognitively he identifies his letters and numbers and shows an emerging ability to copy his name. His work behaviors include good attention span, good organizational skills, the ability to discriminate effectively, and a rigid approach to tasks.

The parents corroborated the major PEP findings and added that their son enjoys coloring. An important goal for them would be to have their child learn how to write. Writing also seemed reasonable from the perspective of long-term goals for this child. The ability to master this skill is realistic given his high level of cognitive functioning.

After combining the PEP information, parental input, and long range goals to identify writing as a realistic, appropriate and desirable objective, the strategies of naturalistic observation and task analysis are used as our assessment–teaching–reassessment process evolves. We start with one of the standard developmental sequences of writing skills and then make adjustments according to the considerations outlined in this chapter. For example, copying diamonds is generally one of the steps in the developmental sequence for writing skills. However, although it might be at his level developmentally, this is a meaningless task for most autistic youngsters. On the other hand, writing numbers is developmentally higher than copying diamonds but more meaningful for many autistic children and usually an area of strength. Therefore, the normal developmental sequence of first copying diamonds and then numbers might be altered by eliminating the diamonds for most autistic youngsters.

During our naturalistic observations, we also look for information that will help us to adopt appropriate teaching strategies. For most children, the ability to write horizontal and vertical lines comes before the ability to write diagonal and curved lines. This was also true of Ted, so we directed him to write the letter T. However, he was unable to do this. Our next step was to add cues as both a teaching strategy and an assessment strategy because they provided us with additional information about his skill level. The first cue was the teacher's writing the letter T and asking Ted to copy it. He was still unable to do this and was then given dots to trace in the form of the letter T. He was successful at this level.

The next step was to begin programming. We began with a teaching objective of copying two-stroke configurations. Alphabet letters fitting into this category were T, L, V. As these letters were mastered, the next steps were to include writing three-stroke straight line letters (H, I, F, N), adding a curve or circle (P, B, D), and copying a longer sequence of mastered letters. This sequence of assessing, developing objectives, teaching, reassessing, and revising the objectives and teaching strategies is a dynamic process that continues and is used for all areas of a child's individualized curriculum.

A second example of this assessment process in the area of language and communication is a low-functioning nonverbal 5-year-old student named Alan. The most relevant PEP information is that he has no imitation skills but does some babbling. During the administration of the PEP, he led the examiner to the door to get out of the room (a form of communication), responded to verbal commands and gesturing to "sit down," and was inhibited by "no." Cognitively, the child has no matching skills. His relating and play skills suggested minimal interest in materials, some exploration of the room, crying when demands were made to sit down, and giggling in response to swinging, physical play, and bubbles.

The parents reported that he moves their hands to request desired objects and cries out in protest to reject undesirable objects. They also provided the teacher with a list of preferred activities including eating, outside play, sand, and water. The parents wanted their child to make his wishes known to others in order to reduce his frustration level.

In terms of long range needs, a functional communication system is essential if one is to have any meaningful contacts in community-based living and working environments. The development of such a system, no matter how basic, is always a major priority for a lower-functioning child.

Having collected the information on Alan's deficits, parental perspectives, and long-range needs, the next step is to combine naturalistic observations with the task analysis process. While there is considerable information available about the natural development of language and usual developmental sequences, much of it is not applicable to autistic children because of their atypical language development. Division TEACCH has developed a communication curriculum for low functioning children, emphasizing communicative intent, which is the basis of our naturalistic observations and task analyses in this area (Watson, 1985). The system examines the autistic child's attempts at communication and builds upon those, rather than imposing a communication structure that is inconsistent with the minimal communication ability the child already has.

In our initial analysis of this young boy's attempts at communication, we observed only crying and hand-leading behaviors, generally consistent with the parents' reports and the PEP. Our analysis of these communicative intents showed their function to be either rejecting or requesting objects. Additional observations suggested situations involving food were most likely to elicit communication from Alan. These observations suggested to us that the focus of our initial programming efforts should be on replacing crying and pushing away with more acceptable modes of communication in contexts involving food.

The next step was to determine an acceptable mode of communication (e.g., pictures, speech, signs, objects). Because our goal was to change Alan's mode of communication to a more acceptable one, it was especially important to keep the content and situations the same. Autistic children become confused quite easily, so it is essential to keep as many aspects of a situation as consistent as possible. Once Alan is able to use an alternative communication system (e.g., pictures), we will move on to teaching other concepts (e.g., asking to play with sand, water, or a favorite toy), and to other settings (e.g., outside).

CONCLUSION

The assessment of any child, whether in the classroom or the clinic, does not have to be an irrelevant or nonfunctional activity. If done thoughtfully and reasonably, it can be a crucial ingredient of an educational program, especially for autistic children demonstrating such widely scattered skills and abilities. This chapter has explored some of the issues around the classroom assessment process and emphasized the need to examine characteristic deficits, parental desires, and long-range needs. We have also argued for a dynamic process of assessment, development of objectives, teaching, reassessment, and adjustment of the teaching objectives and strategies as needed. Professionals working with autistic children in classroom situations should find this process extremely helpful in developing the truly individualized curricula and teaching approaches that are essential for autistic children to achieve their full potential.

REFERENCES

Donnellan, A. M. (1980). An educational perspective of autism: Implications for curriculum development and personnel development. In B. Wilcox & A. Thompson (Eds.), *Critical issues in educating autistic children and youth*. Washington, D.C.: U. S. Department of Education.

Brown, L., Branston, M., Hamre-Nietupski, S., Pumpion, I., Certo, N., & Gruenewald, L. (1979). A strategy for developing chronological age appropriate, functional curriculum for severely handicapped adolescents and adults. *Journal of Special Education, 13*, 81–90.

Loovas, O. I. (1977). *The autistic child*. New York: Irvington.

Mesibov, G. B., Schopler, E., Schaffer, B., & Landrus, R. (1988). *Individualized assessment and treatment for autistic and developmentally disabled children. Vol. 4. Adolescent and adult psychoeducational profile (AAPEP)*. Austin, TX: Pro-Ed.

Schopler, E., & Mesibov, G. B. (Eds.) (1983). *Autism in adolescents and adults*. New York: Plenum.

Schopler, E., & Reichler, R. J. (1971). Parents as co-therapists in the treatment of psychotic children. *Journal of Autism and Childhood Schizophrenia, 1*, 87–102.

Schopler, E., & Reichler, R. J. (1979). *Individualized assessment and treatment of autistic and developmentally disabled children. Vol. I: Psychoeducational profile (2nd ed.)*. Austin, TX: Pro-Ed.

Schopler E., Reichler, R. J. & Lansing, M. (1980). *Individualized assessment and treatment of autistic and developmentally disabled children. Vol. 2, Teaching strategies for parents and professionals* (2nd ed.). Austin, TX: Pro-Ed.

Watson, L. R. (1985). The TEACCH communication curriculum. In E. Schopler & G. B. Mesibov (Eds.), *Communication problems in autism*. (pp. 187–206). New York: Plenum.

18

Diagnosis and Assessment of Preschool Children

LINDA R. WATSON and LEE M. MARCUS

INTRODUCTION

Our purpose in this chapter is to provide a clinically useful discussion of the diagnosis and assessment of preschool children with autism and related disorders. The syndrome of autism is by definition a disorder which is first manifested during the preschool years, usually prior to thirty months of age (American Psychiatric Association, 1980; National Society for Autistic Children, 1978; Rutter, 1978). Thus, child development professionals in various fields need to recognize the symptoms of the condition in preschool-age children, and be prepared to assess the skills and needs of these children and their families.

It is our belief that an early diagnosis of autism has potential benefits for both children and parents. The discussion in this chapter draws heavily on our experiences in Division TEACCH (*T*reatment and *E*ducation of *A*utistic and related *C*ommunication-handicapped *CH*ildren), a statewide program in North Carolina established to provide services to children with autism and related handicaps and their families (Schopler & Olley, 1982). In the vast majority of cases, preschool children referred to Division TEACCH have been previously identified as exhibiting some developmental disability. The most typical prior diagnoses are language delay, pervasive developmental disorders, and mental retardation or global developmental delay. Such diagnoses are also accompanied by a recognition of the need for services. At times questions are raised about the desirability of further labeling the child with a diagnosis of autism. If the diagnosis is appropriate, several benefits can be identified.

In the case of the child, a diagnosis of autism implies the need for emphasizing the assessment of certain skills and deficits which might not be addressed as areas of particular concern in a child diagnosed as mentally retarded or language delayed. For the family, there are the benefits of coming to a better understanding of the nature and cause of their child's developmental problems. For both child and family, there is little to be gained through diagnosis and assessment, however, unless there is meaningful intervention available based

---

LINDA R. WATSON and LEE M. MARCUS • Division TEACCH, The University of North Carolina at Chapel Hill, Chapel Hill, North Carolina 27599-7180.

on assessment. Detailed information on the way in which assessment and intervention are linked in the TEACCH program is available in Schopler, Reichler, and Lansing (1980), and Schopler, Lansing, and Waters (1983). Determining what intervention is appropriate and finding such services early is the most important potential benefit of diagnosing a child as autistic during the preschool years.

Although there is relatively little information available to date on the effectiveness of preschool intervention with autistic children, we believe firmly that such intervention can be very effective in facilitating the adaptation of the child to everyday life, and the adaptation of the family to the child. In a recent review of the available studies in this area, Simeonsson, Olley, and Rosenthal (1987) concluded that the most successful intervention programs had the following characteristics: (1) treatment at an early age, (2) intensive behavioral programming, (3) parental involvement, and (4) a focus on communication and social skills. A relatively greater effectiveness of preschool versus later intervention in terms of longer range outcomes is suggested by the results of Fenske, Zalenski, Krantz, and McClannahan (1985). Further program evaluation and research on preschool intervention with autistic children will be helpful in optimizing services for this age group. We suggest that such evaluation and research will probably lead to refinements of the basic characteristics of successful programs as described by Simeonsson et al. (1987), rather than to vastly different models of intervention.

The first sections of this chapter discuss the diagnosis of the autistic syndrome during the preschool years. We have expressed our belief that an early diagnosis is desirable in terms of potential benefits for both the child and the family. An issue that follows from this is the feasibility of early diagnosis of the syndrome, and we begin our discussion of diagnosis by addressing this question.

In the next section on diagnosis, we discuss developmental indices in autism. The preschool period is a time of marked developmental change for nonhandicapped children as well as for children with autism. The child is developing physically as well as cognitively and socially. The implication for diagnosis of the autistic syndrome is that it will be manifested in somewhat different ways, depending on the developmental status of the child. In order to diagnose the syndrome reliably, clinicians need to understand how development normally progresses during the preschool years, and also how the syndrome of autism may be exhibited in children at various ages across this time period.

The third section of the chapter is concerned with different courses of development in autism. Different patterns of onset of autistic characteristics occur in preschool children with this syndrome. Being aware of these different courses will reduce confusion in diagnosing the condition which could otherwise result from being confronted with children who have markedly different early developmental histories.

In the sections on assessment of autistic children, we address assessment in different developmental domains, including social, communicative, cognitive, and motoric development, as well as the assessment of medical factors and family needs. Each assessment area is first discussed in terms of the content of assessment for that domain. Then strategies which can be used to assess the domain are described, including both formal test instruments where appropriate and informal assessment strategies.

The last major section of the chapter is concerned with some of the clinical implications of the diagnosis and assessment of preschool children with autism. There are some special opportunities and challenges of working with children in this age group and their families, which are considered in this section.

DIAGNOSIS

Early Identification and Diagnosis

Related to the issue of the importance of early diagnosis is the question of the feasibility of identifying this condition before the age of two or three years. Kanner's original group was diagnosed at age 5 and up, even though the symptoms were described as present during the preschool years (Kanner, 1943). Developmental and mental health specialists often complain that autism is difficult to distinguish from other developmental or related problems in the early years. Yet, clinical experience within TEACCH and other programs and empirical evidence (Volkmar, Cohen & Paul, 1986) indicate that the primary characteristics of autism are apparent before 30 months in the large majority of later diagnosed cases, and that typically parents are aware of a significant problem in development by 18 months. Retrospective reports and clinical data suggest that delays and deviancies in language development and impairments in social relatedness differentiate autistic children from other referred children during the preschool years (Rescorla, 1986). In addition, a high proportion of children later diagnosed autistic show a range of bizarre behavioral patterns typical of this population. It is evident, then, that with appropriate methods and an understanding of the basic problems in autism, professionals should be able to make a reliable diagnosis during the preschool years.

One possible source of confusion are the different diagnostic categories for children with severe developmental problems, an issue not unique to the preschool-aged population. While DSM-III has somewhat simplified and objectified the classification, the inclusion of Childhood Onset Pervasive Developmental Disorders and Atypical Pervasive Developmental Disorders has served to cloud the diagnostic picture of autism. The Yale studies (Dahl, Cohen & Provence, 1986) suggest that the main differences among these groups, based on data of the preschool population, are degrees of impairment rather than qualitative distinctions. It may be clinically more useful to consider these different groups of "atypical" children along a continuum with a common set of basic dysfunctions rather than as suffering from disparate conditions requiring completely unique interventions.

The diagnosis of autism should be based on direct observation of the child during both structured and unstructured periods, parent report, and information from related sources, such as medical records, school observations, and other professionals. In the TEACCH program, the Childhood Autism Rating Scale (Schopler, Reichler & Renner, 1986; see Chapter 11) has been especially useful in assisting in the diagnosis of autism in the preschoolers. This observational scale can be used in conjunction with formal testing and enables the diagnostician to organize data in a clinically objective way. If, through the diagnostic process the child scores in the autism range of the CARS and has manifested the cardinal features of impairments in social relatedness, communication and response to the environment, then a diagnosis of autism can be firmly established.

Developmental Indices

While the broad characteristics and specific symptoms of autism have been widely discussed, less is understood or documented about developmental parameters. Distortions or deviancies in language and social relatedness cannot be assumed to be comparable from infancy through early childhood. The need for age-related indices has been raised by Ritvo and colleagues (Freeman, Ritvo & Schroth, 1984) and attempts to chart developmental steps have been made (Freeman & Ritvo, 1984). Examples of such a sequence involve the consideration of areas of sensorimotor development, speech and language, and relating to people, objects, and events. For example, at 0–6 months the area of speech and language may be characterized by lack of vocalization, and crying not related to needs; by 36–60 months this area may be marked by lack of speech, echolalia, pronoun reversal, abnormal tone and rhythm in speech or unusual thoughts—the major diagnostic features of the disorder as commonly described. With regard to relatedness, at 0–6 months the child may be described as failing to attend to mother and crib toys, and showing no anticipatory social responses, whereas by 36–60 months characteristics may include being upset by changes in routines.

Wing (1981) described "the triad of social and language impairment" seen in children with autism and related disorders, a triad that includes impairments of social interaction, language development, and imaginative abilities. The characteristics of autism described in various diagnostic systems (American Psychiatric Association, 1980; Creak, 1961; National Society for Autistic Children, 1978; Rutter, 1978; Schopler, Reichler & Renner, 1986) can each be related to one of the three major categories of impairment discussed by Wing (1981). Thus, we use Wing's triad as an organizing construct to present the diagnostic characteristics of preschool children with autism. Using this framework, Table I presents information on the development of nonhandicapped children in social interaction, language and communication, and imaginative abilities over the preschool age range. In parallel fashion, Table II summarizes developmental changes in the symptoms of autism during the preschool years, using information from Freeman and Ritvo (1984), DeMyer (1979), Hoshino, Kumashiro, Yashima, Tachibana, Watanabe, and Furudawa (1982), and other sources.

For both nonhandicapped children and autistic children, there are large degrees of individual variation in both rate and specific characteristics of development in these areas. In Table I, we have tried to list markers conservatively; that is, most children would have achieved a given skill by the age at which the marker is listed. For children with autism, there are even wider variations in development. Some children show more extreme overall delays than other children, and the children differ from one another in the developmental profile across areas as well. Also, there is relatively little information available on early development in these children. Thus, neither the markers nor associated ages in Table II should be construed as universals of development in autism. However, even though the empirical evidence is sparse on the issue of developmental markers, clinicians need to be sensitive to both what is expected of normal youngsters in the preschool years, and what constitutes significant deviations from the norm in the major areas of communication, social relatedness, and response to the environment.

Courses of Development

Investigators have usually noted two types of course of early development in the autistic child: either slow and/or deviant development from the outset with delayed milestones and the presence of a range of unusual features; or fairly normal development (at least no strikingly atypical patterns), until the mid- to latter part of the second year of life (DeMyer, 1979; Harper & Williams, 1975; Rutter & Lockyer, 1967). With the second group there is

Table I. Aspects of Normal Development during Preschool Years

Age (mo.)	Social interaction	Language and communication	Imaginative abilities
2	Turns head and eyes to locate sound Social smile	Cooing, vocalic sounds	
6	Reaches in anticipation of being picked up Repeats actions when imitated by adult	Vocal "conversations" or turntaking in face-to-face position with parent Consonant sounds emerging	Undifferentiated actions on one object at a time
8	Differentiates parents from strangers "Give-and-take" object exchange games with adults Peek-a-boo and similar games with a script Shows objects to adults Waves bye-bye Cries and/or crawls after mother when she leaves room	Varies intonation in babbling including questioning intonation Repetitive syllable babbling (ba-ba-ba, ma-ma-ma) Pointing gesture emerging	Actions differentiated in terms of characteristics of objects Use of two objects in combination (not socially appropriate use)
12	Child initiates games with increasing frequency Agent as well as respondent role in turn-taking Increased visual contacting of adults during play with toys	First words emerging Use of jargon with sentencelike intonation Language most frequently used for commenting on environment and vocal play Uses gestures plus vocalizations to get attention, show objects, and make requests	Socially appropriate actions on objects (functional use of objects) Two or more objects related appropriately

(continued)

Table I. continued

Age (mo.)	Social interaction	Language and communication	Imaginative abilities
18	Peer play emerging: showing, offering, taking toys Solitary or parallel play still more typical	3 to 50 word vocabulary Beginning to put two words together Overextension of word meanings (e.g., "daddy" refers to all men) Uses language to comment, request objects and actions, and get attention Also pulls people to get and direct attention May "echo" or imitate frequently	Frequent symbolic acts (pretends to drink, to talk on the toy telephone, etc.) Play tied largely to child's own daily routine Child is agent in pretend play
24	Peer play episodes are brief Peer play more likely to revolve around gross motor activity (e.g., chasing games) than sharing of toys	3 to 5 words combined at times ("telegraphic" speech) Asks simple questions (e.g., Where Daddy? Go bye-bye?) Uses "this" accompanied by pointing gestures Calls self by name rather than "I" May briefly reverse pronouns Cannot sustain topic of conversation Language focuses on here and now	Applies pretend play routines to dolls, stuffed animals, adults (e.g., "feeds" doll) frequently Pretend actions not limited to own routine (e.g., pretends to iron) Sequences of pretend actions develop (feeds doll, rocks, and puts it to bed) Pretend play triggered by available objects
36	Learning turntaking and sharing with peers Episodes of sustained cooperative interaction with peers Altercations between peers are	Vocabulary of about 1000 words Most grammatical morphemes (plural, past tense, prepositions, etc.) used appropriately Echoing infrequent by this age	Symbolic play preplanned—announces intention and searches for needed objects Substitutes one object for another (e.g., block for car)

Age			
	frequent Enjoys helping parents with household chores Enjoys showing-off to make others laugh Wants to please parents	Language increasingly used to talk about "there-and-then" Much questioning, often more to continue interaction than to seek information	Objects treated as agents capable of independent activity (e.g., doll is made to pick up own cup)
48	Negotiates roles with peers in sociodramatic play Has preferred playmates Peers verbally (and sometimes physically) exclude unwelcome children from play	Complex sentence structures used Able to sustain topic of conversation and add new information Will ask others to clarify utterances Adjusts quality of language depending on listener (e.g., simplifies language to 2-year-old)	Sociodramatic play–pretend play with two or more children Use of pantomime to represent needed object (e.g., pretends to pour from absent teapot) Real-life and fantasy themes Child can sustain role for extended period
60	More peer- than adult-oriented Intensely interested in forming friendships Quarreling, name-calling with peers common Able to change role from leader to follower in peer play	More appropriate use of complex structures Generally mature grammatical structure (some problems still with subject/verb agreement, irregular forms, pronoun case, etc.) Ability to judge sentences as grammatical/ungrammatical and make corrections Developing understanding of jokes and sarcasm, recognition of verbal ambiguities Increasing ability to adjust language according to listener's perspective and role	Language is important in establishing theme, negotiating roles, and playing out drama

Table II. Early Development in Autism

Age (mo.)	Social interaction	Language and communication	Imaginative abilities
6	Less active and demanding than non-handicapped infant Minority are extremely irritable Poor eye contact No anticipatory social responses	Crying is difficult to interpret	
8	Difficult to soothe when upset About 1/3 are extremely withdrawn, and may actively reject interaction About 1/3 accept attention but initiate little	Limited or unusual babbling (e.g., squeals or screeches) No imitation of sounds, gestures, expressions	Repetitive motor movements may predominate waking activity
12	Sociability often decreases as child begins to walk, crawl No separation distress	First words may appear, but often not used meaningfully Frequent, loud crying, remains difficult to interpret	
24	Usually differentiates parents from others, but little affection expressed May give hug, kiss as automatic gesture when asked Indifferent to adults other than parents May develop intense fears Prefers to be alone	Fewer than 15 words, usually Words appear, then drop out Gestures do not develop; few point to objects	Little curiosity/exploration of environment Unusual use of toys—spins, flips, lines up objects

	Social	Language/Communication	Play
36	Failure to accept other children Excessive irritability Failure to understand meaning of punishment	Word combinations rare May echo phrases, but no creative language use Odd rhythm, tone, or stress Poor articulation in about half of speaking children 1/2 or more are without meaningful speech Takes parent by hand and leads to object Goes to customary location, and waits to be given object	Mouthing of objects often persists No symbolic play Continuation of repetitive motor movements—rocking, spinning, toewalking, etc. Visual fascinations with objects—stares at lights, etc. Many show relative strength in visual/motor manipulations, such as puzzles
48	Unable to understand rules in peer play	A few combine two-to-three words creatively Echolalia persists; may be used communicatively Mimics TV commercials Makes requests	Functional use of objects Few acts directed to dolls or others; most involve child as agent Symbolic play, if present, limited to simple, repetitive schemes As more sophisticated play skills develop, still spend large amounts of time in less sophisticated activity Many do not combine toys in play
60	More adult than peer-oriented Frequently becomes more sociable, but interactions remain odd, one-sided	No abstract concepts expressed or understood (e.g., time) Failure to carry on conversation Pronouns rarely used correctly Echolalia persists in children with speech Questions rare; if used, repetitive questioning predominates Abnormal tone and rhythm persist	Unable to pantomime No sociodramatic play

often reported a setback, loss of skills, or regressions, especially in the speech and language. Associated with the problems in language come social withdrawal and odd responses to the environment. DeMyer (1979) describes a third possible developmental course: approximately 20% of her sample were described as fairly normal during the first year but then began to lag behind or fail to keep up with normal milestones. This group seems to differ somewhat from the setback group by having a more subtle shift into the developmental disorder. A consistent finding from the literature is the loss of previously acquired speech, including reportedly meaningful language, in a large percentage of autistic children (Creak, 1961; Kurita, 1985; Usudu & Koizumi, 1981). It appears that the prognosis for these children may be poorer than for children who have not shown such regressions in language development (Kurita, 1985; Usuda & Koizumi, 1981).

While many parents suspect early developmental problems, even during the first year, few are sufficiently worried to seek out professional help. It is common for a mother to report retrospectively that her child was a nondemanding, "perfect" baby, only later realizing that this pattern was a sign of social unresponsiveness and lack of alertness to the environment. More typically parents become more concerned during the second year and, according to DeMyer, years 2–4 are the most difficult; probably due to the combined effect of severity of the autistic characteristics, parental worry and feelings of helplessness, and the exhausting search for appropriate professional support.

ASSESSMENT

The purpose of assessment is to provide the information that will form the basis of an intervention plan for the individual child and family. Thus, while in diagnosis we look for a set of features (or syndrome) children with autism have in common, in assessment we look at all areas of development whether they are uniquely affected in autism or not. The goal in assessment is to gain as complete information as possible on the characteristics of the individual child and family. A coherent intervention plan is possible only after detailed information is available on the strengths, weaknesses, and prioritized needs of the child and family.

Although we separate our discussion of assessment conceptually into the domains of social, communication, cognitive, and motor development, these distinctions are somewhat arbitrary. Each domain overlaps with the other domains in significant ways, and it is important both to cover all domains thoroughly in assessment and also to integrate the information from across domains. For example, the information from the social assessment of the child should be considered in light of the child's communication, cognitive, and motoric skills before interpreting the results and formulating recommendations for intervention.

Social Assessment

We consider two major areas in assessing social skills (Olley, 1986). First, we are interested in the motivation and skills of the child in initiating and responding to social interaction. Second, we examine the child's ability to conform to social expectations regarding appropriate behavior, whether interactive or not.

In assessing the child's initiation and response to social interaction, it is relevant to know what devices are at the child's disposal for initiating or maintaining an interaction. We would also like to know how consistent the child's social interaction is in different situations and with different people serving as social partners.

Gaze

One important device normally used by infants and young children for initiating and maintaining social interactions is gaze. There are indications that eye contact is important from the beginning in the formation of bonds of attachment between parent and child, at least from the parent's point of view (Argyle & Cook, 1976; Robson, 1967; Stern, 1974). Eye contact continues to be an important device through which babies get adults to interact with them (Brazelton, 1982; Stern, 1971). Thus, it is important to determine how the autistic child is using gaze, not only for what it says regarding the child's social development, but also for the implications it has for effects on the child's caregivers. Some children may avoid gaze or fail to gaze at others (Richer, 1978; Rutter, 1978; Wing, 1976; Wolff & Chess, 1964). Others may gaze unflinchingly at another person. Still others may use their gaze in a way that is not synchronous with the rest of their interaction (Mirenda, Donnellan & Yoder, 1983).

Unusual eye contact is often just one manifestation of generally unusual patterns of visual attention. Additional social impacts may be observed in the ways the child uses gaze with respect to establishing a joint focus of attention with another person. Does s/he look at an object that is held up or manipulated by the other person? Does s/he follow a pointing gesture, look only at the other person's hand, or fail to attend to the gesture at all? The issue of visual attention should also be considered in the cognitive domain with respect to the child's use of gaze in nonsocial contexts.

Facial Expression

A second device that figures importantly in interactions between parents and their babies and young children is the child's facial expression. Before babies have the ability to intentionally influence the actions of others, parents interpret facial expression such as smiling and frowning or crying, and respond as though their babies are intentionally communicating something (Brazelton, Koslowski & Main, 1974; Oster, 1978). It is believed that this process of attributing intentionality by parents is important in helping babies become intentional in their actions (Schaffer, 1977). The child who has an "expressionless face," a common characteristic of young autistic children as reported by Hoshino *et al.* (1982), or whose facial expressions are at odds with what is expected in a given situation, are at a disadvantage in eliciting and maintaining interaction with others. Showing enjoyment in the approaches of and interaction with others is also important feedback which encourages the child's partners to repeat their efforts to engage him in interaction.

Vocalizations

Vocalizations and verbalizations are also important in initiating and maintaining interaction. As with facial expressions, parents (at least in our culture) attribute meaning to their babies' vocalizations and treat them as conversational "turns" long before there is any reason to believe that the babies intend to communicate something through their vocalizations (Bateson, 1975; Snow, 1977; Stern, 1977). Thus, if a given autistic child vocalizes little as a baby and young child, s/he is lacking prelinguistic behaviors important in regulating early social interactions. In the DeMyer study (1979), many parents reported that their autistic children babbled noticeably less than nonautistic siblings or peers. The assessment of language and communication will be discussed in greater detail later.

Use of Body

The child's body can also be used in a number of ways that facilitate or discourage interaction with others. For instance, Kubicek (1980) described the videotaped interactions between a mother and her 16-week-old twins, one of whom was later diagnosed autistic. In contrast to his brother, this twin turned away and cut off the mother's approach with an abrupt arm movement when his mother attempted to initiate an interaction. In addition, his back was arched, and his arms flexed rigidly.

Some ways in which the child might use his or her body to initiate or respond to social interaction include approaching a person, standing close to a person, molding to another person's body when held, touching another person, leading someone by the hand, pointing at objects in order to direct another person's attention, and so forth. In general, children with autism show fewer such social contacts with both parents and other adults than is the case with normal children (e.g., Sigman & Ungerer, 1984; Sigman, Mundy, Sherman & Ungerer, 1986), but it is important in assessment to observe the behaviors characteristic of the individual child.

Social Attachments

In addition to determining what devices the child has available to use in social interactions with others, another aspect of assessment in this area is to consider the child's interaction with various people. Reports on autistic children are varied in this regard. Most parents report that they have reason to believe their autistic children recognize them and consider them important. However, it is important to assess if and how the child shows that parents are distinguished from other people. Are signs of anxiety apparent upon separating? Does the child show pleasure or other acknowledgement of the parents' return? Is the child more likely to approach and initiate interactions with parents than with unfamiliar adults, and is the child more responsive to parents than to others? (See Sigman & Ungerer, 1984.)

Peer Relations

Impairments in social relations with peers are reported even more consistently among autistic children than impaired relations with adults (Howlin, 1986; Sherman, Shapiro & Glassman, 1983). Perhaps this is because peers are less skillful than adults in accommodating the deficiencies and idiosyncracies of an autistic partner. Interest and skills in initiating and responding to interactions with peers is thus another important area to assess.

Social Situations

In addition to assessing the child's interaction with different people, it is also valuable to determine the types of situations in which the child is most/least likely to interact. Is there more responsiveness when rough-and-tumble play is initiated than during an activity involving looking at a book? Does the child initiate interaction when injured? Assessment of situational factors in interaction can be valuable in determining what serve as social motivators for the child.

Interfering Behaviors

A final issue in the assessment of interaction is the type and level of interfering behavior (Olley, 1986; Volkmar, 1986). To what extent does the child exhibit self-stimulatory behaviors or more complex repetitive routines? And, more importantly, how easily can these behaviors be interrupted to engage the child in social interaction? This can vary greatly within the same child. For example, one 4-year-old we know can be easily disengaged from finger posturing to participate in a social interaction, but interrupting his mirror play is considerably more difficult.

Another characteristic of many autistic children which interferes with social adaptation is difficulty in making transitions from one activity to the next. With some children the problem is so extreme that temper tantrums occur at nearly every point of transition. When transitions are observed or reported to be difficult for a child, the assessment should determine the extent to which this is alleviated by establishing routines of consistently following one type of activity with another type of activity, and also determine the effectiveness of using concrete visual cues to indicate to the child what the next activity will be.

Social Conformity

A second type of social assessment is concerned with conformity to social expectations for appropriate behavior. Appropriate social interacfion is certainly part of this, but noninteractive behaviors are also subject to social expectations. Assessment of this should consider the following factors:

1. Ability to stay in a situation and respect its boundaries (e.g., remain at table during meals, in yard during outdoor play)
2. Appropriate handling of objects and materials (e.g., uses spoon to eat but not to flip; looks through book without ripping pages), and inhibiting handling of taboo objects
3. Appropriate use of body (e.g., approaches visitor, but does not try to climb over him; uses hand for self-feeding but not for finger-posturing at meals)
4. Social appropriateness of vocalizations and verbalizations (e.g., are they interactive? meaningfully related to the context? an appropriate volume? inhibited in situations in which quiet is expected?)

For most children, there will be variation in the appropriateness of behavior from one situation to another, so that it is also important to consider the different contexts that are relevant to a given child's life, such as meals, toileting, traveling in a car, indoor and outdoor play, shopping, family gatherings, preschool classroom, and so forth. The assessment should tap both the child's strengths and deficiencies with respect to appropriate social behavior.

Strategies for Social Assessment

The two major strategies for social assessment are observation and parent interview. In making observations, it is useful to have some defined framework or structure to guide the process. This helps not only in organizing the current observation, but also provides a standard for future reference. Ideally the framework can also serve as a guideline for establishing intervention goals.

Much of the assessment content described above is tapped by the observational procedures outlined in the TEACCH Social Skills Curriculum (Olley, 1986). Although designed for use in a classroom or home setting, the same general scheme can be used in organizing observational information about a child's social behavior in a clinical setting with both parents and examiners. Valuable opportunities for observational assessment in clinical settings arise when the child is separated from and reunited with parents. Our clinical assessment procedures in the TEACCH program also include observation of brief parent/child play sessions.

The Psychoeducational Profile (Schopler & Reichler, 1979) uses observational information to assess social behaviors in the areas of relating, cooperating, and human interest, as well as affect displayed during interaction. Sherman, Shapiro, and Glassman (1983) describe an observational assessment of play which includes consideration of the child's social behavior during play.

Because of contextual limitations of clinical (and educational) settings, it is important to supplement observational information with descriptions gained through parental interview. This process will be described in more detail later, but the interviewer should include questions on the dimensions of social behavior described in this section, with particular emphasis on areas which are difficult to observe adequately in clinical settings, such as peer play, social attachment, and social adaptation to the demands of everyday life. The Vineland Adaptive Behavior Scales (Sparrow, Balla & Cicchetti, 1984) provide more formal data based on interview information regarding many aspects of behavior, including social behavior.

Communication Assessment

Important dimensions of communication assessment include communicative purposes or functions, content, means, and context (Watson, 1985; Watson, Schaffer, Lord & Schopler, in press). These dimensions can be applied to the assessment of expressive and comprehension skills.

There are several reasons for choosing "communication" rather than "language" as the domain of assessment for this group. First, most autistic children seen in their preschool years are not verbal and thus have no formal language skills to assess. Second, there is no way to predict with certainty which nonverbal children will eventually acquire language skills and which will not. Assessment of language skills is limited in that it does not tell us where to start an intervention program for many preschool (and older) children with autism.

Although language skills are often not present, it is rarely the case that a child is totally lacking in the ability to communicate. The assessment of communication is thus more likely to provide some information regarding abilities that can be built on in intervention. By contrast, it is widely recognized that autism involves impairment of not only language abilities, but of the broad range of communicative abilities, both verbal and nonverbal.

Communicative Intent

An initial concern in assessing communication skills is to consider the child's communicative intent. As discussed under social assessment, children exhibit many behaviors that adults "read" in order to determine how the child feels, what s/he wants, and so forth. The behaviors of autistic children (e.g., cries, facial expressions) may be difficult to read, reflecting a basic level of social impairment. In assessing communication skills, however, the concern is not only with whether the child's behavior can be interpreted, but also with whether the child intends for a behavior to communicate something to another person (Hermelin & O'Conner, 1985). There is obviously some subjectivity in making this judgment, but cues such as the child's eye gaze, approaching or contacting another person, or repeating some behavior until another person responds, contribute to our confidence that a child is intentionally directing communication toward another person.

Once the judgment is made regarding intentionality, the next area of assessment is to determine the purposes or functions of a child's intentional communicative behavior. Nonverbal children with autism have been reported to communicate in order to "request" objects or actions from other people, but not in order to draw someone else's attention to an object or scene of interest to the child (Curcio, 1978). Both types of behavior are common in normally developing children by the end of the first year of life. Other sorts of communicative purposes include rejecting something or refusing to participate in an activity, seeking information, giving information, expressing one's feelings, or participating in social/communicative routines.

Communicative Means

A second assessment issue is the child's means of communication. Is communication accomplished through motoric means such as pulling on an adult, leading the adult by the hand, or bringing an object to another person? Does the child use vocal signals to get or direct other people's attention? Are gestures used, such as pointing, shaking or nodding the head, or pantomiming actions? Does the child use pictures, printed words, or signs to communicate? Is speech used communicatively by the child? The communicative means a child is able to use will change developmentally. This is partially related to the cognitive skills of the child. Thus, a child must be able to relate pictures to the objects, people, or activities they represent in order to be able to use pictures as a flexible means of communication. Similarly, children must be capable of symbolic behavior in order to use speech or sign language in more than a rote way.

In examining the child's communicative means, it is important to consider how complex and how flexible the child's communicative system is. For instance, for a child using motoric communication, one would like to know if two or more actions are chained together at times in order to communicate some intent, and whether, when the child fails to communicate something effectively with one action, s/he is able to use some alternative action or communicate the same intention through some other means. It is a little easier to address the questions of complexity and flexibility when a child is using language to communicate: one can then look at how many words are combined together, what different types of constructions are present in the child's speech, and whether phrases used are rote repetitions or instead reflect some rule learning so that the child is able to generate word combinations of his or her own.

Communicative Content

As a third consideration, the communication assessment should examine the content of the child's communication, or the type and range of concepts the child communicates. For the nonverbal child, it may be easiest to think about this in terms of the topics of the child's communication (e.g., communicates about wanting soft drinks, peanut butter, and bananas to eat; about wanting to be swung up into the air; and about wanting to go outside). Even for children who are nonverbal it is possible to enumerate the different topics and also group them into categories, which is useful in gaining some picture of how restricted versus rich the child's communication is in its content. For children who use language meaningfully, one can look at the range of vocabulary and the semantic categories represented by that vocabulary, such as objects, actions, locations, actors, and so forth.

Context of Communication

Last, it is important to look at how the child uses communication in relation to context. This includes evaluating whether the child's communication is restricted to a particular person(s) or situation(s), and whether a communicative behavior occurs only in the context in which it was originally learned, or only in the presence of certain cues. It is also the case that when communicative skills are transferred to new contexts by a child with autism, the generalization is often made in such a way that there is a mismatch between the communication and the context (Swisher & Demetras, 1985). For instance, a 4-year-old boy in one classroom was told during the class's morning circle that, "The xylophone is finished." Later in his work session he was observed putting away a puzzle and saying, "Xylophone is finished."

Comprehension

The above discussion has focused on the child's communicative expression. The same dimensions should also be considered in examining comprehension (Lord, 1985). It is important to determine the extent of a child's receptive vocabulary, and ability to understand spoken phrases and sentences of varying complexity level, but to stop there would be far too limited an assessment of a preschool child with autism. We also want to know whether the child understands object cues, gestures, pictures, voice tone, and so forth, and whether s/he understands language in combination with some of these other means of communication, if language is not understood well alone. Some communicative purposes may be more readily processed than others. For instance, a child may understand that people frequently communicate in order to get him to do things, but not understand that sometimes people communicate because they want him to say something. The possible impact of context on comprehension is widely recognized, but in most language assessment the effort is made to eliminate contextual cues in order to assess language comprehension per se. In assessing an autistic preschooler, it is more useful to include contextual cues systematically in order to determine how much meaning a child is able to extract from them. Most autistic children face severe lifelong difficulties in understanding language, so the ability to use contextual cues in processing other people's communicative intent is an important skill to develop.

Communication Assessment Strategies

Formal testing, informal and observational assessment, and parental interview are all useful strategies for assessing communication skills. Even though there is a major developmental impairment of language among children with autism, there are some standardized measures which can be applied. Among the most useful is the Sequenced Inventory of Communication Development (SICD) (Hedrick, Prather & Tobin, 1975), which covers expressive and receptive skills from 4 months to 4 years. This instrument covers such behaviors as intonation, gesture, and nonverbal and verbal imitation as well as the use and understanding of language. Another appropriate instrument is the Reynell Developmental Language Scales (Reynell, 1978), which measures receptive and expressive language skills of children from one to seven years of age. For those children who have an understanding of pictures, the Peabody Picture Vocabulary Test, Revised edition (Dunn & Dunn, 1981) is a satisfactory measure of single-word receptive vocabulary.

The TEACCH Communication Curriculum (Watson, 1985; Watson, Schaffer, Lord & Schopler, in press) includes an observational assessment framework which covers the content described above, and an interview protocol for use with parents. Some elicitation procedures useful in the informal assessment of communication skills are provided in Wetherby and Prutting (1984). Lord (1985) suggested strategies for the assessment of comprehension skills in autistic children and made the clinically useful point that much of the information gathered in the assessment of other skill areas can be regrouped to give a picture of the child's comprehension skills.

Cognitive Assessment

In assessing the cognitive aspects of the preschool autistic child's development, we mainly consider the problem-solving and abstract reasoning abilities inferred from the child's use of objects, play, or capacity to imitate. While understanding the child's cognition cannot be independent of his language system, it is important to analyze the nonverbal components of his/her learning. Unevenness of the developmental profile is characteristic of most autistic children, even in the preschool years, with nonverbal skills such as visuo-motor, visual spatial skills more advanced than language or social skills. Yet there is consistent clinical and research evidence (DeMyer, Hingtgen & Jackson, 1981) that the relatively proficient nonverbal skills are limited to nonsymbolic visual matching or simple decoding abilities. Parents often are struck by what appears to be signs of brightness in their nonverbal autistic child who might do fairly complex puzzles, have a good memory for where a favorite item has been stored away or recognize logos or signs for fast food restaurants. Yet, these apparently normal skills do not necessarily reflect underlying normal intelligence, but more typically a circumscribed set of isolated abilities. DeMyer (1979) asked her mothers each to report the brightest thing her child did. Whereas 57 of 58 mothers of normal children reported an action or skill judged to be at age level, this was the case in only one half of autistic children's reports. Examples often included early reading skills, precise location recall, or puzzle assembly. Again, none of these necessarily indicates potential for average cognitive functioning.

Play with Objects

More relevant dimensions for assessing cognitive potential involve indices of spontaneous and imaginative thinking, flexible problem-solving, and rule-based as opposed to rote learning. How the autistic child plays with objects is a window to the understanding of his/her symbolic development. Does the child use age-appropriate toys as intended by the manufacturer or rather in a repetitive, idiosyncratic manner? Does the play seem governed by sensorimotor interests (e.g., for visual, auditory, or tactile-kinesthetic stimulation) rather than by its pretend qualities? Are toys used in an imaginative way to represent other objects or is their use limited to one or two simple actions? Often even when the autistic child engages in what appears to be make-believe play such as pushing a small car in a garage, it turns out to be fairly uncomplicated or repetitive. Play usually lacks variety and is limited to simple schemes. To the extent to which object play is an index of cognitive functioning, its richness or paucity can help us assess the child's capacity for abstract reasoning and logical thinking. In addition, inadequate or poorly elaborated play may be highly associated with the autistic feature of insistence on sameness, which can be viewed as an indication of cognitive inflexibility.

Preacademic Skills

Some autistic children are able to learn preacademic concepts such as color, shape, and letter discrimination and naming. Names of body parts and the ability to copy some designs may also be present. These "products" of early learning may represent a positive sign of future learning ability, especially as applied to academic instruction, but one needs to be concerned about how the child uses these concepts and if they generalize flexibly across contexts. Were they rotely learned after many repetitions or did they develop in normal sequence? Are they the result of a "peak" skill such as visual memory or are they well integrated with other early childhood abilities?

Imitation

The ability to imitate is a prerequisite for early learning. Many autistic children are significantly delayed or inconsistent in their understanding of the imitation process. What is a natural and spontaneous process for the normal infant and toddler comes either very slowly or with specialized efforts by parents and teachers. To some extent these imitative dysfunctions may be related to inattentiveness to others, part of the social deficits in autism, or to visuo-motor integration difficulties involving the use of the body. The subtle motor disabilities of the autistic child can interfere with the capacity to imitate. Parent reports of suspicions of problems in infancy may reflect the lack of early social reciprocity such as the infant failing to sustain an interaction based on the mother's imitation of the infant. As with some aspects of play, some presumably imitative actions (e.g., echoed speech) may not reflect the basic process, but rather a mechanical repetition of an immediately observed or heard event. Again one needs to assess the variety and elaborateness of the child's imitative actions.

Social Cognition

Finally, cognitive abilities can be inferred from the developing child's understanding of social rules, including peer play. It is increasingly recognized that there is a strong cognitive component to social development in normal children (Rutter, 1983) and the social deficits in autism consequently reflect underlying cognitive deficiencies. Parental reports of their autistic child's failure to learn from normal discipline techniques likely indicate a difficulty in grasping and applying basic rules governing social behavior. The child who is hard to toilet train, to teach socially appropriate habits, or to behave properly in public may be prevented from learning these skills because of limited awareness of contingencies, cause-and-effect relations, or memory for complex sequences. Significant limitation in peer play reflects, in part, a weakness in learning the give-and-take of social rules. An autistic youngster who is perceived as "aggressive" in peer relations may be simply attempting a social approach but lacking the knowledge of how to effectively initiate such an interaction.

Cognitive Assessment Strategies

Measures of cognitive functioning can be derived through formal testing. The earlier notion that valid and reliable formal testing of autistic children was not possible has changed with the increased understanding of the nature of the disorder. With appropriate test selection and knowledge and application of sound behavior management principles in the test situation, the clinician can successfully complete a thorough developmental assessment (Marcus & Baker, 1986). Regardless of the age or functioning level of the child, there are useful test instruments that can be administered.

In the TEACCH program, the primary developmental test given is the Psychoeducational Profile or PEP (Schopler & Reichler, 1979). This instrument is particularly helpful in the assessment of the preschool autistic child because most of the items are developmentally suitable for the 18-month–5-year-old. The PEP has three main purposes: assessment of developmental functioning in the areas of imitation, motor abilities, eye–hand integration, and cognition; measurement of behavioral pathology specific to autism; and educational programming. Because the test is flexible in its administration and allows opportunities for observation of play, the PEP in a relatively brief time provides the examiner with both formal and informal data relevant to many of the areas of assessment described in this chapter.

Psychological testing with the autistic preschooler can be accomplished with careful test selection. In most instances, tests highly dependent on language such as the earlier Stanford–Binet (Terman & Merrill, 1960) should not be given. Typically the administration of such a test will result in behavior problems and lead to false assumptions about the child's abilities. The Bayley Scales of Infant Development (1969) and the Merrill–Palmer Scale of Mental Abilities (Stutsman, 1948) are most frequently used in the TEACCH program with the younger autistic child. Both yield useful information on a variety of skills and behaviors and test cooperation is usually satisfactory. Table III summarizes characteristics of several psychological tests that can be used with the preschool autistic child.

Table III. Summary of General Intelligence Tests for Young Autistic Children

Test	Age range	Description	Children for whom test is best suited	Advantages	Disadvantages
Bayley Mental Scale of Infant Development	2 mo. to 30 mo.	Motor, language, and social skills assessed in tasks designed to measure small increments of ability.	Young or severely delayed children, particularly if attentional and behavioral skills are poor.	Breaks down social and language skills into small components. Tasks require only brief attention.	For children with poor language and social skills, but good visual motor skills, range of visual-motor tasks may be too low; items are not intrinsically interesting.
Merrill-Palmer Test of Mental Abilities	18 mo. to 6 yr.	Wide range of visual motor tasks, smaller number of language items.	Children whose conceptual and language deficits make tests inappropriate but who have relatively good visual-motor skills.	Attractive materials. Language and non-language items fairly well separated.	Language skills not comprehensively assessed. Autistic children with good visual-motor skills may score misleadingly high. No derived IQ.
McCarthy Scales of Children's Abilities (McCarthy, 1972).	2 1/2 yr. to 8 1/2 yr.	Five subscales partially overlapping, measure verbal, perceptual-performance, quantitative, motor, and memory skills.	Children whose language skills are not severely delayed and who have relatively good attentional and behavioral skills.	2 1/2 to 8 1/2 year range better suited to many children than Wechsler tests. Fewer tasks dependent on language. Attractive materials. Administration allows for repeated demonstration, encouragement.	Language and conceptual demands too difficult for many autistic children. Comparison of subtest scores difficult.

Test	Age range	Description	Recommended use/population	Strengths	Weaknesses
Wechsler Preschool and Primary Scale of Intelligence.	4 yr. to 6 1/2 yr.	Verbal and Performance subscales. Emphasis on language skills. Several subtests assess formally acquired knowledge (e.g., Arithmetic, Information).	Higher-level autistic children, whose language skills are only mildly delayed, and who have good attentional and behavioral skills.	Well-designed and well-standardized. Several subtests assess skills emphasized in school. Alternation of Verbal and Performance subtests helps reduce language demands.	Language and conceptual demands too difficult for most autistic children. Receptive language important even on Performance subtest. Administration guidelines fairly rigid.
Kaufman Assessment Battery for Children (K-ABC)	2 1/2 yr. to 12 yr.	Separates abilities from acquired knowledge; format requires simple motor responses or short verbal answers; measures variety of cognitive and achievement skills.	Similar to Wechsler group; need for further study as test becomes more widely used.	Well-designed and standardized; age range wider than Wechsler or McCarthy; teaching items for each subtest allow for flexibility of administration; expressive language demands minimal; visually oriented format; easy to administer.	Does not allow for assessment of language peculiarities and problems picked up by Wechsler; neuropsychology model (sequential-simultaneous dichotomy) of questionable value for autistic group; lack of research and clinic use with this population warrants cautious approach to interpretation.

Play is an area best assessed through observation. A number of observational studies have been carried out with autistic and similar children; these are useful as references for deriving a framework and evaluative methods. Most studies have focused largely on the cognitive aspects of play (e.g., Ungerer & Stigman, 1981; Tilton & Ottinger, 1964; Wing, Gould, Yeates & Brierly, 1977). Sherman, Shapiro, and Glassman (1983) included observation of the child's functional use of objects, level of symbolic play behavior, and diversity of play, as well as social behavior during play.

Motor Assessment

As pointed out by DeMyer (1979) and by Ornitz, Guthrie, and Farley (1977), autistic children as a group show early and marked delays in motor development. This runs counter to the often-presented picture of children with autism as physically agile and well coordinated and points to the importance of assessing motor development in children with autism and similar disorders.

Content of Motor Assessment

Assessment in this area is usually divided into the broad areas of gross motor and fine motor development. The gross motor skills involved in locomotion (walking, running, climbing) are areas of relative strength for most children with autism, but milestones in these areas are nevertheless usually delayed in comparison to normal development. Also, oddities in locomotion, such as toe walking, are common. Skills in gross motor activities such as pedaling a tricycle and throwing and catching a ball are usually even more delayed than locomotive skills.

In the fine-motor area, it is not uncommon to find peak skills in certain perceptual–motor activities, which may be performed close to or at age level. These usually involve fitting pieces together, or matching designs (e.g., puzzles and block design tasks). However, it is important to also assess such perceptual–motor skills as the ability to imitate fine motor movements, to reproduce lines, circles, and other geometric figures in drawing, to cut, fold, and so forth, which are often markedly deficient skills in children with autism. In assessing fine motor skills, it is important to observe how well the child coordinates looking with motoric efforts to perform a task, what level of fine-motor precision is used, and whether sufficient hand strength is applied to accomplish a task.

During the motor assessment, it is also important to look for indications of disturbance in sensorimotor functioning. One frequently noted problem is "tactile defensiveness," a term used to describe a child's reluctance to allow or initiate certain types of physical contact (for instance, related to particular textures, and/or to particular parts of the body such as the palms of the hand or inside of the mouth). Another disturbance seems to be related to vestibular functioning, and is reflected in a resistance to rapid changes in body position (e.g., being turned upside-down in a rough-and-tumble game). Sensorimotor activities observed in nonhandicapped babies, such as hand gazing, mouthing of objects, and repetitive actions with objects, often persist in children with autism even when the child is capable of cognitively more sophisticated actions.

A major goal of assessment should be to determine what the source of an observed and documented deficiency is. Suppose, for example, that a child is found to be unable to unscrew a jar lid in order to obtain a raisin inside. The problem may stem from any one of several sources, or some combination of them, including insufficient muscle tone, insufficient muscle control (e.g., stemming from a neuromotor disorder such as cerebral palsy), dyspraxia, or difficulty in planning and then smoothly executing a coordinated motor movement, insufficient cognitive skills to recognize that one could obtain the raisin by unscrewing the jar lid, and lack of motivation (e.g., child hates raisins, and has no inherent desire to perform tasks in order to please the examiner).

In sorting out these possibilities, it is helpful to use information about motivational factors for the individual child and his or her known cognitive skills in structuring the motor assessment. It is also helpful to obtain as much information as possible about the child's motor performance in functional, everyday activities that are a familiar part of the daily routine.

Motor Assessment Strategies

The motor area can be assessed both formally and informally. The Psychoeducational Profile (Schopler & Reichler, 1979) includes the assessment of both fine and gross motor skills, as well as items designed to assess some of the common disturbances in sensorimotor functioning. Another instrument appropriate for use in motor assessment of this age group is the Peabody Developmental Motor Scales (Folio & Fewell, 1983). When the child fails to attempt an item, or attends only briefly, it is important to try to determine whether the child is unable to perform the skill or simply will not perform it within that specific context. Parent interview can provide information regarding the child's interests, and more or less comparable behaviors observed at home. This might suggest a different format by which the clinician can informally assess the skill in question. It is also important to integrate information from the cognitive, social, and communication assessments with information from the motor assessment before interpreting the results.

Assessing Family Needs

Assessing the family with a young autistic child involves two dimensions: how the child functions at home, especially in the areas of communication, play, behavior, and self-help skills; and the impact of the child's handicap on the family. In addition, parents of young autistic children are relatively inexperienced in communicating with professionals and the assessment process itself may be stressful as well as enlightening as the family begins to understand the developmental irregularities of their child. Thus, by a careful and sensitive review of the primary problem areas associated with autism, the professional can help a family clarify confusing behaviors or learning patterns (e.g., why a 3-year-old can do complex puzzles but cannot speak). In the early stages of finding out about their child's condition, the assessment is a crucial step in giving parents the knowledge and support necessary to enable them to effectively deal with the long-term challenges of raising an autistic child.

Concerns about the Child

The typical major concerns presented by parents which require further exploration involve behavior problems and lack of speech. Parents usually emphasize the failure of verbal communication, so questions pertaining to nonverbal forms of communication and the development of receptive language, both verbal and nonverbal, are necessary to determine the pervasiveness of the communication dysfunction. Behavioral problems often involve lack of compliance and unpredictable tantrums. Assessing these problems should be linked to the possibility of lack of communicative understanding as a cause. Parents often attribute non-compliance to willfulness or "laziness," assuming that the child understands what is being asked. As the child's fundamental impairment in language comprehension is clarified through an assessment, the parental perspective can shift. Methods of discipline, including consistency between parents, should be discussed. It is helpful to know what has or has not worked and to what extent parents have become frustrated. For example, if a child has not responded to spanking, this may indicate either a lack of understanding of cause and effect (a clue to the child's level of cognitive awareness) or relative insensitivity to pain (related to sensory dysfunction). Again, not only does the assessment contribute to a further understanding of the child's condition for the professional but provides the family with alternative perspectives not previously considered.

Discussion of how the child plays helps verify diagnosis as well as give information on how the child occupies his/her time and engages in constructive activities. Assessing this area may make parents more aware of the child's developmental delays and can be compared with the results of formal cognitive testing. For example, the inability of the child to show imaginative play at home may be mirrored in a low score on a standardized cognitive measure. A parent who has not thought of the child as having mental retardation can better recognize the cognitive delays when the clinic and home data are consistent.

How the child is progressing in self-help skills such as toileting, dressing, and feeding is also important to determine. These skills are dependent on adequate motor, language, and cognitive development. Delays in these areas are additional indications of developmental problems as well as targets for interventions. Helping parents teach such skills may be more quickly productive than verbal communication. Thus, it is useful to establish through the assessment process the relevance of exactly how much the child can or cannot do for him/herself.

Impact of the Child on the Family

Assessment should also cover the impact of the child's handicap on the family. When the child is young, the effects may primarily include confusion and worry over why the child is not developing normally. If professionals have not supported the family's perception of a developmental problem, then self-doubt and frustration are likely emotional responses. It is important to know what the parents' understanding is of the child's problems and what they have been told. Parents of the young autistic child are especially seeking a diagnostic label and feel stress during this period of uncertainty regarding the cause of their child's problems.

There are also stress factors unrelated to the handicapped child, such as the needs of other children in the family, financial well-being, and marital status and satisfaction. These potential sources of stress are often exacerbated by the demands of coping with the handicapped child and understanding his/her problems.

The emotional support network available to a family should be assessed. Is there extended family close by and have they been supportive? Understanding the potential sources of support to the family becomes increasingly relevant for long-range planning.

Interviewing Parents

Obtaining information from parents is essential for a comprehensive assessment. Not only is such information valuable for understanding how the child behaves, plays and communicates in his natural environment, but engaging the parents in the assessment process lays the groundwork for future collaboration during intervention.

There are three sources of information from parents typically obtained in the TEACCH program: questionnaires completed prior to the evaluation, information provided during a semistructured interview and more formal data from the Vineland Adaptive Behavior Scales (Sparrow, Balla & Cicchetti, 1984).

There are two reasons why the completion of questionnaires facilitates the assessment process. First, staff is better prepared to help the family when provided with information on the main issues of concern, what services have been provided and what the family's understanding of the problem is. Second, the questionnaires provide the parents with an indication of what is involved in the evaluation. For example, the TEACCH questionnaires include a history form based on factual data, a behavior checklist geared to autistic characteristics, and an open-ended form for each parent that enables them to describe what a typical day is like, what their main concerns are, what is most distressing and satisfying about their child. In combination, these forms orient the parents to the behavioral and developmental focus of the upcoming evaluation. In addition it signals to them the importance of the parental perspective. This can be reassuring to parents who perhaps have not been actively included in prior assessments or whose observation or opinions have not been seriously considered.

The parent interview need not follow a rigid format, but it should be fairly structured and cover relevant areas. It should also allow the parents sufficient time to air out feelings and worries, while still providing as objective a view as possible of the child's life at home. It is useful to initially determine what the parents' main questions and concerns are and what they hope to gain from the evaluation. The interviewer's manner should be conducive to the establishment of trust. The interviewer should also be sensitive to the difficulty of this experience for the family, and understand that there is a natural tendency for the parents to protect their child. It is helpful to know what the parents' expectations of their child's future may be and what they judge to be their child's current level of functioning and explanation for his/her problems. Specific areas to review include behavioral problems, communication skills, play skills, relationships with siblings, daily living and motor skills. Information about informal or formal support networks is also useful to help in planning a program.

The Vineland Adaptive Behavior Scales (Sparrow et al., 1984), the revision of the popular Vineland Social Maturity Scale (Doll, 1965), provides additional objective data in the domains of communication, daily living, socialization and motor skills (for children under 6 years of age). The survey form yields sufficient detail to assess areas of relative strength and weakness and, if significant gaps are indicated, can facilitate decisions about adaptive and self-help skills to work on.

At the conclusion of a parent interview, the clinician should have a clear picture of the family and its relationship to the handicapped child, its worries and hopes, what resources are available and what treatment recommendations for the home should be. In addition, the family should be better prepared for the diagnostic and assessment information that will be presented at the interpretative conference.

Medical Assessment

While this chapter is concerned mainly with the developmental aspects of autism related to problems in learning and behavior, it is important to recognize the possible medical factors associated with autism. A variety of biologic conditions have been documented including congenital rubella, tuberous sclerosis, certain viral infections, abnormalities in purine metabolism and intestinal absorption, and phenylketonuria. The fragile-X syndrome (Coleman &

Gillberg, 1985) and Retts syndrome (Holm, 1985) have been increasingly reported in conjunction with autism. While many such conditions do not respond to any specific treatment, some (such as PKU) do require effective intervention and there may be genetic implications for families (e.g., tuberous sclerosis). Other possible impairments such as hearing or visual problems should be assessed. Comprehensive information on the medical aspects of autism can be found in Coleman and Gillberg (1985) and in Schopler and Mesibov (1987).

CLINICAL IMPLICATIONS

Ideally, the process of diagnosing and assessing children with autism and similar disorders should begin during the preschool years for every child. It is clear that these disorders result in life-long handicaps which are not abated by a "wait-and-see" approach. The preschool years are a period of unique opportunity, with some age-specific issues and challenges.

Diagnostic Clarity

The overlap between autism and other pervasive developmental disorders is not an issue unique to the preschool population. However, it seems particularly crucial to recognize the overlap and similarities among these disorders during the preschool period to avoid unnecessary delays in developing a treatment plan. Establishing the diagnostic primacy of autism in this population enables the professional to take a course of action that is specific to the problems. There is a tendency to be evasive when the diagnosis falls within the other categories of pervasive developmental disorder. Parents are particularly sensitive to this indefiniteness.

Need for Reassessment

Owing to the fluidity of behavior during the preschool years, there is a need for frequent reassessment of the child. Occasionally, an original diagnosis may prove erroneous. Much more frequently, new skills and new problems will emerge which require a revision of the intervention. This is also a period during which initial educational placement decisions are made for children, and assessment makes an essential contribution to these decisions by identifying the child's strengths and needs. Ongoing informal assessment should be a part of every intervention program, to monitor the child's progress toward established goals and aid in decision-making for further intervention.

Integration with Nonhandicapped Peers

Another opportunity of the preschool years is the integration of the child into normal settings, both educationally and socially. During this period, the developmental gaps between children with autism and their nonautistic age-mates are less apparent than will be true in later years. In an educational setting, it is easier during this period to design activities which are developmentally and functionally relevant to both autistic children and nonhandicapped children. Although simply being placed in a setting with nonhandicapped children may be of little value to most preschool autistic children, there is evidence that integration is beneficial for them when social interactions are planned for and facilitated as a part of the curriculum (McHale & Gamble, 1986). The extent to which autistic children can participate in and benefit from integrated activities likely will depend on both the general level of retardation in the autistic child as well as the severity of autism. The type and extent of integrated activities must be individualized to meet the child's needs, just as the rest of the child's educational program is developed on an individualized basis. In addition to positive changes in the autistic children, nonhandicapped children can gain skills which enable them to be more successful social partners for the handicapped children.

Play

Both an opportunity and a challenge for assessment and intervention in the preschool years is the use of play. Play is the primary activity of nonhandicapped children during the preschool years. Thus it is developmentally and functionally appropriate to incorporate play into the intervention program for preschool children with autism and similar disorders. Play offers the opportunity to assess and intervene in the areas of communication, social, cognitive and motor skills. The use of play in assessment and intervention implies a focus on what is fun and interesting for the child. Assessment and intervention are also more rewarding for parents and professionals when the activities are pleasurable for the child.

Like social interaction with peers, however, it would be a mistake to assume that unstructured play will be a developmentally progressive activity for the child with autism or related disorders. The effective use of play in intervention with this population requires careful planning of play activities designed to foster the developmental skills targeted for the individual child in each domain of concern, as well as taking into account the idiosyncratic motivational factors of that child.

Parental Involvement

Perhaps the greatest opportunities during the preschool years lie in the children's parents. For most children, handicapped or not, early childhood is the period during which parents are most intensively involved with their children and fill roles as teachers of their children. Even for children attending day care or preschool programs, the major tasks of early childhood are an integral part of learning to be a member of a family. In diagnosis, assessment, and intervention with preschool autistic children, one challenge is to capitalize on the commitment and energy level of the parents. To this end, professionals need to help parents understand their children's disorders and collaborate with parents in developing the best intervention goals and strategies, while also promoting a healthy self-respect among parents for the value of their expertise regarding their own children.

In our experience at TEACCH, parents who are given an early diagnosis of their child have greatly benefited from this information, largely because it enables them to get appropriate help for their child at an earlier point in time. Families who have been given no or confusing diagnoses are often at a disadvantage in knowing what to do and with whom to consult. While painful, an early diagnosis helps parents understand the reasons for their child's unusual and delayed development. Such information facilitates the long acceptance process. Given the normal denial that parents (and others close to a child) experience

(Marcus, 1984; Searle, 1978), an inadequate or vague diagnosis such as Childhood Onset Pervasive Developmental Disorder only raises doubts in parents' minds and postpones the important process of coming to grips with the actual problem. Parents are potentially the primary source of assistance for their young handicapped child (Marcus & Schopler, 1987). Their need for accurate diagnostic information is a prerequisite to enable them to fully participate in their child's treatment program.

Parents of preschool children diagnosed autistic frequently want answers regarding what their child will be like in the future. The preschool years are the period during which predictions about future development of a given child are the most tenuous. Parents of preschool children diagnosed autistic frequently want answers regarding what their child will be like in the future. It would be a mistake to foster the hope or expectation in parents that their child with autism will eventually function in a completely normal way. However, it is also important to be able to say to parents, "We don't know," regarding the specific long-term outcomes for their child. In recognizing the fluidity of behavior during the preschool years, parents and professionals alike can find reasons for optimism in this period. Although such optimism may later be tempered, it can be a source of increased energy in working with the preschooler, leading to greater developmental gains for the child. Provided the immediate objectives, strategies, and interactions with the child are developmentally appropriate, overly optimistic hopes for the child's future are not harmful to the child. In addition, these may be a helpful coping mechanism for parents during the early stages of understanding and accepting their child's handicap. Thus, the professionals working with such parents must walk a thin line on which they avoid engendering false hopes but also avoid the needless destruction of hopes and optimism.

CONCLUSION

The issues and strategies involved in diagnosis, assessment, and treatment of preschoolers with autism and related disorders versus older children with these handicaps certainly overlap to a substantial degree. However, as we have discussed, work with very young children also entails some issues and strategies which are specific to the age group. More information on young children with autism and related disorders is needed in terms of course of development, diagnostic symptoms, assessment instruments and procedures, and intervention. However, it is currently possible to diagnose the disorder reliably, to make a meaningful assessment of skills and deficits, and to plan effective interventions for preschool children with these disorders. There is little to lose and much potential gain for the children and their parents in taking these steps as early as possible.

REFERENCES

Argyle, M., & Cooke, M. (1976). *Gaze and mutual gaze.* Cambridge: Cambridge University Press.
Bayley, N. (1969). *Bayley Scales of Infant Development.* New York: Psychological Corporation.
Brazelton, T. B. (1982). Joint regulation of neonate-parent behavior. In E. F. Tronick (Ed.), *Social interchange in infancy: Affect, cognition, and communication* (pp. 7–22). Baltimore: University Park Press.
Brazelton, T. B., Koslowski, B., & Main, M. (1974). The early mother-infant interaction. In M. Lewis & L. A. Rosenblum (Eds.), *The effect of the infant on its caregiver* (pp. 49–76). New York: Wiley.

Coleman, M., & Gillberg, C. (1985). *The biology of the autistic syndromes.* New York: Praeger.

Curcio, F. (1978). Sensorimotor functioning and communication in mute autistic children. *Journal of Autism and Childhood Schizophrenia, 8,* 281–292.

Creak, M. (1961). Schizophrenic syndrome in childhood: Progress report of working party. *British Medical Journal, 197,* 889–890.

Dahl, E. K., Cohen, D. J., & Provence, S. (1986). Clinical and multivariate approaches to the nosology of pervasive developmental disorders. *Journal of the American Academy of Child Psychiatry, 25,* 170–180.

DeMyer, M. K. (1979). *Parents and children in autism.* New York: Wiley.

DeMyer, M. K., Hingtgen, J. N., & Jackson, R. K. (1981). Infantile autism reviewed. *Schizophrenia Bulletin, 7,* 388–45.

Doll, E. (1965). *Vineland Social Maturity Scale.* Circle Pines, MN: American Guidance Service.

Dunn, L., & Dunn, L. (1981). *Peabody Picture Vocabulary Test—Revised.* Circle Pines, MN: American Guidance Service.

Fenske, E. C., Zalenski, S., Krantz, P. J., & McClannahan, L. E. (1985). Age at intervention and treatment outcome for autistic children in a comprehensive intervention program. *Analysis and Intervention in Developmental Disabilities, 5,* 49–58.

Folio, M. R., & Fewell, R. R. (1983). *Peabody Developmental Motor Scales and Activity Cards.* Allen, TX: DLM Teaching Resources.

Freeman, B. J., & Ritvo, E. R. (1984). The syndrome of autism: Establishing the diagnosis and principles of management. *Pediatric Annals, 13,* 284–96.

Freeman, B. J., Ritvo, E. R., & Schroth, P. C. (1984). Behavior assessment of the syndrome of autism: Behavior Observation System. *Journal of the American Academy of Child Psychiatry, 23,* 588–94.

Harper, J., & Williams, S. (1975). Age and type of onset as critical variables in early infantile autism. *Journal of Autism and Childhood Schizophrenia, 5,* 25–36.

Hedrick, D. L., Prather, E. M., & Tobin, A. R. (1975). *Sequenced Inventory of Communication Development.* Seattle: University of Washington Press.

Hermelin, B., & O'Connor, N. (1985). Logico-affective states and nonverbal language. In E. Schopler & G. B. Mesibov (Eds.), *Communication problems in autism* (pp. 283–310). New York: Plenum.

Holm, V. A. (1985). Rett's syndrome: A progressive developmental disability in girls. *Developmental and Behavioral Pediatrics, 6,* 32–6.

Hoshino, Y., Kumashiro, H., Yashima, Y., Tachibana, R., Watanabe, M., & Furukawa, H. (1982). Early symptoms of autistic children and its diagnostic significance. *Folia Psychiatrica et Neurologica Japonica, 36,* 367–74.

Howlin, P. (1986). An overview of social behavior in autism. In E. Schopler & G. B. Mesibov (Eds.), *Social behavior in autism* (pp. 103–31). New York: Plenum.

Kubicek, L. F. (1980). Organization in two mother–infant interactions involving a normal infant and his fraternal twin brother who was later diagnosed as autistic. In T. M. Field, S. Goldberg, D. Stern, & A. M. Sostek (Eds.), *High-risk infants and children: Adult and peer interactions* (pp. 99–110). New York: Academic.

Kurita, H. (1985). Infantile autism with speech loss before the age of thirty months. *Journal of the American Academy of Child Psychiatry, 24,* 191–6.

Kanner, L. (1943). Autistic disturbances of affective contact. *Nervous Child, 2,* 217–50.

Lord, C. (1985). Autism and the comprehension of language. In E. Schopler & G. B. Mesibov (Eds.), *Communication problems in autism* (pp. 257–81). New York: Plenum.

Marcus, L. M. (1984). Coping with burnout. In E. Schopler & G. B. Mesibov (eds.), *The effects of autism on the family* (pp. 311–26). New York: Plenum.

Marcus, L. M., & Baker, A. F. (1986). Assessment of autistic children. In R. J. Simeonsson (Ed.), *Psychological assessment of special children.* (pp. 279–304). Boston: Allyn & Bacon.

Marcus, L. M., & Schopler, E. (1987). Working with families: A developmental perspective. In D. Cohen, A. Donnellan, & R. Paul (Eds.), *Handbook of autism and atypical developmental* (pp. 499–512). New York: Wiley.

McHale, S. M., & Gamble, W. C. (1986). Mainstreaming handicapped children in public school settings: Challenges and limitations. In E. Schopler & G. B. Mesibov (Eds.), *Social behavior in autism* (pp. 191–212). New York: Plenum.

Mirenda, P., Donnellan, A., & Yoder, D. (1983). Gaze behavior: A new look at an old problem. *Journal of Autism and Developmental Disabilities, 13,* 397–409.

Olley, J. G. (1986). The TEACCH curriculum for teaching social behavior to children with autism. In E. Schopler & G. B. Mesibov (Eds.), *Social behavior in autism.* (pp. 351–73). New York: Plenum.

Olley, J. G., & Watson, L. R. (May, 1986). Developing a public school-based model for preschool education for children with autism. Paper presented at the annual meeting of the Association for Behavior Analysis, Milwaukee, WI.

Ornitz, E. M., Guthrie, D., & Farley, A. H. (1977). The early development of autistic children. *Journal of Autism and Childhood Schizophrenia, 7,* 207–29.

Oster, H. (1978). Facial expression and affect development. In M. Lewis and L. A. Rosenblum (Eds.) *The development of affect* (pp. 43–75). New York: Plenum.

Rescorla, L. A. (1986). Preschool psychiatric disorders: Diagnostic classification and symptom patterns. *Journal of the American Academy of Child Psychiatry, 25,* 162–9.

Reynell, J. K. (1978). *Reynell Developmental Language Scales, Revised Edition.* Windsor, England: NFER/Nelson.

Richer, J. (1978). The partial noncommunication of culture to autistic children—An application of human ethology. In M. Rutter & E. Schopler (Eds.), *Autism: A reappraisal of concepts and treatment* (pp. 47–61). New York: Plenum.

Robson, K. S. (1967). The role of eye-to-eye contact in maternal–infant attachment. *Journal of Child Psychology and Psychiatry, 8,* 13–25.

Rutter, M. (1978). Diagnosis and definition of childhood autism. *Journal of Autism and Developmental Disorders, 8,* 139–61.

Rutter, M. (1983). Cognitive deficits in the pathogenesis of autism. *Journal of Child Psychology and Psychiatry, 24,* 513–31.

Rutter, M., & Lockyer, L. (1967). A five to fifteen year follow-up study of infantile psychosis. I. Description of the sample. *British Journal of Psychiatry, 113,* 1169–82.

Schaffer, R. (1977). *Mothering.* Cambridge, MA: Harvard University Press.

Schopler, E., Lansing, M. D., & Waters, L. (1983). *Individualized assessment and treatment for autistic and developmentally disabled children. Vol. III.: Teaching activities for autistic children.* Austin, TX: Pro-Ed.

Schopler, E., & Mesibov, G. B. (Eds.). (1987). *Neurobiological issues in autism.* New York: Plenum.

Schopler, E., & Olley, J. G. (1982). Comprehensive educational services for autistic children: The TEACCH model. In C. R. Reynolds & T. R. Gutkin (Eds.), *The handbook of school psychology* (pp. 629–43). New York: Wiley.

Schopler, E., & Reichler, R. J. (1979). *Individualized assessment and treatment for autistic and developmentally disabled children. Vol. I: Psychoeducational profile* (2nd ed.). Austin, TX: Pro-Ed.

Schopler, E., Reichler, R. J., & Lansing, M. D. (1980). *Individualized assessment and treatment for autistic and developmentally disabled children. Vol. II: Teaching strategies for parents and professionals.* Austin, TX: Pro-Ed.

Schopler, E., Reichler, R. J., & Renner, B. R. (1986). *The Childhood Autism Rating Scale.* New York: Irvington.

Searl, S. J., Jr. (1978). Stages of parent reaction. *Exceptional Parent,* April, F27–F29.

Sherman, M., Shapiro, T., & Glassman, M. (1983). Play and language in developmentally disordered preschoolers: A new approach to classification. *Journal of the American Academy of Child Psychiatry, 22,* 511–24.

Sigman, M., Mundy, P., Sherman, T., & Ungerer, J. (1986). Social interactions of autistic, mentally retarded and normal children and their caregivers. *Journal of Child Psychology and Psychiatry, 27,* 647–55.

Sigman, M., & Ungerer, J. A. (1984). Attachment behaviors in autistic children. *Journal of Autism and Developmental Disorders, 14,* 231–44.

Simeonsson, R. J., Olley, J. G., & Rosenthal, S. (1987). Early intervention for children with autism. In M. J. Guralnick & F. C. Bennett (Eds.), *The effectiveness of early intervention* (pp. 275–96). New York: Academic.

Snow, C. E. (1977). The development of conversation between mothers and babies. *Journal of Child Language, 4,* 1–22.

Sparrow, S. S., Balla, D. A., & Cicchetti, D. V. (1984). *Vineland Adaptive Behavior Scales.* Circle Pines, MN: American Guidance Service.

Stern, D. (1971). A micro-analysis of mother–infant interaction: Behavior regulating social conduct between a mother and her 3½ month old twins. *Journal of the American Academy of Child Psychiatry, 10,* 501–17.

Stern, D. N. (1974). Mother and infant at play: The dyadic interaction involving facial, vocal, and gaze behaviors. In M. Lewis & L. A. Rosenblum (Eds.), *The effect of the infant on its caregiver* (pp. 187–214). New York: Wiley.

Stern, D. (1977). *The first relationship: Infant and mother.* Cambridge, MA: Harvard University Press.

Stutsman, R. (1948). *Merrill–Palmer Scale of Mental Tests.* Los Angeles: Western Psychological Services.

Swisher, L., & Demetras, M. J. (1985). The expressive language characteristics of autistic children compared with mentally retarded or specific language impaired children. In E. Schopler & G. B. Mesibov (Eds.), *Communication problems in autism* (pp. 147–62). New York: Plenum.

Terman, L. M., & Merrill, M. A. (1960). *Stanford-Binet Intelligence Scale.* Boston: Houghton-Mifflin.

Tilton, J. R., & Ottinger, D. R. (1964). Comparison of toy play behavior of autistic, retarded, and normal children. *Psychological Reports, 15,* 967–75.

Ungerer, J. A., & Sigman, M. (1981). Symbolic play and language comprehension in autistic children. *Journal of the American Academy of Child Psychiatry, 20,* 318–37.

Usuda, S., Koizumi, T. (1981). Children with abnormal speech development. In P. S. Dale & D. Ingram (Eds.), *Child language* (pp. 353–372). Baltimore: University Park Press.

Volkmar, F. R. (1986). Compliance, noncompliance, and negativism. In E. Schopler & G. B. Mesibov (Eds.), *Social behavior in autism* (pp. 171–88). New York: Plenum.

Volkmar, F. R., Cohen, D. J., & Paul, R. (1986). An evaluation of the DSM-III criteria for infantile autism. *Journal of the American Academy of Child Psychiatry, 25,* 190–7.

Watson, L. R. (1985). The TEACCH communication curriculum. In E. Schopler & G. B. Mesibov (Eds.), *Communication problems in autism* (pp. 187–206). New York: Plenum.

Watson, L. R., Schaffer, B., Lord, C., & Schopler, E. (in press). Teaching spontaneous communication to autistic and developmentally handicapped children. New York: Irvington.

Wetherby, A., & Prutting, C. (1984). Profiles of communicative and cognitive-social abilities in autistic children. *Journal of Speech and Hearing Research, 27,* 364–77.

Wing, L. (1976). Epidemiology and theories of etiology. In L. Wing (Ed.), *Early childhood autism* (2nd ed.). (pp. 65–92). Oxford: Pergamon.

Wing, L. (1981). Language, social and cognitive impairments in autism and severe mental retardation. *Journal of Autism and Developmental Disorders, 11,* 31–44.

Wing, L., Gould, J., Yeates, J. R., & Brierly, L. M. (1977). Symbolic play in severely mentally retarded and in autistic children. *Journal of Child Psychology and Psychiatry, 18,* 167–78.

Wolff, S., & Chess, S. (1964). A behavioral study of schizophrenic children. *Acta Psychiatrica Scandinavica, 40,* 438–66.

19

Assessment of Low-Functioning Children

NANCY M. JOHNSON-MARTIN

INTRODUCTION

Psychologists and educators are sometimes called upon to assess children whose development is sufficiently deviant or delayed to challenge the assumptions of traditional assessment procedures. Some of these children are so physically handicapped that they cannot interact with traditional test materials. Others have markedly delayed development in all areas. They may be too old (beyond 30 months) for the age norms of the most commonly used infant tests, but are functioning at an infant level. Still others, including many autistic children, are delayed in all areas but also have strikingly deviant development. Perhaps their language skills are much more delayed than motor skills, or they have widely scattered skills within one domain (e.g., good vocal imitation without any vocal communication).

Although the number of these children is small, their challenge to our assessment skills is great. It is not sufficient to attempt traditional procedures and describe the children as "untestable" or to assign to them summary scores (e.g., an I.Q. of 9) that are not only statistically unsound but meaningless as descriptors of individual characteristics. These children need and deserve our time and attention. Their appropriate assessment is essential in order to provide access to necessary services, to determine appropriate intervention goals and objectives, and to monitor progress over time.

This chapter does not attempt to address the assessment of physically handicapped children. More pertinent to this volume are the assessment issues involved in the other two groups of difficult to assess children described above. For the want of a better term, these children with very delayed and/or deviant development will be referred to as low-functioning children. They are children with severe to profound mental retardation who may have significant behavioral abnormalities as well. This chapter first reviews the problems in assessment posed by these children, then discusses various assessment materials that are available to help in the solution of these problems and concludes with some recommendations for clinical practice.

NANCY M. JOHNSON-MARTIN • CHILD Project, Duke University Medical Center, Durham, North Carolina 27705.

PROBLEMS IN ASSESSMENT

The basic problems facing professionals charged with assessing low functioning children are somewhat similar to those faced by the professionals who assess other groups of children who, for environmental or other reasons, are significantly different from the general population. These problems include determining which assessment procedures will satisfy the specific goals of the assessment, dealing with inappropriate test norms, accommodating atypical patterns of development, and identifying tests with appropriate content. Each of these problems as it relates to the low-functioning child is discussed.

Goals for Assessment

Psychoeducational assessment of developmentally disabled children serves three basic goals: (1) to provide an estimate of cognitive functioning for purposes of diagnosis and gaining access to services, (2) to describe characteristics that may be used in planning intervention services, and (3) to document development and progress over time. It is important that the person conducting an assessment of any child, but especially a low functioning child, be clear as to the particular goal or goals for a given assessment. The assessment questions determine the problems that will be encountered in the assessment as well as the tests and procedures that will be appropriate.

There are basically two kinds of assessment instruments that one may choose to use: those that are norm referenced and those that are criterion referenced. A norm referenced test is one that is given in a prescribed fashion and provides scores that describe a person's performance relative to the performance of a normative sample of people who were given the test under the same standardized conditions. IQ tests and achievement tests that yield percentile scores and grade levels are examples of norm referenced tests. A criterion-referenced test is a compilation of specific skills to be learned, accompanied by a description of the criteria by which one determines that each skill has been mastered. Instead of producing a summary score, the test provides a profile of skills that have been mastered and a list of skills that must yet be taught to reach some defined goal (e.g., walking independently). Most developmental curricula include a criterion-referenced assessment.

Norm-referenced tests are essential for diagnostic purposes and often for meeting the legal requirements that provide access to services. Criterion-referenced tests may be more appropriate for planning particular treatment goals. Both are useful for charting progress over time, although each provides somewhat different information. The norm-referenced test will describe progress in terms of increasing mental age or developmental level or in terms of changes in standing relative to the normative sample (e.g., an increase in IQ). The criterion-referenced test will describe progress in terms of specific skills mastered since the previous assessment. For children whose development is slow, criterion-referenced assessments are generally better instruments for documenting progress over time.

The lines between norm- and criterion-referenced tests often become blurred, particularly when designed for children functioning under the 3-year level, where the content of all tests is very similar. Although not intended for such use, norm-referenced tests are often used to describe specific skills a child has mastered and to outline the goals for treatment. Since most of the items on criterion-referenced tests have been drawn from norm-referenced tests, these items may be assigned age levels and normative statements can be made about a child (e.g., "his language skills are between the 3rd- and 4th-month level"), again putting the test to a use for which it was not intended. It is important to remember that these kinds of evaluation tools were developed in different ways to serve different purposes. The norm-referenced test is a sampling of representative skills and therefore does not include all the important skills that should be considered for intervention. It is necessarily a limited programming guide. The criterion-referenced test should include the important skills for a programming guide but, at best, is accompanied only by estimates of developmental levels for each of the skills. Therefore, one must exercise extreme caution in making normative statements based on a criterion-referenced test. Anyone planning an assessment of a low-functioning child should first determine the critical goals of the assessment and then use an instrument or a combination of instruments that will make it possible to reach those goals.

Inappropriate Test Norms

One of the major dilemmas that confronts the individual charged with assessing a low-functioning child is the need for a valid IQ score, when there is no test available to provide such a score. What is required is a standardized, norm referenced test appropriate to the age and handicapping conditions of the child. In some instances, the low-functioning child may not have sufficient skills to be testable on the Stanford Binet (Terman & Merrill, 1972) or other traditional childhood tests but he/she is too old for the norms of an infant test. In practice such a child is frequently assessed with an infant test, a mental age is estimated, and a ratio IQ is computed using the traditional formula (MA/CA × 100). This may be the only alternative available to meet the requirement for an IQ, but the limitations of this practice should be recognized. Ratio IQs are somewhat less stable than deviation IQs (a deviation IQ is based on where the child's score falls on a normalized distribution of scores from other children his/her age). In addition, ratio IQs are less comparable between different tests than deviation IQs; very low IQ scores (e.g., below 20) probably have little meaning; and there is always a question as to the appropriateness and/or value of assessing only infant skills in a child who is no longer an infant.

In other instances, the low-functioning child may be at an appropriate age for the test chosen, but the normative tables do not go sufficiently low to provide a score. For example, the Bayley Scales of Infant Development (Bayley, 1969) and the McCarthy Scales of Children's Abilities (McCarthy, 1972) do not provide scores below 50. Again, mental ages can be estimated and ratio IQs computed. However, a more statistically defensible procedure may be to use extrapolated scores based on the standard deviations of the tests. Naglieri (1981) and Harrison and Naglieri (1978) provided scores down to 28 for the Bayley Scales and the McCarthy Scales, respectively. It must still be recognized, however, that these scores are based on statistical manipulations rather than on observations of low-functioning children within the normative sample.

Atypical Development

Norm-referenced assessment procedures for children functioning under the 3-year level are almost always age scales. The items were chosen both because they were considered important and because they distinguish between children of different ages. As such, they are compilations of developmental milestones observed in normally developing children. Underlying these assessment procedures are the twin assumptions that development takes place in a particular order within a developmental domain (e.g., language or sensorimotor skills) and that development is reasonably even across domains, i.e., a child with 6-month skills in language will have approximately 6-month skills in sensorimotor development (Johnson, 1982; Gaussen, 1984). These assumptions are invalid for many low-functioning children. These children are not just slow. They cannot be understood by presuming that they are like children younger than themselves. Rather, their development is often characterized by scattered skills both within and across domains. This is especially true of autistic children. For example, a child may have no spoken speech at all, perhaps not even the babbles of a 6-month-old, but may be able to put together puzzles like a 3-year-old or understand instructions like a toddler. Another may not demonstrate understanding the meaning of any words but may be able to repeat complex sentences. Still another may read words but be unable to talk meaningfully.

Atypical patterns of development may make it difficult to obtain basal and ceiling levels on standardized tests, may render summary IQ or mental index scores relatively meaningless and may therefore, make diagnostic conclusions about mental ability questionable. Similarly, this atypical development may make it difficult to plan intervention programs and chart developmental progress effectively.

Criterion-referenced tests are often touted as being preferable to norm-referenced tests for children with atypical development because they divide development into several domains that are assessed separately (e.g., gross motor, fine motor, social, language) and therefore do not assume even development across domains. A close look at most of these tests, however, will show that both the variety of items included in each domain and the suggested profile analysis of strengths and weaknesses indicate that these tests also operate on the assumption of relatively even development within and across domains (Johnson, 1980; Gaussen, 1984; Johnson-Martin, Jens & Attermeier, 1985). When a child's development is atypical, the data from such tests may suggest inappropriate treatment goals (e.g., promoting cognitive development by teaching "block stacking" to a child with significant motor problems). Similarly, such tests may not be sensitive to progress that does not follow traditional development sequences.

Test Content

Norm and criterion referenced tests that are based on normal developmental milestones have another underlying assumption that is often not recognized. This is the assumption that the important behaviors of the developing child are those that are correlated highly with chronologic age (Gaussen, 1984). Yet, behaviors that are not age specific are important to the understanding of any child and may be critical to the planning of treatment or remediation for the low functioning and/or autistic child. Some examples of such behavior are: preferences for certain stimuli; social responsiveness; modes of social and communicative interaction; temperament qualities such as irritability, soothability, motivation, persistence, and fatiguability; free play characteristics; and self-stimulatory or other "aberrant" activities. One of the goals in planning an assessment for a low functioning child, therefore, is to determine means for assessing critical variables that are not included in commonly used norm or criterion referenced tests. It is not enough that attention is paid to these variables informally and that they be mentioned in the "behavioral observations" section of an assessment report. Observations should be refined sufficiently that they can be repeated reliably and can serve as yardsticks for measuring change over time.

APPROACHES TO SOLVING ASSESSMENT PROBLEMS

The first step in assessing a low-functioning child is to determine the specific goals of the assessment. If the goal is diagnostic assessment, i.e., to determine the degree of retardation or the level of skills relative to the general population, different approaches to assessment should be considered than if the goal is to plan treatment or educational intervention. If the goal is to establish a baseline so that progress may be measured over time, still other considerations may determine the choice of instruments. If two or all three goals are to be met, a variety of instruments will be required. If time is limited, it may be necessary to determine which goal is paramount and choose instruments appropriate to that goal while recognizing their limitations in meeting the other goals.

Diagnostic Assessment

In requiring that adaptive behavior measures as well as IQ tests be used to document the presence and level of mental retardation, the American Association for Mental Deficiency (Grossman, 1973) recognized that diagnosis requires more than one kind of assessment and that assessment for diagnostic purposes should be based both on direct observations of the child and on reports of caretakers familiar with his/her behavior in daily surroundings. In both cases, however, standardized, norm referenced instruments should be used for diagnosis. The choice of instruments will be based on the particular characteristics of the child.

Direct Assessment

The most commonly used assessment instruments for low functioning children are the Bayley Scales of Infant Development (Bayley, 1969), for children developmentally under 30 months, and the Stanford Binet Intelligence Scale, L-M, for children developmentally over 24 months. These tests have the most representative norms of tests available for children functioning in the 0–36-month range and the results are reported in deviation IQs. However, the language demands on the Binet and both the language and speed demands of the Bayley at its upper levels make these tests problematic for low functioning children with significant limitations in language, motor dexterity, and/or motivation. A number of other instruments are available that may be appropriate for particular children although none have norms as adequate as the Bayley and Binet.

Merrill–Palmer Scale of Mental Tests

The Merrill–Palmer Scale (Stutsman, 1931) was developed for the evaluation of children between the ages of 18 and 71 months. This age range is an advantage for many low functioning children who are too old for the Bayley norms but are functioning in the age range of the Bayley. The test consists primarily of sensorimotor items, an advantage for nonverbal children. The items are varied and intrinsically interesting for most children. The scoring system provides for an adjustment to account for refusals, a major accommodation for children with attentional and motivational deficits. For these reasons, the Merrill–Palmer is particularly appropriate for use both with low functioning children and with other autistic children. The test provides a mental age table from which a ratio IQ can be computed.

Gould (1975) reported that scores on the Merrill–Palmer are higher than those obtained on the Vineland Social Maturity Scale and on the Reynell Developmental Language Scale, perhaps reflecting more outdated norms or differences in the kinds of skills tapped by each test. This potential for overestimating cognitive ability should be kept in mind when using the test for diagnostic purposes. Its limited sampling of both receptive and expressive language skills, while an advantage for determining the level of retardation in a nonverbal child makes the test problematic as a programming guide. Accurate determination of language skills is an important aspect of assessment for treatment purposes. Likewise, the test's value as a measure of progress will be limited in the language and verbal conceptual areas.

Griffiths Mental Development Scales

The Griffiths Scales (Griffiths, 1970) consist of two scales, a birth to 2 years scale and a birth to 8 years scale. The babies' scale is much more detailed for that early period than is the children's scale. The children's scale, however, has the advantage of a wider age range than other tests for young children, thereby accommodating the widely scattered skills sometimes observed in low functioning and autistic children. Both include the following scales: Loco-motor, Personal–social, Hearing and Speech, Hand and Eye, and Performance. A practical reasoning scale is included only on the children's scale. A mental age is derived from the norms for each scale and a scale quotient is computed (MA/CA × 100). The General Quotient is an arithmetic average of the subquotients.

The primary limitation of these scales as a diagnostic instrument lies in the unavailability of U.S. norms. In this author's experience, the scores obtained on the Griffiths have generally been higher than those obtained from the Bayley or the Binet. The advantage of having a test that crosses the age ranges of the Bayley and the Binet and that divides abilities into different domains of development may outweigh that limitation in some assessment situations, however. The inclusion of more items than are included on most norm referenced tests and the division of abilities into different domains with norms for each domain, make this test more useful as a programming guide and as a means of documenting developmental progress than most other norm-referenced tests.

Cattell Infant Intelligence Scale

The Cattell was standardized for children between 2 months and 4½ years of age (Cattell, 1960). It was developed as a downward extension of the Stanford Binet and may be useful for those children whose skills fall on the borderline of the Bayley and the Binet. Its items are very similar to those of the Bayley but it has the advantage that there are no time limits. This advantage is particularly useful for the low functioning children who are difficult to engage in test tasks. Test results are reported in terms of a mental age and a ratio IQ. Perhaps because the test is based on older norms than the Bayley scales, the IQs obtained on the Cattell have been found to be higher than those obtained on the Bayley Scales (Erickson, Johnson & Campbell, 1970). Thus, caution must be taken in interpreting the scores. The test has the same limitations as the Bayley as a programming guide and as a measure of progress, i.e., a relatively limited number of skills are sampled, skills are not divided according to domains of development, and only summary scores are available.

Leiter International Performance Scale

Developed for children aged 2–18 years, the Leiter requires no understanding of verbal instructions, although it makes significant demands on attention and motor coordination (Leiter, 1936). Only the earliest items would be appropriate for the low functioning children described in this chapter, but these items are often useful for determining matching and discrimination abilities not sampled by other tests. Testing procedures at the lower levels also allow teaching the child to do the task. This teaching is often instructive for evaluating the child's ability to profit from demonstration. Many professionals choose the Leiter for autistic children because it is a nonverbal test. It should be noted, however, that the attentional demands are great and that although it begins with simple matching, it rapidly becomes highly conceptual. This leads to abrupt ceiling scores and provides little help in identifying strong and weak areas in the low functioning or autistic child.

The Leiter yields a mental age and a ratio IQ. The normative sample is small and not representative by current standards. Reports have been mixed about its relationship to other tests, making it problematic as a genuine diagnostic instrument. It also has very limited usefulness as a programming guide or as a means of documenting developmental progress.

Reynell–Zinkin Developmental Scales for Young Visually Handicapped Children, Part 1: Mental Development

Although these scales were developed for visually impaired children between the ages of 3 months and 5 years, norms are provided for sighted children (as well as for partially sighted and blind children) (Reynell, 1979). The scales are useful for low-functioning children with or without visual impairment because they are scored both on the basis of parent report and direct observation and include areas often neglected by other tests but important to the understanding of the low-functioning child. The subscales included are Social Adaptation, Sensorimotor Understanding, Exploration of Environment, Response to Sound and Verbal Comprehension, and Expressive Language. Developmental ages are derived for each subscale and may be compared with chronological age but the test author does not recommend a summary IQ as the aim of the test is to identify skills in several areas of development rather than to provide an overall estimate of ability. Normative data is limited to a small British sample. Although norm referenced, this instrument is probably more useful as a programming guide and as a means of documenting progress than as a diagnostic assessment.

Assessment by Parent Interview

Any child may demonstrate different abilities in different situations. The low functioning child, particularly one with autistic features, however, may be even more affected by environmental differences. Lichstein and Waller (1976), for example, documented significant differences in stereotypic behaviors and attention to the environment in an autistic child under different environmental influences. It is always important to have a caretaker who is very familiar with the child observe any direct assessment and to comment on how comparable the performance is both to the child's usual performance and his/her optimal performance in familiar settings. In addition, structured interview techniques should be used to get information about the child to corroborate direct observations and to provide data about behaviors not observed during the testing session. There are a number of structured interviews that may be used effectively with low-functioning children.

Wisconsin Behavior Rating Scale

This is an adaptive behavior scale for children functioning in the 0–3-year developmental range (Song, Jones, Lippert, Metzgen, Miller & Borreca, 1980). It was developed to provide a more comprehensive assessment of skills at these lower levels than is provided by other adaptive behavior scales that cover a wider age range. Items are assessed on a 3-point rating scale in the following areas: Gross Motor, Fine Motor, Expressive Language, Receptive Language, Play Skills, Socialization, Domestic Activities, Eating, Toileting, Dressing and Grooming. Data are reported in terms of a behavioral age for the total scale and age equivalents for the subscales. Preliminary data suggest that this instrument will be very useful for assessing development in low functioning children (Song, Jones, Lippert, Metzgen, Miller & Borreca, 1984). It may prove to be very useful not only as an aid to diagnosis but as a guide for intervention and a means of documenting progress.

Children's Handicaps, Behavior, and Skills Schedule

The HBS schedule consists of 35 sections falling into two categories: (1) those indicating the stage of development reached in the areas of mobility, feeding, continence, dressing, comprehension and use of language, levels of play, academic and practical skills and (2) those concerning abnormal or difficult behavior (Wing & Gould, 1978). Items are rated on a 3-point scale with provisions made for computing scores when evidence is unobtainable or equivocal. Data indicate good reliability between parents and professionals as reporters on the developmental items with less agreement on the behavioral abnormalities items (Bernsen, 1980). This instrument should be an excellent aid in diagnostic, programming, and progress assessment, but its use may be limited by the requirement that those who administer it have training by the authors (Wing & Gould, 1978).

Vineland Adaptive Behavior Scales

There are two forms of the new Vineland Scales—revisions of the long-used Vineland Social Maturity Scale developed by Doll and published in 1935 (Sparrow, Balla & Cicchetti, 1984). Both forms are designed to assess adaptive skills in individuals from birth to 18 years 11 months through the interview of a parent or other caretaker familiar with the client. The Survey Form contains 297 items and is the form generally used in a diagnostic assessment. The Expanded Form with 577 items is more comprehensive and may be more useful in planning remedial programs. Both provide excellent normative data. Behavior is assessed in four domains—Communication, Daily Living Skills, Socialization, and Motor Skills—and 11 subdomains. Standard scores are available for each of the four domains and for an Adaptive Behavior Composite. For each of the subdomains, adaptive levels and age equivalents can be derived. A maladaptive behavior domain is included for optional use with individuals over 5 years. This "new Vineland" should prove to be an excellent addition to available assessments, not only for low-functioning children but for older higher-functioning autistic children.

Developmental Profile

The Developmental Profile is a well-standardized inventory of skills designed as a screening instrument to assess developmental skills from birth through 12 years (Alpern and Boll, 1972). It is administered by interview to the primary caretaker to identify the level of a child's functioning in five areas: Physical, Self-Help, Social, Academic, and Communication. Normative data indicate no racial or sex biases. This is a useful instrument to supplement direct assessment of a child, particularly if the child responds very differently in a familiar environment than in the test environment, a problem often noted in low-functioning and autistic children. Furthermore, it is useful because it assesses areas often neglected by many direct assessment instruments. Because it is a screening instrument, however, it has a relatively limited number of items at each level. Therefore, its use as a programming guide and measure of developmental progress in slowly developing children is limited.

Assessment for Planning Intervention and Charting Developmental Progress

Information from diagnostic instruments may serve as a basis for planning an intervention program and for charting progress over time. These uses are limited, however, by the kinds and numbers of items included. For low functioning and/or autistic children more extensive criterion-referenced assessments will be necessary.

Assessments from Infant Curriculum Materials

Many criterion referenced assessment materials for children functioning within the 0–3-year level have been developed in the last ten years. These assessments are either part of a more comprehensive curriculum or are meant to be used as curriculum guides. The reader is referred to Bailey, Jens, and Johnson (1983) for a discussion of problems in curriculum development for children in this developmental range, as well as for a listing of representative curricula and guidelines for evaluating curricula. They note that the primary differences among curricula are in layout, design, or organization of domains rather than in content. Among the more comprehensive curricula evaluated by these workers are the Vulpe Assessment Battery (Vulpe, 1977), the Hawaii Early Learning Profile (HELP) (Furuno, O'Reilly, Hosaka, Inatsuka, Ailman & Zeisloft, 1979), and the Carolina Curriculum for Handicapped Infants and Infants at Risk (CCHI) (Johnson-Martin, Jens & Attermeier, 1985). Although the CCHI makes more provisions for atypical development due to physical and sensory impairments than do the other two curricula, all three are based primarily on a developmental milestones approach. As such they are good programming guides and are effective for measuring developmental progress in children functioning at the infancy level. All provide age estimates for items to allow for estimates of developmental levels in the various domains although the estimates are based on the normative data from other tests (e.g., the Bayley), not on normative samples of their own. They were not designed to be used as primary diagnostic instruments.

These curricula, as well as other available infant curricula may neglect important behavioral characteristics that should be considered if programming is to be effective for the low functioning and/or autistic child. Among those that should be considered are social, affective and interactional behaviors (including pre-language skills); Learning, attention and problem solving; temperament; and spontaneous play behaviors. Most examiners assess these characteristics informally through observations during testing. A number of instruments or procedures have been developed, however, which may make such observations more systematic (i.e., make the characteristics measurable) and therefore provide not only objective descriptions but a means of documenting change over time.

Assessments Designed Specifically for Autistic and Other Developmentally Delayed Individuals

It is often difficult to capture the social, learning, and other behavior characteristics of autistic and/or low functioning children through formal assessments based on normal or common developmental characteristics. There are few instruments that have been developed specifically for atypical populations. Division TEACCH (*T*reatment and *E*ducation of *A*utistic and related *C*ommunications-handicapped *CH*ildren) at the University of North Carolina at Chapel Hill has been responsible for the production of two such instruments, one for younger children and one for adolescents and adults.

The *Psychoeducational Profile* (Schoper & Reichler, 1979) is an inventory of behaviors and skills for use with children functioning at the preschool age level within the age range of 1–12 years. It was designed to identify uneven and idiosyncratic learning patterns. It provides assessment in the areas of Imitation, Perception, Fine-Motor, Gross Motor, Eye–Hand Integration, Cognitive Performance, and Cognitive Verbal Skills. It also provides a means for identifying the degrees of behavioral pathology in the areas of affect; relating, cooperating, human interest; play and interest in materials; sensory modes; and language. Each skill is assessed on a pass, fail or "emerging" basis, making it particularly useful for identifying the best foci of intervention. The administration is flexible and language is minimized to accommodate the characteristics of autistic and many other developmentally disabled children. This is an exceptionally valuable assessment to use for designing treatment programs and evaluating progress for children whose skills fall above the 12-month level. The behaviors assessed in the pathology scale could readily be assessed during other infant assessments with the use of a few additional materials and would increase the effectiveness of such evaluations for low-functioning children. The test was not designed to yield an IQ or other summary score, but it does provide a test profile with developmental scores in the various domains assessed.

For older low-functioning and/or autistic individuals, the Adolescent and Adult Psychoeducational Profile (AAPEP) (Mesibov, Schopler & Schaffer, 1984) provides an alternative to the questionable practice of using infant and toddler test items as program or intervention goals. The APEP includes three scales: a Direct Observation Scale administered to the client by a professional in a clinical setting, a Home Scale based on behavioral reports from parents or group home managers, and a School/Work Scale based on a similar interview with the client's work supervisor or teacher. Each of the three scales is divided into six functional areas, making it possible to evaluate the strengths and weaknesses of a client across environments: vocational skills, independent functioning, leisure skills, vocational behavior, functional communication, and interpersonal behavior. Like the PEP, the AAPEP is scored on a pass–fail–emerging basis. Each of the AAPEP functional scales includes tasks representing a wide range of difficulty. There are some simple tasks that could probably be mastered by a normal child around 2 years old but are appropriate to the interests of an adolescent or adult (e.g., sorting washers, bolts, nuts and buttons; opening a package of crackers independently). Some examples of the more difficult tasks are: collating cards with numbers on them, reading signs, operating a pinball machine after demonstration, and follows simple written instructions.

The AAPEP is clearly preferable to the usual developmental assessments for planning treatment or intervention for older low functioning clients and for assessing progress related to that intervention. Developmental scores are not available, but the information obtained is more meaningful for understanding and finding appropriate environments for the client than age equivalents or IQ scores.

Assessment of Social, Affective, and Interactional Behaviors

The ability of a child to respond affectively to his/her caretakers has a major impact on maintaining the relationships essential to early learning and emotional growth. Fraiberg's (1977) descriptions of the impact of the blind child's inability to establish eye contact with the parent is pertinent to our understanding of how missing or deviant signals from an infant may stress the relationship with his/her parent and set the stage for a mutually unsatisfying interaction. Many low-functioning children respond in unusual ways or develop the ability to respond so slowly that parental responses are "extinguished" before good interaction is attained. Other children may process information at such a slow rate as to be "out of sync" with their parents to the extent that mutual attention is not maintained (Jens & Johnson, 1982). In recent years, a number of procedures have been developed that facilitate systematic assessment of affective expressions, attachment, and other social behaviors that may be critical to our understanding of the low-functioning child.

Cicchetti and Sroufe (1976) asked mothers of children with Down syndrome to stimulate their infants with a series of behaviors that had been demonstrated to produce smiling and laughter in normally developing infants. These infants appeared to develop positive affective responses to the stimuli in approximately the same sequence as normally developing infants, but their ability to respond was delayed and was related to mental age. In addition, their best responses were less intense than those of normally developing children. Since that report, there have been a number of efforts to use this Smile Procedure to study affective and cognitive development in handicapped children. For example, in a study of a mixed group of handicapped children, Gallagher (1979) found that smiling responses were related to mental age, but also that handicapping conditions appeared to affect both the latency and the intensity of responses. Anderson (1980), using a similar sample of children found that scores on the Smile Procedure correlated positively with both mental age and a number of care-provider ratings on the Carolina Record of Individual Behavior (Simeonsson, 1979). Among these were social orientation, goal directedness, endurance, receptive language, object orientation, reactivity, and responsiveness to the examiner. She also found that the primary contributors to these correlations were the scores on the social and visual items in the Smile Procedure (as opposed to the tactile and auditory items).

As a clinical tool, the Smile Procedure may be useful for demonstrating the kinds of stimuli that produce positive affect in a low-functioning child, for helping to identify asynchronies in a mother's speed of stimulus presentation and a child's ability to respond, and for charting changes in a child's affective responses over time. Although there is currently no literature on its use with autistic children, it should be considered for this population, particularly as a means of identifying changes in affective responsiveness over time.

The Infant Clinical Assessment Procedure (ICAP), developed by Solyom, Horner, and Hoffman (1983), was designed to evaluate the emotional development of infants. It focuses on the quality of attachment and on the characteristics of affective expressions and states. It was developed for use with children aged 3–30 months and is designed to be integrated into a regular developmental assessment, adding approximately 30 min to the time necessary for assessment. It includes eight brief episodes: infant free play, the examiner's approach to the child, directed mother–child interaction, developmental testing, free play, mother–infant separation, mother–infant reunion, and neuromuscular screening. The ICAP does not provide scores but systematizes observations in such a way that the child's behaviors can be described objectively and compared from one assessment to another. It has been found to be helpful in planning infant intervention (Solyom et al., 1983) and is promising as a procedure for assessing important emotional and behavioral characteristics in children who may no longer be infants but who are functioning in that range of development.

In an effort to develop an assessment that included domains not included in traditional assessment, that evaluated generic characteristics and traits rather than task specific responses, and that capitalized on clinical insights and judgments, Simeonsson (1979) developed an observational instrument based on the Infant Behavior Record of the Bayley Infant Scales. The Carolina Record of Individual Behavior (CRIB) was designed to be completed in conjunction with another developmental assessment. This rating scale consists of three parts. Section A assesses social orientation, participation, motivation, endurance, communication, object orientation, and consolability. Section B assesses activity, reactivity, goal directedness, response to frustration, attention span, responsiveness to caretaker, tone or tension of body, and responsiveness to examiner. Section C lists specific behaviors (e.g., nonverbal vocalization, rhythmic habit patterns) rated according to the frequency with which they are exhibited. The CRIB has been used with many young handicapped children and has been found useful for documenting unique characteristics of children with varying handicapping conditions (Simeonsson, Huntington & Short, 1982), for comparing mothers' and intervention staff members' perceptions of young handicapped children (Beckman, 1984) and for rating social responsiveness and atypical habit patterns in neurologically impaired and normal children (Stahleeker & Cohen, 1985).

Assessment of Prelanguage Communication Skills

Most criterion- and norm-referenced tests suitable for low-functioning children assess communication skills through items that focus on speech and on an understanding of speech. Very little attention is paid to other forms of communication, such as gestures, eye gaze, and leading an adult. Yet, for the low-functioning child, these may be the primary means of communication for many years. It is therefore important to consider ways to assess these additional forms of communication systematically and to promote their development through intervention. The Carolina Curriculum for Handicapped Infants and Infants at Risk (Johnson-Martin et al., 1985) is the only curriculum-based assessment that makes specific provision for the assessment of some early alternative communication skills, such as watching the person talking and gesturing, imitating gestures, and understanding gestures. Two other more comprehensive sources of assessment of these important skills in low-functioning children are: How to Recognize and Assess Prelanguage Skills in the Severely Handicapped (Mount & Shea, 1982) and Prerequisites to the Use of Augmentative Communication Systems (Porter, Carter, Goolsby, Johnson-Martin, Reed, Stowers & Wurth, 1984).

Assessments of Learning, Attention, and Problem-Solving

Developmental assessment is directed toward determining what skills a child has mastered rather than at examining the processes by which he or she learns. Yet, it is the learning processes that are the routes of intervention. Some examiners include short teaching sessions as part of their developmental assessments. They take one or more items a child has failed and try to teach, observing carefully how readily the child learns, how much support is necessary for learning, whether the child is active or passive in the learning process, which prompts (physical or verbal) are most effective, and so forth. This is certainly an effective assessment technique if careful notes are made on the observations so that comparisons can be made over time.

Other means of examining the learning process might also be considered. For especially low functioning children it may be necessary to focus assessment on the identification of reinforcers and spontaneous behaviors that might be used to build functional skills (e.g., self-feeding), and on determining the ease with which simple functional skills can be taught. For those who are less handicapped, it may be useful to use a Piagetian-based assessment (e.g., Uzgiris & Hunt, 1975) to evaluate some of the conceptual and learning processes.

Evaluating Learning through Structured Play

If a child is especially passive, negativistic, or inattentive or is otherwise functioning at such a low level that usual assessment procedures are not applicable, a structured "play" session may be the only means of evaluation. In other instances a play session may provide additional information that could not be obtained in other assessments. In either case, it is important to specify the goals of the assessment and to develop means for recording systematically the observations of the assessment.

Materials for a structures play assessment need not be elaborate but should include toys and other objects that have a variety of sensory characteristics, such as different textures, shapes, colors, sounds, and odors. There should also be a number of toys responsive to simple behaviors under the child's voluntary control (e.g., a toy that moves and jingles when pushed slightly) and toys that produce sound and/or spectacles when activated by an adult.

For the most unresponsive children, the goals of the assessment may primarily be to identify preferences that could be used as potential reinforces and to determine if the child will "learn" through the pairing of something he/she appears to prefer with a voluntary behavior. In such an assessment, the child is stimulated by rubbing objects with various textures over his hands, limbs, or body and by presenting various sights, sounds, tastes, and smells. The kind of stimulation is varied. The child's response to each stimulating event is recorded. Then an attempt is made to teach the child by identifying some voluntary behavior of the child and systematically following it with one of the stimuli that appeared to produce a positive response. An example might be activating a music box every time the child vocalizes. Data are collected to record changes in the rate the child makes the identified response. In the course of the assessment, different apparently positive stimuli can be paired with different child behaviors, making it possible to identify effective reinforcers. Figure 1 is an example of a form that could be used to record the information from such a play session and the data that might be obtained.

For the somewhat less handicapped child, the goals of the structured play session might

Stimulus	Positive responses				Negative responses			No response
	Quiets	Smiles	Moves	Explores	Cries	Withdraws	Other	
Rattle			*reaches*	*Shakes*				
Puppet		*x*	*Follows*			*When app. face*		
Pudding (smell)	*x*		*Reaches*					
Pudding	*x*	*x*						
Rocking clown	*x*	*x*	*Hits*					
Hedgehog			*Reaches*			*When touches*		
Spinner	*x*							
Bell			*Reaches*	*Shakes*				
Ball				*Mouths*				
Cloth				*Fingers*				
Cloth (peek-a-boo)					*x*			
Cup								*x*

Comments: Alert; responds positively to many stimuli. Withdraws from or cries to tactile stimuli, particularly on the face. Brightly colored, noisy objects should be used as reinforcers.

Fig. 1. Sample form. Responses to potential reinforcers.

be to identify the child's reinforces and his spontaneous play behaviors, to evaluate his responsiveness to environmental change, and to evaluate his responsiveness to adult efforts to demonstrate or physically prompt new behaviors. For this evaluation, it is useful to present objects and toys one by one to the child, and to observe and record spontaneous behaviors (e.g., means of exploration and manipulation, repetition of behaviors that produce interesting results). The objects may then be presented in pairs to the child to observe his/her choice behaviors. As the child reaches for one object, the second is removed and he/she is allowed to play with the chosen object for several minutes. Subsequent trials involve systematic pairings of each object with every other. The child's pattern of choices will indicate whether choices are random or whether the child has definite preferences. Preferences identified in this way may be considered potential reinforcers in planning an intervention program for the child. Finally, several objects may be selected and attempts made to teach functional behaviors first through demonstration and then through physical prompts.

Throughout such an assessment, it is important to keep an accurate record of the child's responses so that the child's behavior is quantifiable and can be compared with subsequent observations.

Piagetian-Based Assessments

Infant scales based on Piagetian theory are often very useful for evaluating learning and problem solving skills in low functioning children who have reasonable motor skills. The Ordinal Scales of Psychological Development (Uzgiris & Hunt, 1975) is probably the most commonly used instrument of this sort. One of the advantages of these scales is that the materials used in them are flexible and can accommodate the unique preferences of many retarded and autistic children. The scales are designed to focus on the process of problem solving as well as on accomplishment. The areas assessed include object permanence (searching for objects that can no longer be seen), the development of means to obtain desired environmental events, vocal and gestural imitation, the development of an understanding of cause and effect, and the ways in which the child relates to objects. Even if the scales are not given in their entirety, an examiner who is familiar with them and with Piagetian theory can integrate the concepts and procedures into other developmental assessments and can use these controlled observations for planning intervention programs and documenting change.

RECOMMENDATIONS FOR CLINICAL PRACTICE

Too often, the clinician's initial response to seeing a low functioning child is that he/she is untestable or that nothing in the clinician's's usual repertoire is appropriate. Certainly, the assessment of these children challenges the creativity of the examiner. No single assessment instrument is likely to be effective for even one of the assessment goals, i.e., diagnosis, planning intervention, and documenting change. Furthermore, the child's behavior may make direct assessment of his/her skills improbable. Thus, a combination of direct assessment and indirect assessment through parent and teacher report will be necessary. The practice of making observations of a child through several kinds of direct and indirect assessment procedures enhances the likelihood that the variables most relevant to understanding the child's development and unique characteristics will be sampled.

It is also important, however, to avoid ''overassessing'' a child. Low functioning children do, after all, have limited response repertoires. Two, three or four procedures are probably adequate to meet the goals of the assessment and to provide an understanding of the child's skills and behavioral characteristics. Collecting information about the child before the evaluation and then planning the evaluation thoughtfully to address the issues raised in the referring information are essential parts of the assessment process. One should consider the available procedures and select those that are most likely to produce the desired information. New assessment procedures continue to be developed and should be added to those discussed in this chapter as potentially useful techniques. Viewing the assessment of any low-functioning child as a unique problem to be solved will increase the flexibility and creativity of the clinician in meeting the challenge of the assessment and will ultimately determine his/her effectiveness in serving this small but important population.

REFERENCES

Alpern, G. D., and Boll, T. J. (1972). *Developmental profile*. Aspen, CO: Psychological Development Publications.

Bailey, D. B., Jens, K. G., & Johnson, N. M. (1983). Curricula for handicapped infants. In S. G. Garwood and R. R. Fewell (Eds.), *Educating handicapped infants* pp. 387–416. Rockville, MD: Aspen.

Bayley, N. (1969). *Bayley scales of infant development.* New York: Psychological Corporation.

Beckman, P. J. (1984). Perceptions of young children with handicaps: A comparison of mothers and program staff. *Mental Retardation, 22* (4), 176–81.

Bernson, A. H. (1980). An interview technique in assessing retarded children. *Journal of Mental Deficiency Research, 24,* 167–79.

Cattell, P. (1940). *The measurement of intelligence of infants and young children.* New York: The Psychological Corporation.

Cicchetti, D., & Sroufe, A. (1976). The relationship between affective and cognitive development in Downs' syndrome infants. *Child Development, 47,* 920–9.

Doll, E. A. (1965). *Vineland Social Maturity Scale: Manual of directions* (rev. ed.). Minneapolis: Educational Test Bureau (now American Guidance Service).

Erickson, M. T., Johnson, N. M., & Campbell, F. A. (1970). Relationships among scores on infant tests for children with developmental problems. *American Journal of Mental Deficiency, 75,* 102–4.

Fraiberg, S. (1977). *Insights from the blind: Comparative study of blind and sighted infants.* New York: Basic Books.

Furuno, S., O'Reilly, K. A., Hosaka, C. M., Inatsuka, T. T., Allman, T. L., & Zeisloft, B. (1979). *Hawaii Early Learning Profile.* Palo Alto: VORT Corporation.

Gallagher, R. J. (1979). Positive affect in physically handicapped mentally retarded infants: Its relationship to developmental age, temperament, physical status and setting. Unpublished dissertation, University of North Carolina at Chapel Hill.

Gaussen, T. (1984). Developmental milestones or conceptual millstones? Some practical and theoretical limitations in infant assessment procedures. *Child Care Health and Development, 10* (2), 99–115.

Gould, J. (1975). The use of the Vineland Social Maturity Scales, the Merrill-Palmer Scale of Mental Tests (non-verbal items) and the Reynell Developmental Language Scales with children in contact with the service for severe mental retardation. *Journal of Mental Deficiency Research, 21,* 212–26.

Griffiths, R. (1970). *The Abilities of Young Children: A comprehensive System of Mental Measurement for the First Eight Years of Life.* London: Child Development Research Centre.

Grossman, H. (Ed.). (1973). *Manual on Terminology and Classification in Mental Retardation, 1973 Revision.* Washington, D.C.: American Association of Mental Deficiency.

Harrison, P. I., & Naglieri, J. A. (1978). Extrapolated General Cognitive Indexes on the McCarthy Scales for gifted and mentally retarded children. *Psychological Reports, 43,* 1291–6.

Jens, K. G., & Johnson, N. M. (1982). Affective development: a window to cognition in young handicapped children. *Topics in Early Childhood Special Education, 2,* 17–24.

Johnson, N. M., Jens, K. G., Gallagher, R. J., & Anderson, J. D. (1980). Cognition and affect in infancy: Implications for the handicapped. In J. J. Gallagher (Ed.) *New directions for exceptional children: Young exceptional children* (Vol. 3, pp. 21–36). San Francisco: Jossey-Bass.

Kaufman, A. S., & Kaufman, N. L. (1983). *Kaufman Assessment Battery for Children.* Circle Pines, MN: American Guidance Service.

Leiter, R. G. (1936). *The Leiter International Performance Scale* (Research Publication No. 13). Honolulu: The University of Hawaii.

Lichstein, K. L., & Wahler, R. (1976). The ecological assessment of an autistic child. *Journal of Abnormal Child Psychology, 4,* (1), 31–54.

McCarthy, D. (1972). *McCarthy Scales of Children's Abilities.* New York: The Psychological Corporation.

Mesibov, G. B., Schopler, E., & Schaffer, B. (1984). *Adolescent and Adult Psychoeducational Profile.* Hillsborough, NC: Orange Industries.

Mount, M., & Shea, V. (1982). *How to Recognize and Assess Pre-language Skills in the Severely Handicapped.* Austin, TX: Pro-Ed.

Naglieri, J. A. (1981). Extrapolated developmental indices for the Bayley Scales of Infant Development. *American Journal of Mental Deficiency, 85*(4), 548–50.

Porter, P. B., Carter, S., Goolsby, E., Johnson-Martin, N., Reed, M., Stowers, S., & Wurth, B. (1984). *Prerequisites to the Use of Augmentative Communication Systems*. Chapel Hill, NC: Division for Disorders of Development and Learning, Biological Sciences Research Center.

Reynell, J. (1979). *Manual for the Reynell-Zinkin Scales. Developmental Scales for Young Visually Handicapped Children. Part 1. Mental Development*. Windsor Berks, Great Britain: NFER.

Schopler, E., & Reichler, R. J. (1979). *Individualized Assessment and Treatment for Autistic and Developmentally Disabled Children. Vol. 1; Psychoeducation Profile*. Baltimore: University Park Press.

Simeonsson, R. J. (1979). Carolina Record of Infant Behavior (CRIB Experimental Version) Chapel Hill, NC: Carolina Institute for Research on the Early Education of the Handicapped (revised as the Carolina Record of Individual Behavior).

Simeonsson, R. J., Huntington, G. S., & Parse, S. A. (1980). Expanding the developmental assessment of young handicapped children, in J. J. Gallagher (Ed.), *New directions for exceptional children: Young exceptional children* (Vol. 3, pp. 51–74). San Francisco: Jossey Bass.

Simeonsson, R. J., Huntington, G. S., & Short, R. J. (1982). The Carolina Record of Individual Behavior: Characteristics of handicapped infants and children. *Topics in Early Childhood Special Education, 2* (2), 43–55.

Solyom, A. E., Horner, T. M., & Hoffman, P. (1983). Infant clinical assessment procedure: applications of a new tool for diagnosis and treatment. *Infant Mental Health Journal, 4*, (2), 104–15.

Song, A., Jones, S., Lippert, J., Metzgen, K., Miller, J., & Borreca, C. *Wisconsin Behavior Rating Scale*. Madison, WI: Central Wisconsin Center for the Developmentally Disabled.

Song, A., Jones, S., Lippert, J., Metzgen, K., Miller, J., & Borreca, C. (1984). Wisconsin Behavior Rating Scale: Measure of adaptive behavior for the developmental levels of 0–3 years. *American Journal of Mental Deficiency, 88*(4), 401–10.

Sparrow, S. S., Balla, D. A., & Cicchetti, D. V. (1984). *Vineland Adaptive Behavior Scales*. Circle Pines, MN: American Guidance Service.

Stahleeker, J. E., & Cohen, M. (1985). Application of the Strange situation attachment paradigm to a neurologically impaired population. *Child Development, 56*, 502–7.

Stutsman, R. (1931). *Merrill-Palmer Scale of Mental Tests*. New York: Harcourt, Brace and World.

Terman, L. M., & Merrill, M. A. (1972). *Stanford-Binet Intelligence Scale*, Form L-M. Boston: Houghton-Mifflin.

Uzgiris, I. C., & Hunt, J. M. (1975). *Assessment in infancy: Ordinal scales of psychological development*. Urbana: University of Illinois Press.

Vulpe, S. G. (1977). *Vulpe assessment battery*. Toronto: National Institute on Mental Retardation.

Wing, L., & Gould, J. (1978). Systematic recording of behaviors and skills of retarded and psychotic children. *Journal of Autism and Childhood Schizophrenia, 88*, 79–97.

Index

Adaptive Behavior Scale, 134
Adolescent and Adult Psychoeducational Profile (AAPEP), 233–237, 266–267, 312–313
Adolescents with autism, 227–232, 233–238, 252
Adults with autism, 46–47, 227–232, 233–238, 252
  designing programs for children's needs as, 265–266
Affect: *See* Empathy; Social interaction and emotional functioning
Age
  ability to differentiate, 22, 242
  changes with, 100–101
  and diagnosis, 77
  inapplicability of scales, 305–306
Age of onset, 16, 18–19, 29, 82, 100
  as age of recognition, 79–80
  classification of psychoses by, 56
  difficulty of establishing, 105
American Association for Mental Deficiency, 307
American Psychiatric Association: *See* Diagnostic and Statistical Manual
Anxiety, 98, 231
Arousal, 81
Asperger's syndrome, 25, 73, 83, 83–84, 100, 102, 105, 241, 257
Assessment
  components of, in classroom, 263–270
  definition of, 6, 228
  as dynamic process, 296
  disagreement re, 4–6, 261–262
  emphasis on emerging skills, 263–265
  and engagement with environment, 185
  purposes of, 231–233, 262–263, 304–305, 317
  See also Behavior
Attention deficit, 74, 98
Attentional studies, 85

Autism
  basic defect in, 20–23, 241–243
  "core" diagnostic criteria for, 18–20, 76–77, 84–85
  differential diagnosis of, 24–28, 129–130, 131, 134, 228, 258
  differentiated from other developmental disorders, 18, 85, 101–102, 130, 296
  differentiated from normality or mental retardation, 25, 127
  differentiated from other psychoses, 15–16, 72–73, 74–75, 91, 111–112, 124, 126
  early diagnosis of, 271, 272, 273
  etiology of, 17, 28–30, 85–86, 91, 106–107, 112, 240–241
  history of concepts of, 15–16, 72–73
  infantile (*see also* Kanner's syndrome), 46, 75, 105
  most common profile in, 103
  statistical studies of, 76, 115
  subgroups of, 82–83, 85, 103, 130, 211–212
  as syndrome (*see also* Kanner's syndrome), 16–17, 71–72, 113, 211–212
  See also Developmental disorders, pervasive
Autism Behavior Checklist, 129, 130, 153, 156–157
Autism Descriptors Checklist, 152, 155
Autism Screening Instrument for Educational Planning (ASIEP), 129, 131–132, 156–157
Autistic Diagnostic Interview, 243–247, 256–258
Autistic Diagnostic Observation Schedule, 240–253, 257–258

Babbling, 19, 281–282
Bayley Scale of Mental Development, 168, 170, 171, 176–178, 178–179, 289, 290